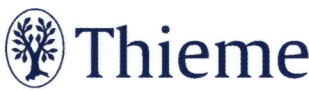

A need for specialized services in foot and ankle surgery has been on the increase for the last few years... Dr Rajiv Shah has utilized his vast knowledge of the subject with his ability to teach in a very effective and erudite manner to offer this creation...The principles of foot and ankle practice are very well illustrated (in this handbook) in meticulous tabulations and algorithms which are essential to the understanding (of the subject)...

Kartik Hariharan, FRCS, FRCS(Ortho),
Consultant Orthopaedic and Foot and Ankle Surgeon,
Newport, South Wales, United Kingdom

This book is 'just what the doctor ordered' in India and other places in the world where foot and ankle surgery is taking roots as a specialty...Dr Rajiv Shah's classic, to-the-point teaching style is reflected in this book which helps busy trainees and surgeons get enriched with the state-of-the-art information in no time.

Vinod K Panchbhavi, MD, FACS,

Professor of Orthopedic Surgery,
Chief, Division of Foot and Ankle Surgery,
University of Texas Medical Branch, Texas, USA

Foot and ankle problems and their management in India is largely different from those in Western countries...In this handbook, he (Dr Rajiv Shah) has taken on the herculean task of providing updated information on the subject in a very lucid manner...I strongly recommend it to all orthopedic surgeons treating foot and ankle problems.

G. S. Kulkarni, MS (Gen Surg), MS (Ortho), FRCS,
Director, Postgraduate Institute of Swasthiyog Pratisthan,
Miraj, India; Former President, Trauma Society of India

The Handbook of Foot and Ankle Orthopedics... is compact, robust and the perfect size for a handbook. It covers all the major foot and ankle conditions that you will encounter in you daily practice. It is presented in a simple, logical and easy-to-grasp format that is not overly lengthy, and is packed full of information...I recommend this book as a must read for all orthopaedic surgeons...

Ashish Shah, MD,

Assistant Professor, Orthopaedics Foot and Ankle,
University of Alabama, USA

Handbook of Foot and Ankle Orthopedics

Rajiv Shah, MS (Ortho),

Managing Director,
Sunshine Global Hospitals, Gujarat, India;
National Chairman,
Indo-US Foot and Ankle Courses, India;
Former President,
Indian Foot and Ankle Society, India

First Reprint, 2017

Thieme
Delhi • Stuttgart • New York • Rio de Janeiro

Publishing Director: Dr. Sonu Singh
Development Editor: Dr. Gurvinder Kaur
Head, Editorial Services: Rachna Sinha
Assistant Manager - Editorial Production:
Kumar Kunal
Sales and Marketing Director: Arun Kumar Majji
Chief Executive Officer: Ajit Kohli

Thieme Medical and Scientific Publishers
Private Limited.
A - 12, Second Floor, Sector - 2, Noida - 201 301,
Uttar Pradesh, India, +911204556600
Email: customerservice@thieme.in
www.thieme.in

Cover design: Thieme Publishing Group
Page make-up by Cerebrum Cross Media
Services

Printed in India by Gopsons Papers Limited

First Reprint, 2017

Handbook of Foot and Ankle Orthopedics

ISBN 978-93-85062-23-0

eISBN 978-93-85062-28-5

This book is dedicated to my dearest wife Dr Bina Shah
whose love, support and tolerance nurtured this book!

Rajiv Shah

Contents

Foreword

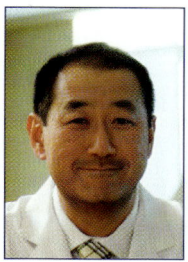

"Education is the most powerful weapon which you can use to change the world."
–Nelson Mandela

India is in the midst of one of the most rapidly changing environments in health care history. With almost 1.3 billion people today and expected to exceed China's population shortly, India spent almost US \$78 billion in health care in 2012 and this is projected to exceed US \$280 billion by 2020. Diabetes is one of the most rapidly rising disease conditions in India, growing at a rate of almost 8% of the population. But because of poor access to primary care physicians and data collection, it is estimated that the rate of diabetes in the country may grow to almost 30%. India also has one of the fastest-growing segments of people aged over 65 years and with degenerative arthritis. And due to very high motor vehicle accident rates and industrial accidents, posttraumatic deformities approach epidemic rates here.

These are formidable times for an orthopedic surgeon in India.

This brilliant handbook written by Dr Rajiv Shah, MS, helps make sense of an overwhelming environment. Rather than running away from the most difficult diabetic foot condition or the worst of a traumatic deformity, the lone orthopedic surgeon can now analyze almost every common foot and ankle condition with logic and reason. With this handbook, the surgeon will get help in identifying common conditions, avoiding frequent mistakes, and imparting a degree of confidence to their patients as they grow within the field of specialized foot and ankle surgery.

The need for this knowledge is pressing. Treated accurately, diabetes and infection can result in limb salvage instead of amputation. Complex deformity can be treated with precise osteotomies if they are recognized in the correct plane and the patient will be returned to an active lifestyle.

As the surgeon's interest in foot and ankle grows, this elegant handbook even guides the reader to building their own specialized practice. Impressively, the book has almost a full year's fellowship within its covers!

As the world of orthopedic surgery changes in developing countries, this handbook will be a valuable guide for all surgeons to learn the art and science of foot and ankle surgery.

Thomas H. Lee, MD,
Vice President,
American Orthopedic Foot and Ankle Society,
United States

Foreword

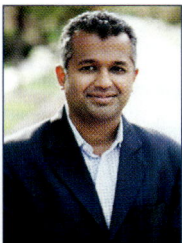

Dr Rajiv Shah has established himself as an eminent foot and ankle surgeon and a respected educator in the field. He has the expertise to analyze and explain foot and ankle surgery in a precise, simple-to-follow and easy-to-remember way.

This handbook is a must-have, quick reference resource for trainees and practicing orthopedic surgeons who are evaluating patients with foot and ankle problems. Dr Shah has consolidated all essential facts about foot and ankle management in this to help orthopedicians evaluate and care for the patients better.

Selene G. Parekh, MD, MBA,
Partner, North Carolina Orthopaedic Clinic,
North Carolina, United States;
Associate Professor,
Department of Orthopaedic Surgery;
and Adjunct Faculty,
Fuqua Business School,
Duke University, North Carolina, United States

Preface

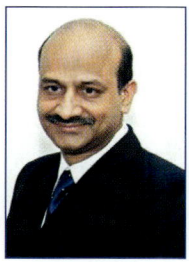

Nine years ago, when I specialized to become the first foot and ankle surgeon of India, I realized that there is a lack of availability of foot and ankle literature as well as expert guidance in the field in our country. I had to heavily rely on Western literature and experts for my guidance and training. What makes practicing foot and ankle orthopedics in developing countries more challenging is the large number of untreated or poorly treated cases, quite a few of whom suffer utter neglect even at the hands of medical practitioners.

The most pressing problems for practicing foot and ankle orthopedicians are lack of resources and nonavailability of equipment, instruments, and implants. These hurdles are further compounded by the financial limitations of patients. In this context, applying Western solutions to indigenous problems led to failures and I had to face many difficulties initially. Gradually, I realized that solutions for our problems have to emerge out of our own innovations and experiences. Doing that was a challenge and I accepted it as a mission.

This work is a step forward in that mission.

This handbook discusses every aspect of foot and ankle orthopedic problems in a concise yet comprehensive manner. In order to serve as a ready reckoner for orthopedic surgeons, it has its content organized in a point-wise format, supported by algorithms, tables, illustrations and real clinical pictures. It offers implementable solutions to both common and complex foot and ankle problems suggested by authors of international repute.

I am certain that this handbook will have a unique and significant place in the armamentarium of every practicing orthopedic surgeon, and it will facilitate the growth of foot and ankle orthopedics as a separate subspecialty of orthopedics in developing countries.

Rajiv Shah

Acknowledgments

This book is a consequence of extensive efforts, both direct and indirect, of many individuals. I would like to recognize and thank them for their significant contributions.

I have been honored by the contributions made to the book by legends in the field like Dr Arun Bal, Dr Vikas Agashe, Dr Ravi Mahajan, and Dr Milind Chaudhary. Notwithstanding hectic work routines, each of their chapters is an extremely sincere effort and would impart invaluable learning to practitioners in the field.

Dr Selene Parekh, Dr Thomas H. Lee, Dr Ashish Shah, Dr G. S. Kulkarni, Dr Mandeep Dhillon, Dr Vinod Panchbhavi, Dr Sudhir Babhulkar, and Dr Hariharan have always been my mentors and source of inspiration. This book is also a result of their influences in no uncertain terms.

Dr Bhikhubhai Patel, Dr Tushar Shah, Dr Nikesh Shah, Dr Jayesh Solanki, Dr Jaykrishna Mekhiya, Dr Suresh Rathwa, and Dr Vakhat Parmar have helped me tremendously by sharing my work obligations cheerfully. It would have been very difficult for me to work on this book without their cooperation.

Last but not the least, I can never have appropriate expressions to thank my family and my patients for their unflinching support and confidence in me.

Rajiv Shah

Contributors

Arun Bal, MS, PhD,
Consultant Diabetic Foot Surgeon,
Founder President, Diabetic Foot Society of India;
Raheja Hospital, Hinduja Hospital, Nanavati Hospital,
Mumbai, India;
Visiting Professor, Amrita Institute of Medical Sciences, Kochi, India

Milind Chaudhary, MS (Ortho),
Director,
International Deformity and Lengthening Institute, Akola, India;
Consultant Orthopaedic Surgeon,
Jaslok Hospital, Mumbai, India

Rajiv Shah, MS (Ortho),
Foot and Ankle Orthopedics,
Director, Foot and Ankle Centre,
Sunshine Global Hospitals, Vadodra, Surat, Gujarat, India

Ravi Mahajan, MS, MCh (Plastic surgery),
Head, Department of Plastic and Reconstructive Surgery,
Amandeep Hospital, Amritsar, India

Vikas Agashe, MS (Ortho), D Ortho,
Orthopedic Surgeon,
P D Hinduja, Kohinoor Hospital and Dr Agashe's Maternity and Surgical Nursing Home,
Mumbai, India

Foot and Ankle Examination

Foot and ankle examination means rule of three!

Precise clinical examination of foot and ankle is the first step toward successful treatment of foot and ankle ailments. Three important rules to be followed by the examiner are listed in **Box 1.1**.

Box 1.1 **Rules for the examiner.**

♦ Gait examination
♦ Foot and ankle examination
♦ Footwear examination

Similarly, there are three important rules to be followed by the patient for proper evaluation, which would allow the examiner to interpret the condition of the disease correctly. Three important rules meant for the patient are listed in **Box 1.2**.

Box 1.2 **Rules for the patient.**

♦ Enters walking
♦ Enters with footwear
♦ Enters with trousers up

Gait Examination

For proper examination of the gait, the following points are to be observed:

♦ Symmetry of parts
♦ Toe versus patella position
♦ In or out toeing
♦ Arches
♦ Foot posture and position
♦ Heel posture and position
♦ Type of gait

Foot and Ankle Examination

Examination should be performed in three positions. **Box 1.3** illustrates the three rules for patient's positions during examination. Examination of the foot is divided into three parts (**Box 1.4**) and is performed in three basic steps, which are listed in **Flowchart 1.1**.

Box 1.3 Rules for patient's positioning during examination.
♦ Examination while walking ♦ Examination while standing ♦ Examination while sitting

Box 1.4 Parts of examination of the foot.
♦ Ankle and hindfoot examination ♦ Midfoot examination ♦ Forefoot examination

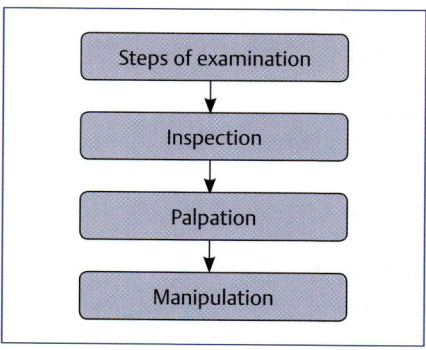

Flowchart 1.1 Steps of examination.

Inspection

Consider the following while inspecting foot and ankle:

♦ Alignment and position of foot with respect to ankle as well as alignment of ankle and foot with respect to leg, knee, and hip
♦ Shape and size of the foot
♦ Deformities, deviations, and prominences
♦ Skin
♦ Callosities and corns
♦ Varicosities
♦ Nails and hair

Palpation

Palpation is done by using the index finger, either self or that of the patient (**Fig. 1.1**), beginning sequentially from the medial aspect to the plantar, to the lateral, followed by the anterior, and finally ending at the posterior aspect.

The three important parts of palpation are mentioned in **Box 1.5**.

For the right foot, start clockwise, and for the left foot start anticlockwise (**Figs. 1.2 and 1.3**).

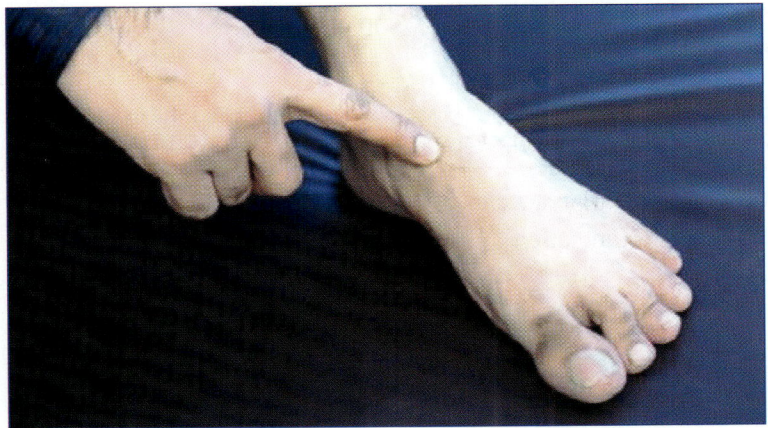

Fig. 1.1   Patient pointing at the painful area with his index finger.

Box 1.5	**Parts of palpation.**

♦ Topographical palpation
♦ Neurological palpation
♦ Vascular palpation

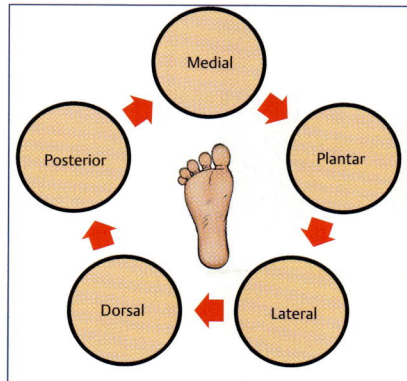 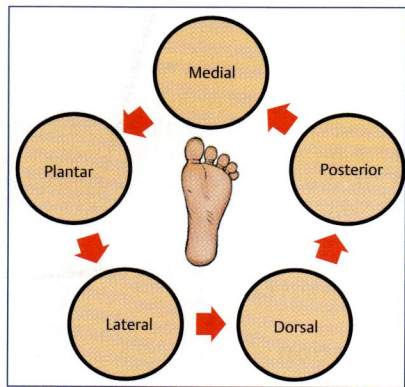

Fig. 1.2   Palpation of the right foot.   **Fig. 1.3**   Palpation of the left foot.

Topographical Palpation

Structures to be palpated in sequence are as follows:

♦ Skin
♦ Bone and joints
♦ Ligaments
♦ Muscles and tendons
♦ Arches

Topographical palpation areas of (1) ankle are depicted in **Figs. 1.4** to **1.8** and are described in **Table 1.1**; (2) midfoot are depicted in **Figs. 1.9** and **1.10** and are described

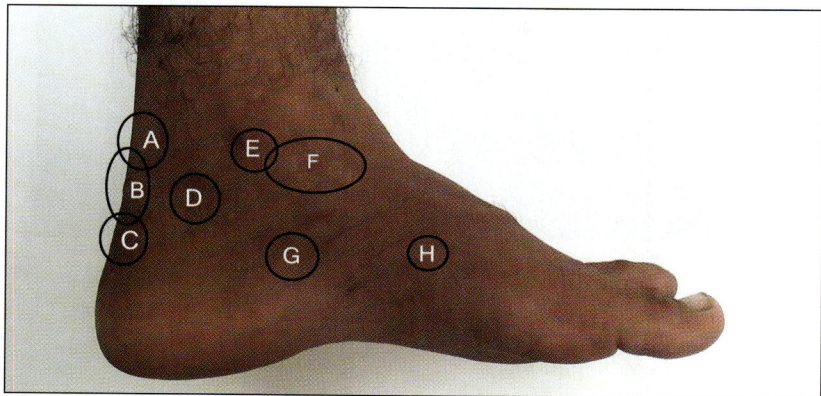

Fig. 1.4   Medial aspect of the foot and ankle. A, Achilles rupture/noninsertional tendonitis; B, insertional Achilles tendonitis; C, calcaneal apophysitis/pump bump; D, retrocalcaneal bursitis; E, tarsal tunnel syndrome/ tibial posterior tendon; F, medial/deltoid ankle sprain; G, entrapment of first branch of lateral plantar nerve; H, accessory navicular/master knot of Henry/medial plantar nerve entrapment.

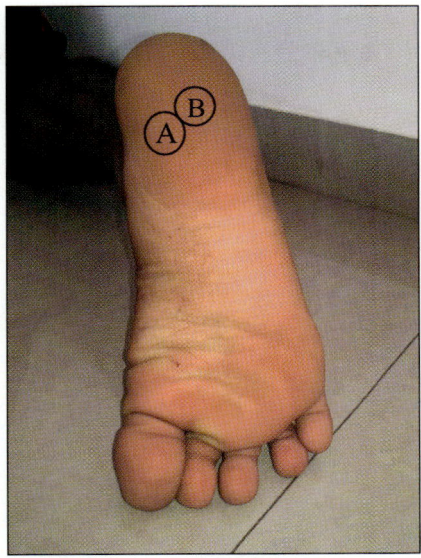

Fig. 1.5 Plantar aspect of the foot. A, plantar fasciitis; B, fat pad atrophy.

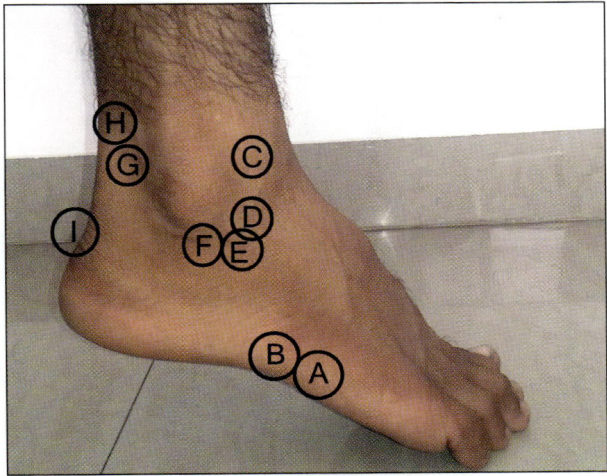

Fig. 1.6 Lateral aspect of the foot and ankle. A, Jones fracture; B, avulsion fracture of the fifth metatarsal; C, anterior ankle impingement; D, anterior talofibular ligament; E, sinus tarsi syndrome; F, calcaneofibular ligament; G, retrocalcaneal bursitis; H, Achilles tendonitis; I, calcaneal apophysitis/Sever's disease/pump bump.

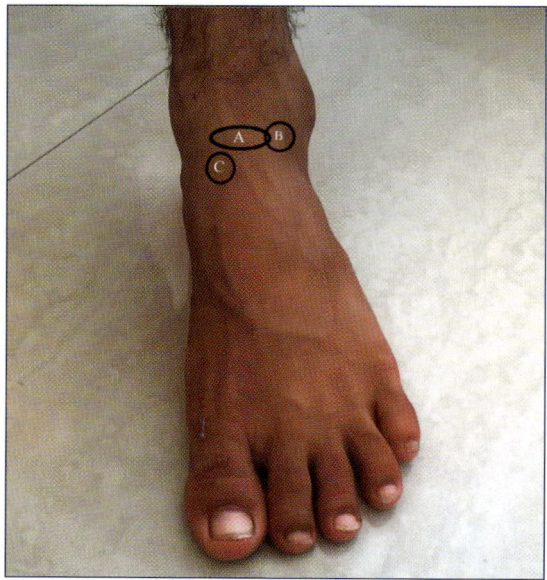

Fig. 1.7 Anterior (dorsal) aspect of the foot and ankle. A, anterior ankle impingement; B, osteochondral defect of talar dome medial or lateral; C, the n spot: navicular stress fracture.

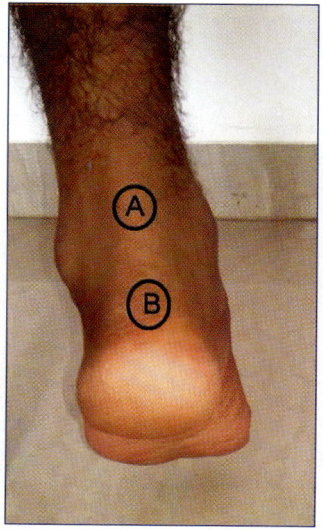

Fig. 1.8 Posterior aspect of the foot and ankle. A, tendo Achilles; B, insertion of tendo Achilles.

Table 1.1   Areas for topographical palpation of ankle

Medial	Plantar	Lateral	Anterior	Posterior
Medial malleolus	Abductor hallucis	Tip of fibula	Tibialis anterior	Achilles tendon
Medial joint line	Plantar fascia	Shaft of fibula	Extensor hallucis longus	Insertion of Achilles
Medial gutter	Abductor digiti minimi	Lateral gutter of ankle	Extensor digitorum longus	Retrocalcaneal
Navicular	Fat pad	Syndesmosis	Tibia	
Talar head		Lateral wall of calcaneus	Talus dome	
Tibialis posterior		Peroneal tubercle	Superficial peroneal nerve	
Flexor digitorum longus		Sinus tarsi	Peroneus tertius	
Flexor hallucis longus		Extensor digitorum brevis	Ankle joint	
Posterior tibial artery		Lateral talar process		
Sustentaculum tali		Peroneal tendons		
Deltoid ligament		Anterior talofibular ligament		
Medial tibia		Calcaneofibular ligament		
Medial talus		Sural nerve		

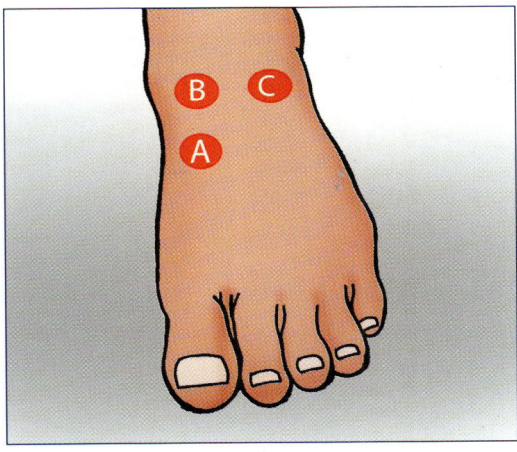

Fig. 1.9 Dorsum of the midfoot. A, naviculo-cuneiform joint; B, talo-navicular joint; C, calcaneo-cubiod joint.

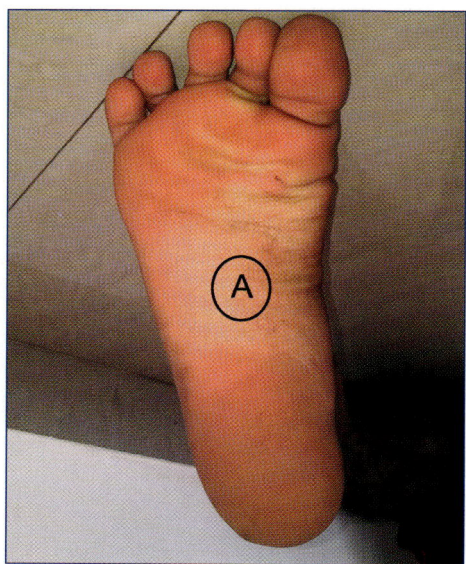

Fig. 1.10   Plantar aspect of the midfoot. A, plantar fascia.

in **Table 1.2;** (3) forefoot are depicted in **Figs. 1.11** and **1.12** and are described in **Table 1.3**.

Table 1.2 Areas for topographical palpation of midfoot	
Dorsal	**Plantar**
Talonavicular joint	Plantar fascia
Calcaneocuboid joint	
Naviculocuneiform joint	
Base of first metatarsal	
Bases of second, third, and fourth metatarsals	
Base of fifth metatarsal	
Insertion of tendon of tibialis posterior	
Insertion of tendon of tibialis anterior	
Insertion of tendon of peroneus brevis	

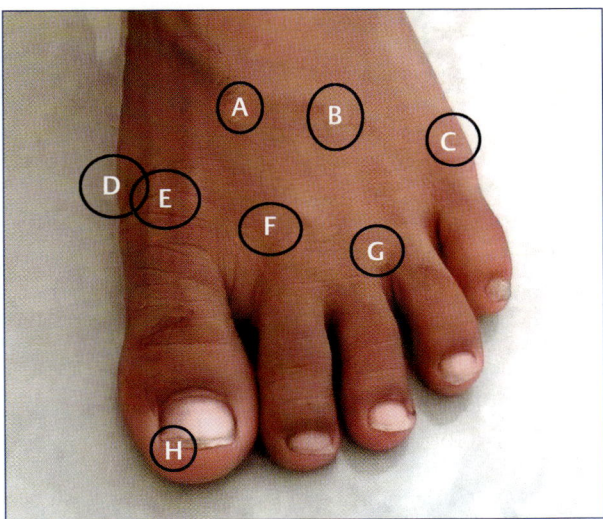

Fig. 1.11   Dorsum of the forefoot. A, lisfranc sprain; B, anterior tarsal tunnel syndrome; C, bunionette; D, bunion/gout; E, hallux rigidus; F, Freiberg infarction; G, Morton neuroma; H, paronychia.

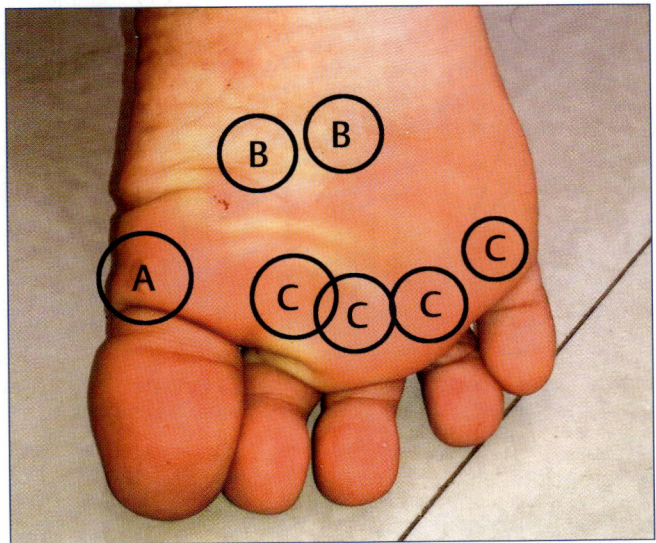

Fig. 1.12   Plantar aspect of forefoot. A, sesamoiditis/stress fracture/sports injury; B, stress fractures of metatarsals; C, metatarsalgia.

Table 1.3	Areas for topographical palpation of forefoot
Hallux	**Lesser toes**
Head of first metatarsal	Metatarsal shafts
Medial sesamoid	Head of metatarsals
Lateral sesamoid	Metatarsophalangeal joints
Dorsalis pedis artery	Extensor digitorum longus
Extensor hallucis longus	Flexor digitorum longus
Extensor digitorum brevis	
Metatarsophalangeal joint	
Flexor hallucis longus	

Neurological Palpation

Nerve supply of foot is shown in **Figs. 1.13** and **1.14**. Neurological palpation includes testing of the following elements:

♦ Sensations
♦ Reflexes
♦ Motor strength
♦ Monofilament testing

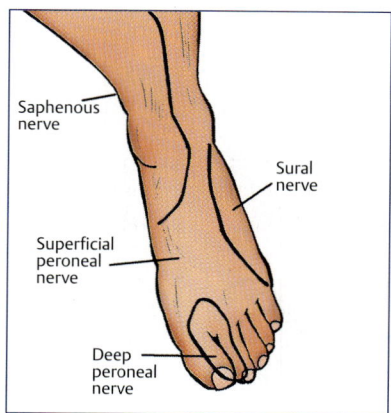

Fig. 1.13   Pattern of nerve supply on the dorsal aspect of the foot.

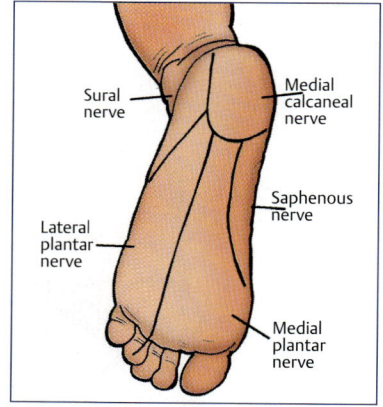

Fig. 1.14   Pattern of nerve supply on the plantar aspect of the foot.

Vascular Palpation

This includes examination of the following:

♦ Dorsalis pedis artery
♦ Posterior tibial artery
♦ Nail bed circulation

Manipulation

Both active and passive manipulations are important!
The following are manipulated:

♦ Joints
♦ Pulses
♦ Neurological examination includes sensations, power, and reflexes
♦ Motor examination includes tone, tightness, snapping, tenderness, fullness, and strength of every muscle of foot and ankle
♦ Plantar fascia
♦ Arches
♦ Deformities and correctability

Footwear Examination

This includes examination of the following:

♦ Wear and sites of wear
♦ Creases
♦ Size and shape
♦ Laces
♦ Heel and heel counter
♦ Forefoot impression
♦ Shoe versus foot shape
♦ Flexion test (**Fig. 1.15**)
♦ Torsion test (**Fig. 1.16**)

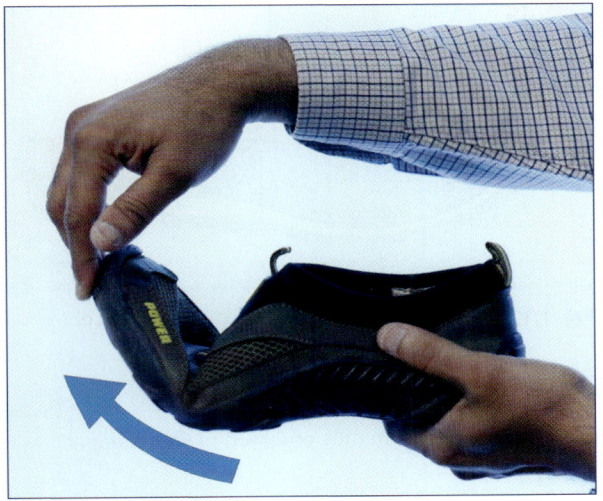

Fig. 1.15   Grossly flexible and deformed footwear on flexion test.

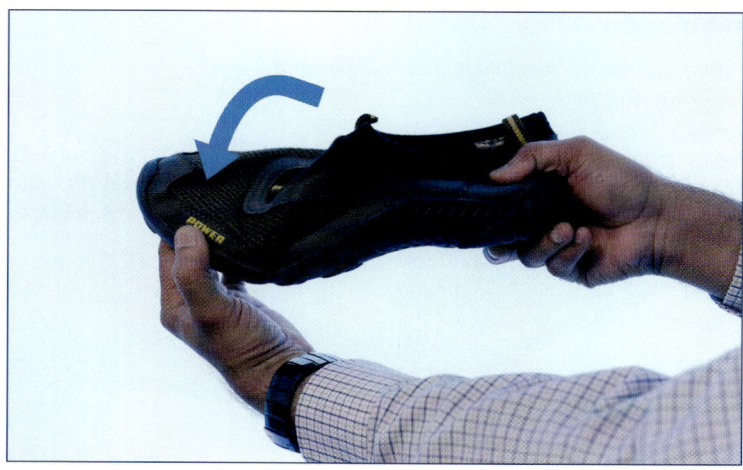

Fig. 1.16 Torsion test. Grossly deformed footwear on twisting front portion over the back portion of footwear.

♦ *Orthosis examination*: Look for the type of orthosis. Fitting of orthosis in the footwear and precise positioning of offloading by orthosis over and above wear and tear of orthosis should be noted (**Fig. 1.17**).

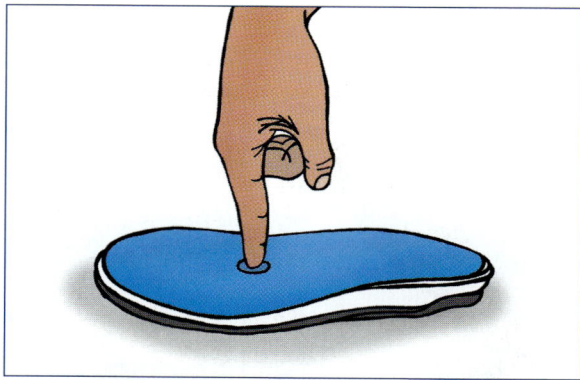

Fig. 1.17 Orthotic examination.

Examination while Standing

The following points are to be carefully observed in foot and ankle in the standing position:

♦ Arches
♦ In toeing/out toeing

- Foot position in relation to ankle and leg
- Shortening
- Toe position
- Heel position
- Tendo Achilles
- Too many toes sign: More than two toes are seen in a patient of flat foot in standing position when examined from behind (**Fig. 1.18**).

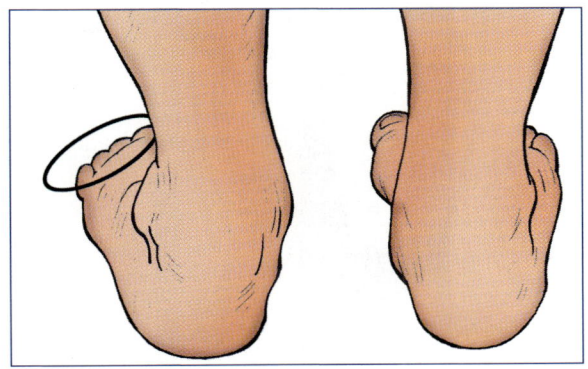

Fig. 1.18   Too many toes sign.

Examination While Sitting

This forms the major part of examination where all the aforementioned examinations are done with the patient sitting on a table with legs hanging. The examiner sits in front of the patient on a low stool (**Fig. 1.19**).

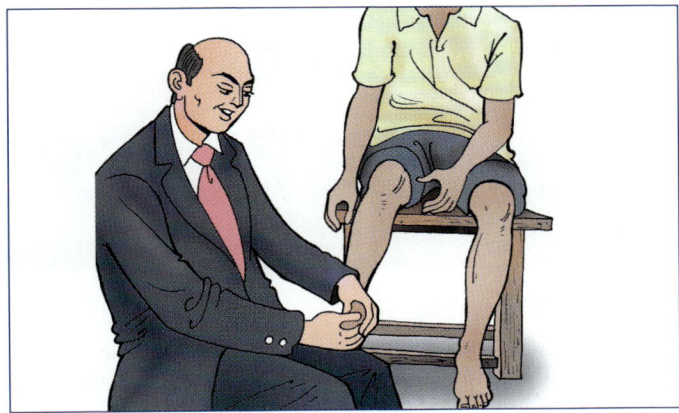

Fig. 1.19   Examination while sitting.

Special Tests for Foot and Ankle Examination

Some special tests are illustrated in **Figs. 1.20** to **1.35**.

♦ *Thompson's test*: This test is performed by squeezing of the calf, which shows plantar flexion of the heel. This means that the tendo Achilles is intact and not ruptured (**Fig. 1.20**).

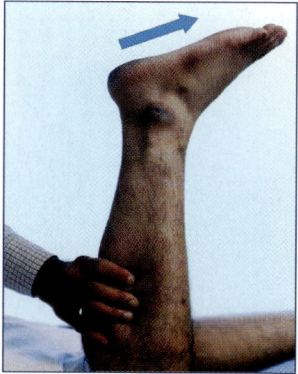

Fig. 1.20   Thompson's test.

♦ *Silfverskiold's test*: This test is done for passive ankle dorsiflexion with knee in extension and in flexion to differentiate tightness or contracture of only the gastrocnemius or both gastrocnemius and soleus (**Fig. 1.21**).

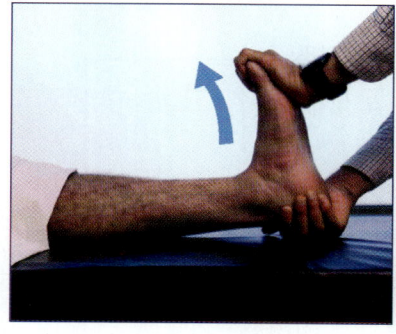 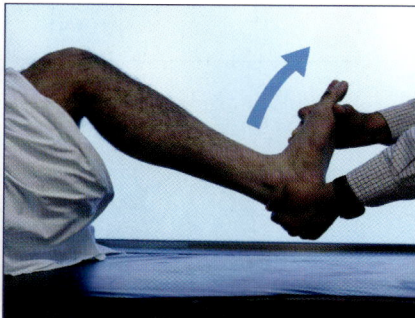

Fig. 1.21   Silfverskiold test.

♦ *Coleman block test*: This test is demonstrated in **Fig. 1.22**, where the forefoot is allowed to drop, while the hindfoot is on a board. The test is used to differentiate whether the varus of the foot is driven by hindfoot or by forefoot, where in the latter case the varus does not get corrected. In **Fig. 1.22**, the varus is corrected because it was driven by the hindfoot.

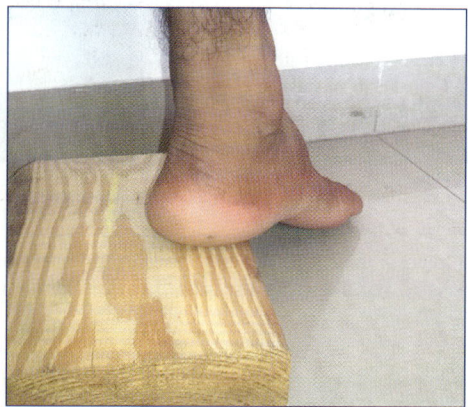

Fig. 1.22   Coleman block test.

◆ *Single heel raise test*: **Fig. 1.23** illustrates the single heel raise test, where it is negative as the patient is able to raise himself on a single heel. A positive test suggests the insufficiency of tibialis posterior tendon as in cases of acquired flat feet.

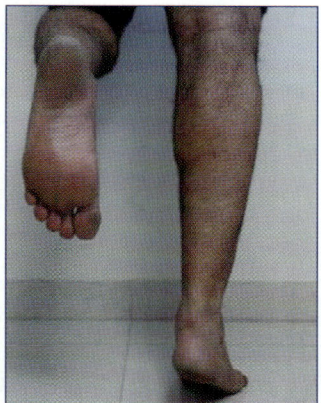

Fig. 1.23   Single heel raise test.

◆ *Mulder's click*: In this test, the metatarsals are rolled with pressure against each other; holding the foot with both the hands, the presence of painful click is checked (**Fig. 1.24**).

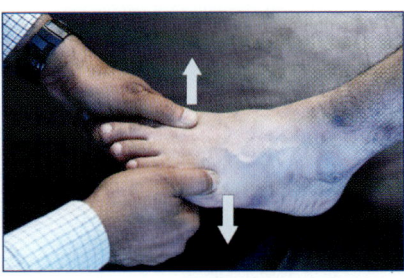
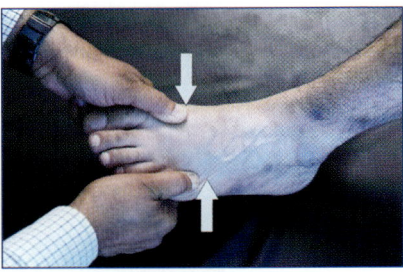

Fig. 1.24   Method of eliciting Mulder's click in a case of Morton neuroma.

♦ *First metatarsal hypermobility*: In this test, the first metatarsal is held with one hand and is rocked up and down against other firmly held metatarsals (**Fig. 1.25**).

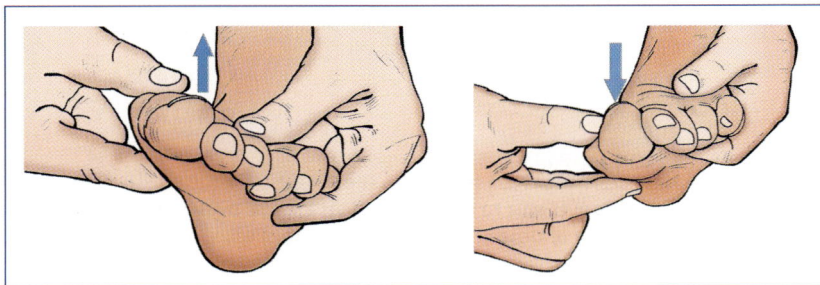

Fig. 1.25   Method of examining hypermobility of the first ray.

♦ *Squeeze test*: This test is for the diagnosis of syndesmotic injury where the calf is squeezed to look for pain at the level of syndesmosis (**Fig. 1.26**).

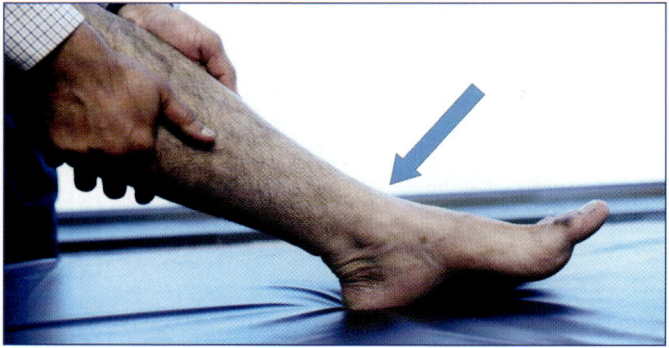

Fig. 1.26   Squeeze test.

♦ *External rotation test*: This test is demonstrated for the diagnosis of syndesmotic injury; it is being done with a foot being rotated externally against a firmly held leg with the other hand. Presence of pain at syndesmosis is diagnostic (**Fig. 1.27**).

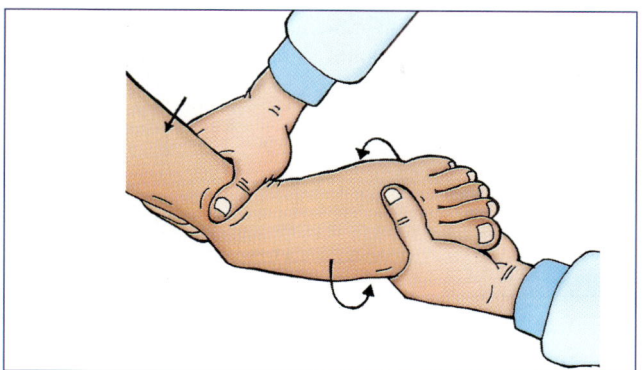

Fig. 1.27   External rotation test.

♦ *Tinel's sign*: **Fig. 1.28** shows percussion of the posterior tibial nerve to elicit Tinel's sign. Such a percussion would elicit tingling sensations in the course of the nerve.

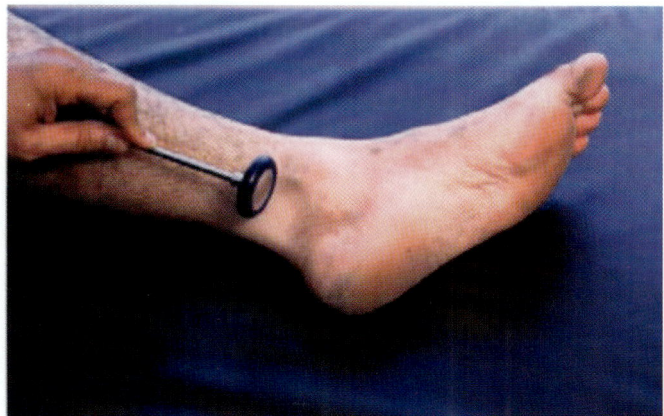

Fig. 1.28   Tinel's sign.

♦ *Stretch test*: It is performed for the diagnosis of tarsal tunnel syndrome. The ankle is fully dorsiflexed and everted with full dorsiflexion of all toes. Presence of pain and paresthesia suggests diagnostic of tarsal tunnel syndrome (**Fig. 1.29**).

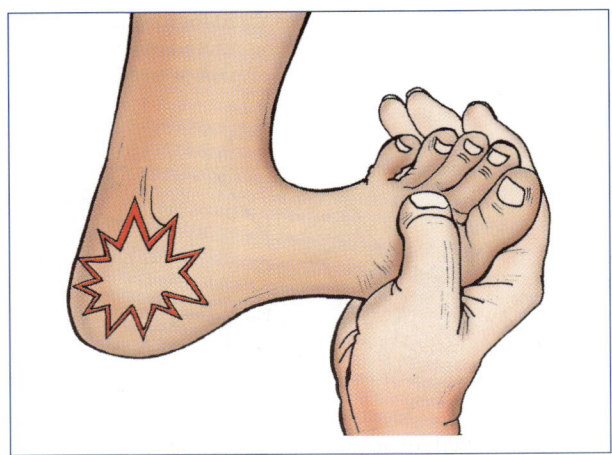

Fig. 1.29 Stretch test.

♦ *Calcaneal compression test*: It is performed by applying pressure of both the fists at the body of the calcaneus. Stress fracture of calcaneus would be tender (**Fig. 1.30**).

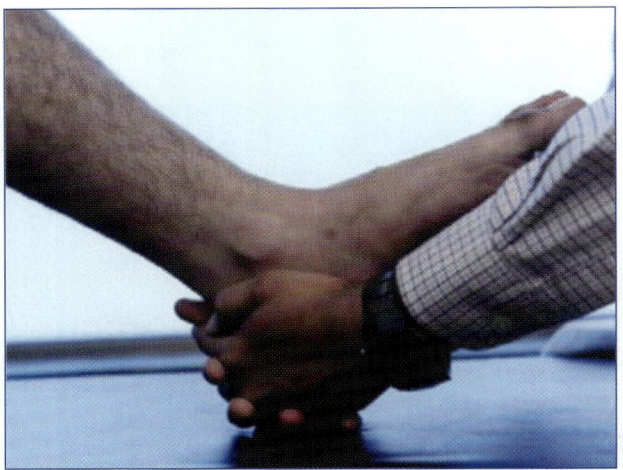

Fig. 1.30 Calcaneal compression test.

♦ *Instability tests*: These tests are shown in **Figs. 1.31** to **1.33**.
  • *Instability test for metatarsophalangeal joint*: This test is done by holding the foot proximal to the joint being tested with one hand and rocking the distal portion of the joint over it with the other hand (**Fig. 1.31**).

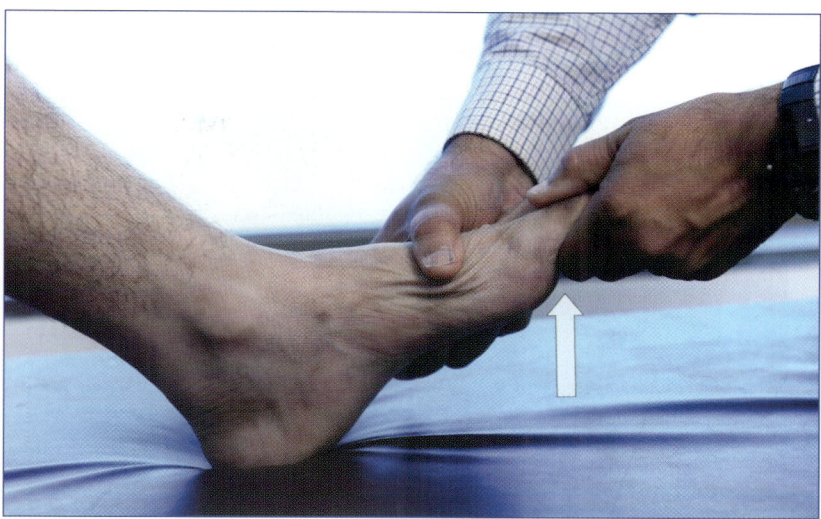

Fig. 1.31   Instability test for metatarsophalangeal joint.

- *Instability test for interphalangeal joint*: This test is done by holding the foot proximal to the joint being tested with one hand and rocking the distal portion of joint over it with the other hand (**Fig. 1.32**).

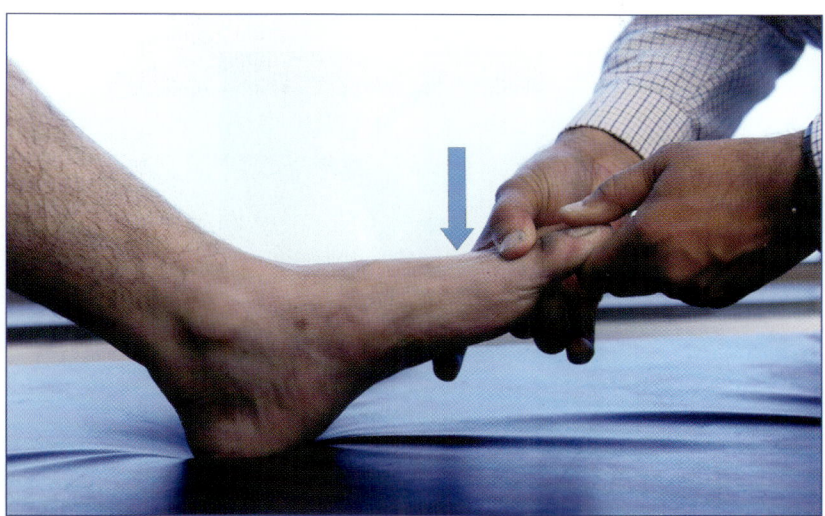

Fig. 1.32   Instability test for interphalangeal joint.

- *Midfoot instability test*: This test is performed with manipulation in abduction and adduction of forefoot against hindfoot (**Fig. 1.33**).

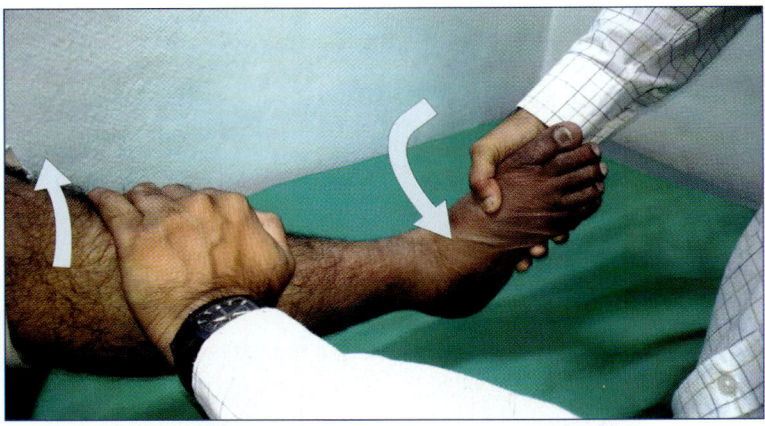

Fig. 1.33   Midfoot instability test.

♦ *Stress tests*: This includes anterior drawer test (**Fig. 1.34**) and talar tilt test (**Fig. 1.35**).
  - *Anterior drawer test*: This test is performed for the diagnosis of ankle instability. A plantarflexed foot held by one hand is pulled anteriorly against tibia stabilized with the other hand and the presence of excessive mobility is evaluated.

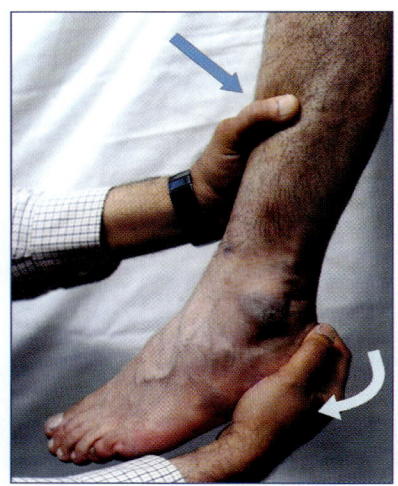

Fig. 1.34   Anterior drawer test.

- *Talar tilt test*: This test is performed where the talus is tilted with one hand against firmly held tibia with the other hand. Any excessive movements are suggestive of positive test when compared with the opposite side (**Fig. 1.35**).

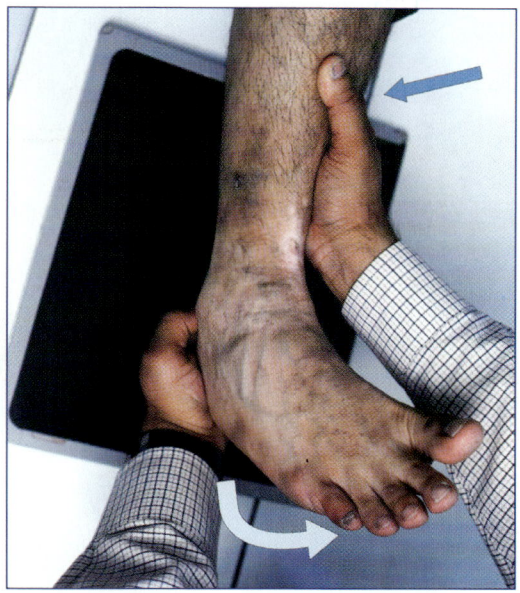

Fig. 1.35   Talar tilt test.

Chapter 2

Radiology in Foot and Ankle

Radiological examination of foot and ankle is not the substitute to clinical examination!

Interpretation of Radiographs

The following points need to be carefully observed and analyzed for correct evaluation of the radiographs:

♦ Position and alignment of bones
♦ Spacing or overlap of bones
♦ Continuity or breech in continuity of bones
♦ Outline of the articular surfaces
♦ Quality of bones
♦ Angles, lines, and radiological signs

In total, there are four types of radiographs. These are listed in **Box 2.1**.

Box 2.1   Types of radiographs

♦ Routine radiographs
♦ Specialized radiographs
♦ Weight-bearing radiographs
♦ Stress radiographs

Routine Radiographs

These include a series of ankle and foot X-rays.

♦ Ankle series X-rays
  • Anteroposterior (AP) (**Fig. 2.1A**)

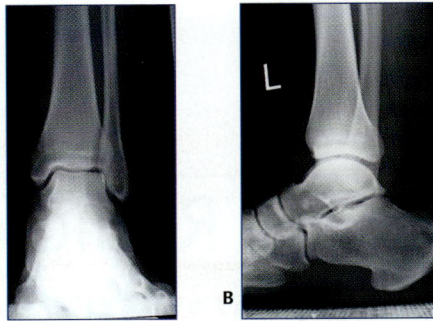

Fig. 2.1 (A and B)   **(A)** Anteroposterior (AP) and **(B)** Lateral (LAT) views of ankle.

- Lateral (LAT) (**Fig. 2.1B**)
- *Oblique (mortise) views*: Mortise view is 15-degree internal rotation view, which clearly shows ankle mortise in its true plane. Mortise view eliminates overlap of fibula over tibia so that position and alignment of both bones can be evaluated (**Fig. 2.2**).
◆ Foot series X-rays
  - Dorsoplantar (AP) (**Fig. 2.3A, B**)
  - Lateral (LAT) (**Fig. 2.3C**)
  - *Oblique (internal oblique or lateral oblique) views*: This view shows lateral column of foot, cuboid, and fourth and fifth metatarsals (**Fig. 2.4A, B**).

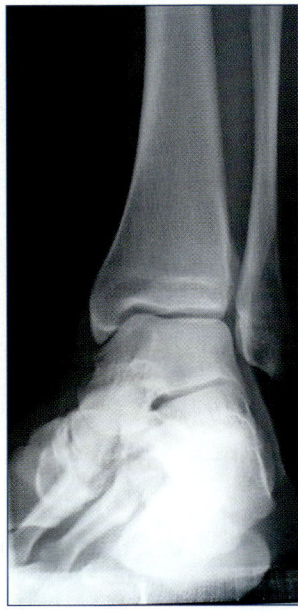

Fig. 2.2   Mortise view of ankle.

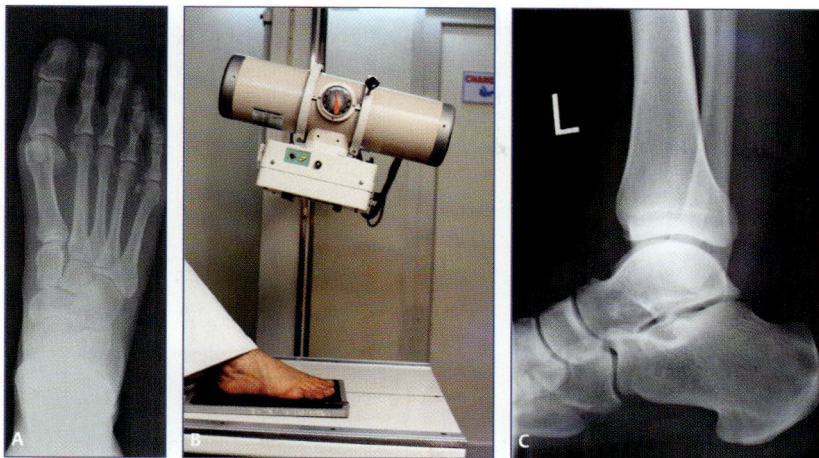

Fig. 2.3 (A-C) **(A)** Dorsoplantar (AP) view of left foot, **(B)** method of obtaining AP view of foot, and **(C)** Lateral (LAT) view of left foot.

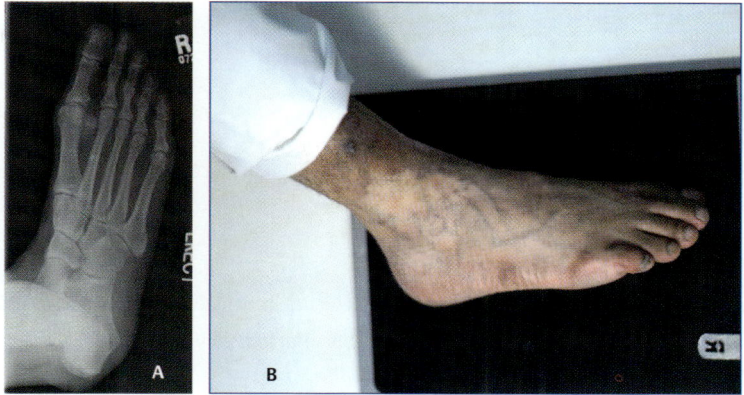

Fig. 2.4 (A and B) **(A)** Internal oblique or lateral oblique view of foot, and **(B)** method of obtaining internal oblique or lateral oblique view of foot.

Specialized Radiographs

♦ *Medial oblique or external oblique view of foot*: This view shows the medial column of foot, navicular, medial cuneiform, first metatarsal and its articulations (**Figs. 2.5 and 2.6**).
♦ *Harris axial view of heel*: This view shows calcaneus and subtalar joint (**Figs. 2.7 and 2.8**).

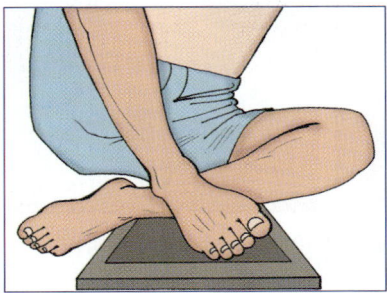

Fig. 2.5 Positioning for taking external oblique or medial oblique view of foot.

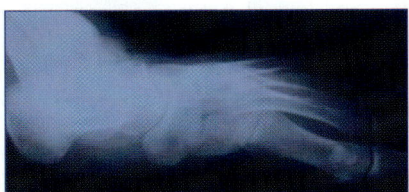

Fig. 2.6 External oblique or medial oblique view of foot.

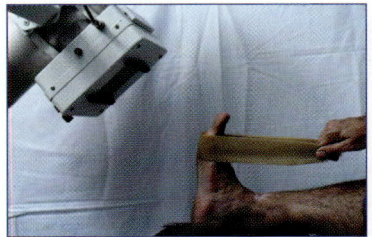

Fig. 2.7 Method of taking Harris axial view.

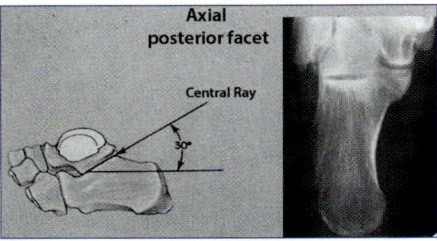

Fig. 2.8 Harris axial view of heel.

♦ *Sesamoid view*: This view is needed for diagnosing the problems of sesamoids (**Figs. 2.9 and 2.10**).
♦ *Broden's views*: These views are taken with 10, 20, 30, and 40 degrees cranial angulation of an X-ray beam focused at the tip of the fibula, with ankle rotated 45 degrees internally. Excellent view of posterior subtalar joint given by these views helps in intraoperative monitoring of calcaneus fracture reduction and assessment of postoperative fusion status of subtalar joint (**Figs. 2.11 and 2.12**).
♦ *Canale and Kelly's view*: This view is taken with foot plantar flexed and pronated to 15 degrees and it delineates medial column along the talus. This view is used

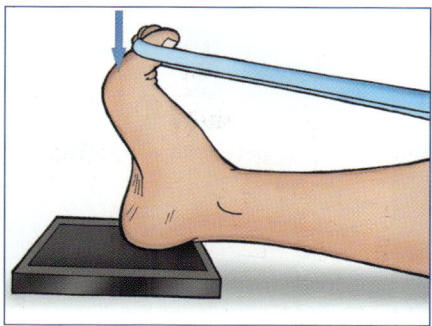

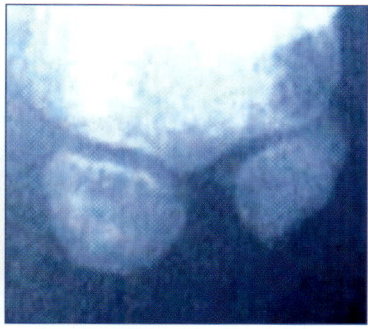

Fig. 2.9 Method of obtaining Sesamoid view.

Fig. 2.10 Sesamoid view of foot.

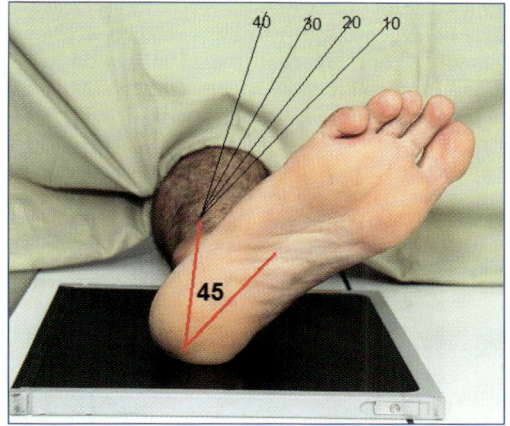

Fig. 2.11 Ankle and foot positioning for obtaining Broden's view.

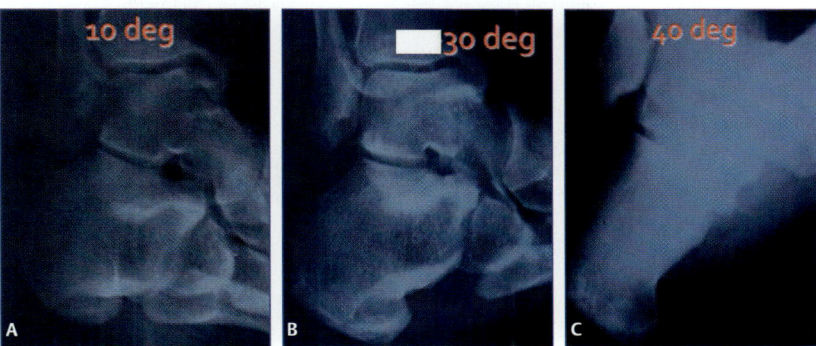

Fig. 2.12 Broden's view at 10°, 30°, and 40° rotation.

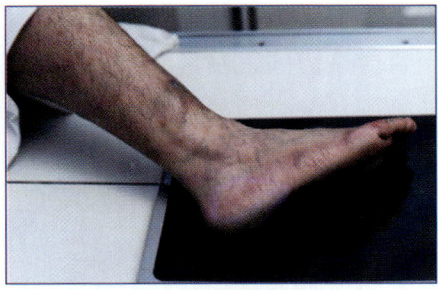
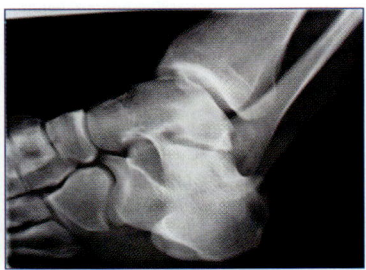

Fig. 2.13 Method of obtaining Canale and Kelly's view.

Fig. 2.14 Canale and Kelly's view.

for assessing the amount of comminution and displacement of fracture neck talus (**Figs. 2.13** and **2.14**).

♦ *Comparative views*: Because of extensive overlap and typical articulating pattern of foot and ankle bones, comparative views are needed. Important information regarding the length of bones, spaces between bones, and pattern of articulation of bones is gained from comparative views. Comparative views are commonly used for planning as well as intraoperative analysis of ankle, midfoot, and Lisfranc injuries.

♦ *Midfoot X-ray projection*: It is mandatory to keep the X-ray beam perpendicular to the midfoot and not to the floor for precise projection of midfoot. This can be done using a special stand or by tilting the X-ray tube (**Fig. 2.15**).

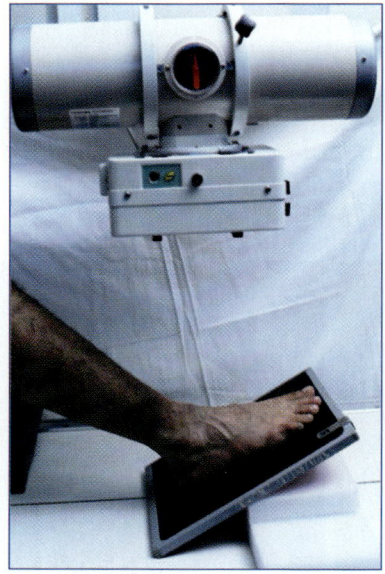

Fig. 2.15 Method of midfoot X-ray projection.

Weight-Bearing Radiographs

Radiographs of the weight-bearing foot and ankle can demonstrate the foot and ankle in a more functional situation and may provide insight into the relationship among the soft tissues, bones, and the joints under physiologic loads. Some important points of consideration are as follows:

♦ Majority of problems in foot and ankle are noticed or aggravated during weight bearing or walking. This justifies the study and analysis of bones and joints during weight-bearing posture. Any alterations seen on weight bearing X-ray views will give information about the integrity of bony and ligamentous structures.

♦ *AP, LAT, and oblique weight-bearing views of ankle*: These views give an idea about the deformation on weight bearing and are useful for defining the stages of flat foot and defining the integrity of deltoid ligament.

♦ *AP, LAT, and oblique weight-bearing views of foot*: These views are important to define subtle injuries of the midfoot, stages of flat foot, and deformation in neuropathic foot. Measurements of various angles for treating hallux valgus are also done through these views (**Figs. 2.16** and **2.17**).

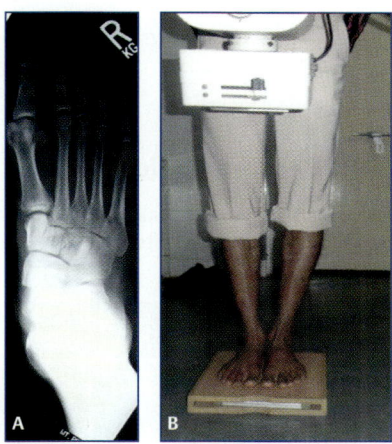

Fig. 2.16 (A and B) (A) Weight-bearing AP image of foot and (B) method of obtaining weight bearing view of foot.

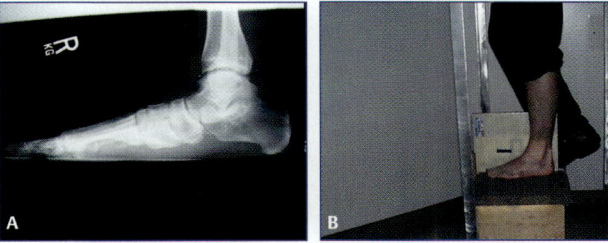

Fig. 2.17 (A and B) (A) Weight-bearing lateral view of foot and (B) method of obtaining weight-bearing lateral view of foot.

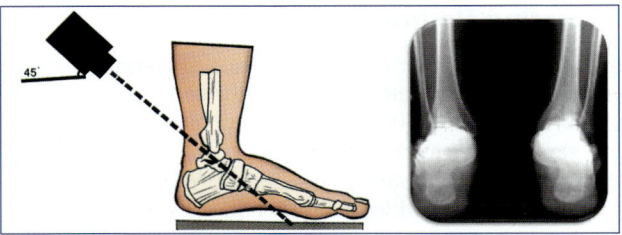

Fig. 2.18 Method of obtaining Saltzman view.

♦ *Saltzman view*: It is a tangential weight-bearing postero-anterior view of the hindfoot and leg, demonstrating weight-bearing relationship of the hindfoot with the leg (**Fig. 2.18**).
♦ Comparison of non–weight-bearing X-ray views with weight-bearing X-ray views is a must.
♦ Interpretation notes on weight-bearing X-rays focuses on the following points:
  • Change in position and alignment of bones
  • Opening of bony spaces
  • Angulation of bones
  • Articular space
  • Angles, lines, and radiological signs

How to Take Weight-Bearing Radiographs?

♦ A special stand with steps is required to take weight-bearing view of the ankle (**Fig. 2.19**). A 1-inch-deep slot on the top step of this stand is used for inserting

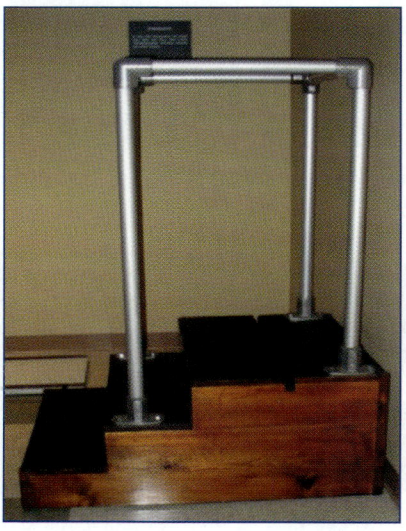

Fig. 2.19 Stand for obtaining weight-bearing AP, oblique, and lateral views of ankle.

the X-ray cassette. The stand needs to be wide enough (2–2.5 feet) for the patient to stand comfortably. The height of the step should not be more than 6 inches. There should be a holding rail attached to the X-ray stand for support.

♦ The patient stands in various positions on the step of the stand in front of the cassette, and the X-ray beam is projected from the front.

♦ The same stand can be used for taking weight-bearing lateral view of the foot where the patient stands on the step and the cassette is inserted in the slot.

♦ For weight-bearing X-rays of foot, a special wooden box is needed where a slot for X-ray cassette is provided (**Fig. 2.20**).

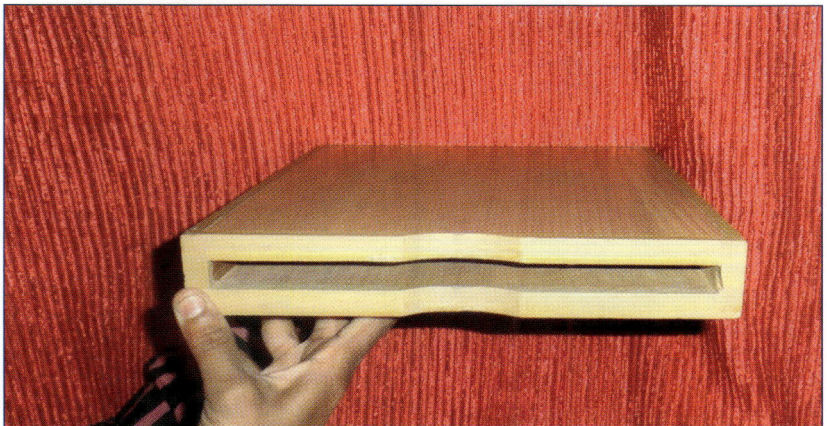

Fig. 2.20   Stand for putting X-ray cassette for obtaining weight-bearing AP and oblique views of foot.

♦ The patient stands on the wooden box, and the beam is centered on the foot in different positions.

Stress Radiographs

♦ Plain radiography has the following limitations:
  • Interobserver variations
  • Variations of exposure
  • Variations due to distance

♦ Stress radiography is the gold standard for analyzing integrity of the capsule-ligamentous structures. Stress radiography is used for the diagnosis and evaluation of trauma as well as disorders of ankle and midfoot.

♦ In painful conditions, stress radiography can be done after injecting local anesthetic in the area of pain.

♦ C-arm-guided intraoperative stress radiography of foot can be done by putting the foot on a firm, flat plate and applying vertical pressure over the foot from above and below.

♦ *Gravity stress view*: is taken through cross-table projection of an externally rotated foot and ankle, with the affected side lying upward. This view would show widening of the medial space and would help to diagnose syndesmotic injuries (**Fig. 2.21**).

♦ *Talar tilt stress view*: helps in manipulation of the talus in inversion and evaluation of opening of ankle joint laterally. This view is used to assess lateral ligament

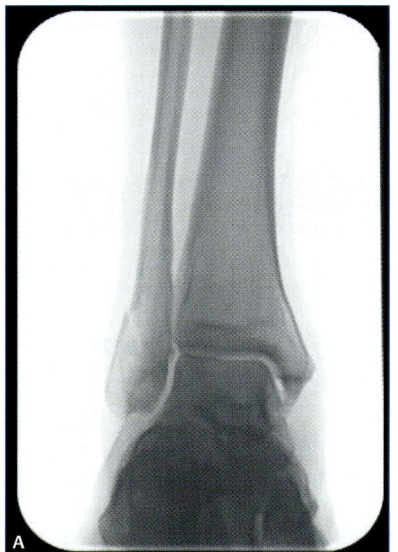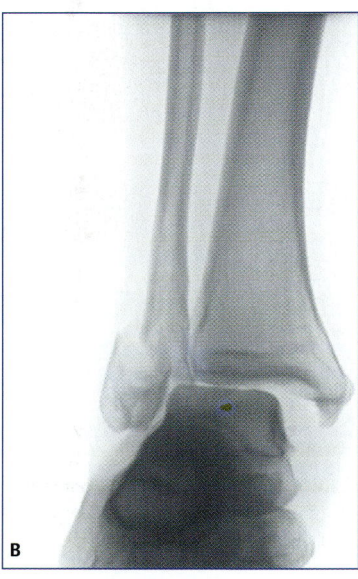

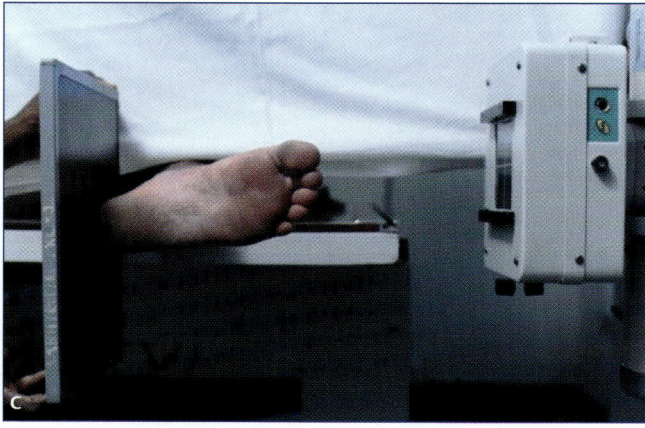

Fig. 2.21 (A-C)   (A and B) Opening up of ankle on gravity stress view of ankle, and **(C)** positioning for gravity stress view.

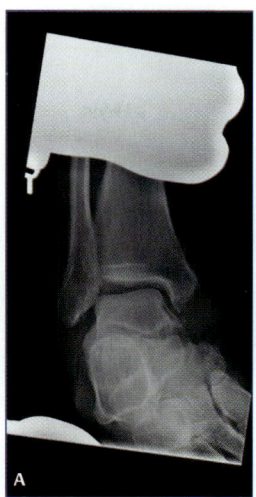
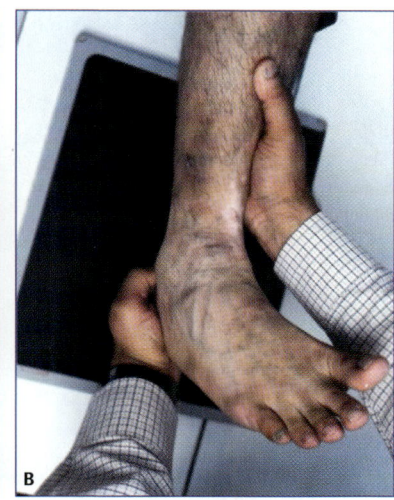

Fig. 2.22 (A and B) **(A)** Talar tilt stress view showing opening of ankle laterally and **(B)** method of obtaining talar tilt stress view.

insufficiency. View is taken by holding talus and tibia. Comparative views may also be required (**Fig. 2.22**).

♦ *Anterior drawer stress view*: assesses the manipulation of the stabilized foot against leg dorsal or plantar wards. This view is useful to assess ankle joint's instability. Lower limb is suspended from the edge of table and the ankle lies in gravity-assisted plantar flexion, while the foot is either pushed or pulled against a stabilized tibia (**Fig. 2.23**).

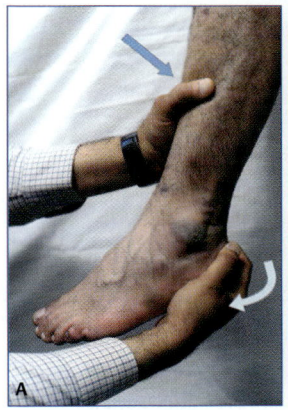
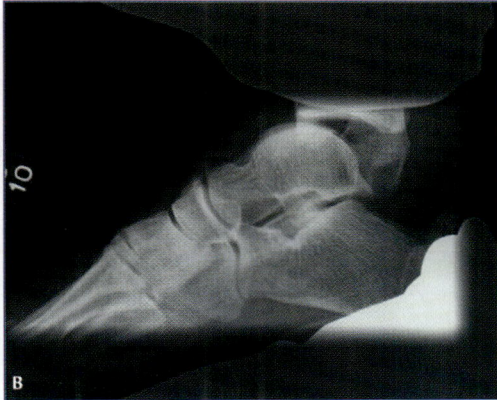

Fig. 2.23 (A and B) Anterior drawer stress view showing instability and the method of taking this view.

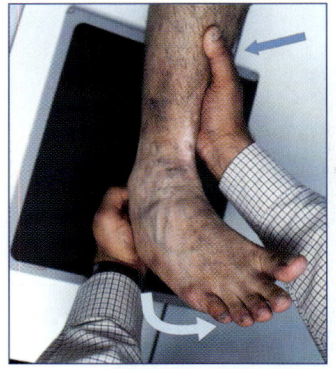

Fig. 2.24 Method of obtaining external rotation stress view.

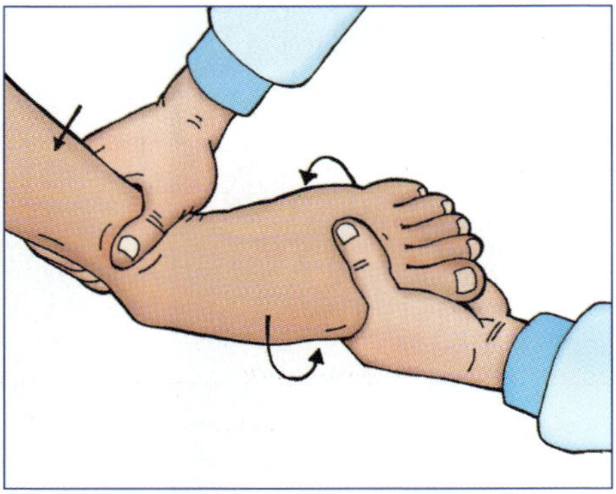

Fig. 2.25 Method of obtaining midfoot stress view.

♦ *External rotation stress view*: is taken by externally rotating the foot against the stabilized leg (**Fig. 2.24**). In cases with syndesmotic injury, there would be pain at syndesmosis.

♦ *Abduction/adduction stress views*: are taken for evaluation of Lisfranc injury where the forefoot is manipulated against the stabilized hindfoot (**Fig. 2.25**).

Radiological Parameters for Ankle

Nine radiological signs are observed for ankle assessment (**Table 2.1**).

Table 2.1   Radiological signs for ankle assessment

S. No.	Radiological view	Radiological sign
1	AP view	Tibiofibular overlap
2	AP view	Tibiofibular clear space
3	AP view	Talar tilt angle
4	AP view	Lateral talar shift
5	AP view	Shenton's line
6	AP view	Dime sign/Arcuate line
7	Mortise view	Medial clear space
8	Mortise view	Talocrural angle
9	Mortise view	Ankle instability sign

Tibiofibular Overlap

It is the distance between the medial border of the fibula and the lateral border of the distal tibia (1 cm above the ankle joint) on AP view. Normal value is 10 mm. This is a syndesmotic reduction parameter (**Fig. 2.26**).

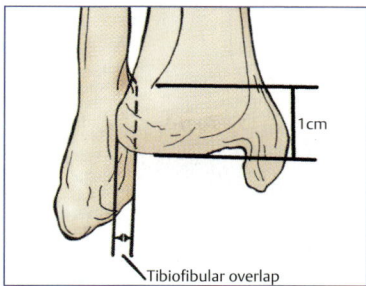

Fig. 2.26 Figure shows how to measure tibiofibular overlap.

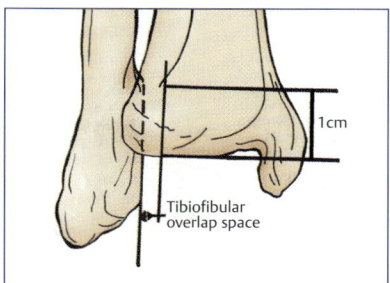

Fig. 2.27 Figure shows how to measure tibiofibular clear space.

Tibiofibular Clear Space

It is the distance between the medial border of the fibula and incisura border of the distal tibia (1 cm above ankle joint). It is normally 5 mm or less. Widened tibiofibular clear space means malreduction of fibula (**Fig. 2.27**).

Talar Tilt Angle

It is the angle between a line parallel to the upper surface of the talus and a line parallel to the long axis of the tibia and is normally less than 2 degrees. Compare it with the opposite side. Talar tilt more than 2 degrees angulation may indicate medial or lateral disruption at the ankle (**Fig. 2.28**).

Lateral Talar Shift Sign

This is an insignificant sign where the lateral border of the talus does not match with that of the inner border of the fibula on comparative views, it suggests talar malposition or shift (**Fig. 2.29**).

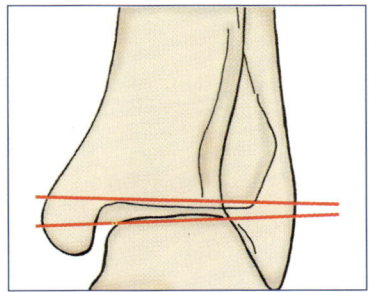

Fig. 2.28 Figure shows how to evaluate talar tilt angle.

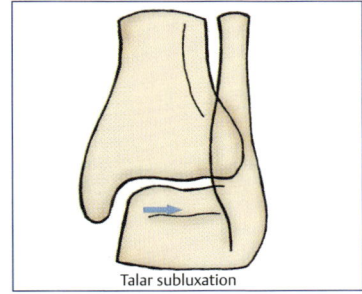

Fig. 2.29 Figure shows how to evaluate lateral talar shift sign.

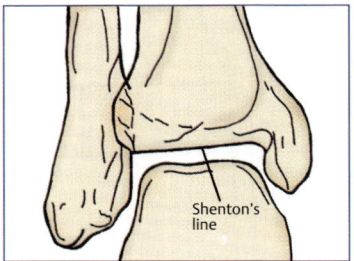

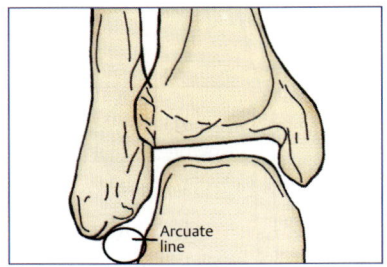

Fig. 2.30 Figure showing the Shenton's line of ankle.

Fig. 2.31 Figure showing the Dime sign or Arcuate line of ankle.

Shenton's Line

Shenton's line is the line of articular surface that runs from articular surface of medial malleolus to ankle and then to lateral malleolus. This line is seen as a dense bone. It must be compared with that of the opposite side (**Fig. 2.30**).

Dime/Ball Sign or Arcuate Line

When a line connecting the medial inferior surface of the lateral malleolus to the lateral inferior talar surface is drawn, it forms a complete ball. This is called Dime sign or Arcuate line of ankle. Arcuate line disruption is suggestive of fibular shortening and malunion (**Fig. 2.31**).

Medial Clear Space

This is the space between the lateral border of the medial malleolus and medial border of talus in a mortise ankle view, which normally is 4 mm or less. More than 4 mm indicates lateral talar shift (**Fig. 2.32**).

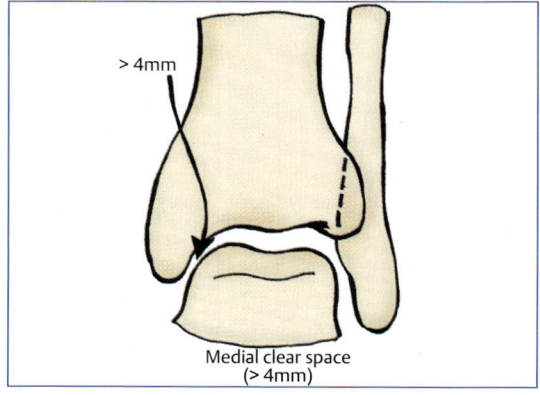

Fig. 2.32 Figure shows medial clear space evaluation.

Talocrural Angle

It is the angle between the distal tibial articular surface and a line from tips of medial and lateral malleoli, which is normally 83 ± 4 degrees. It should also be compared with the opposite side (**Fig. 2.33**).

Ankle Instability Sign

Comparison of medial clear space to the width of ankle joint space between superior surface of the talus and inferior surface of the tibia is done. Whenever a larger medial clear space than the superior clear space is seen, it signifies instability (**Fig. 2.34**).

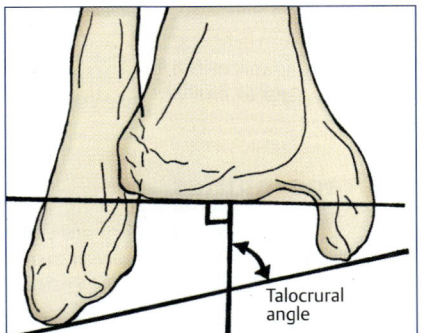

Fig. 2.33 Figure showing the measurement method for talocrural angle of ankle in a mortise view.

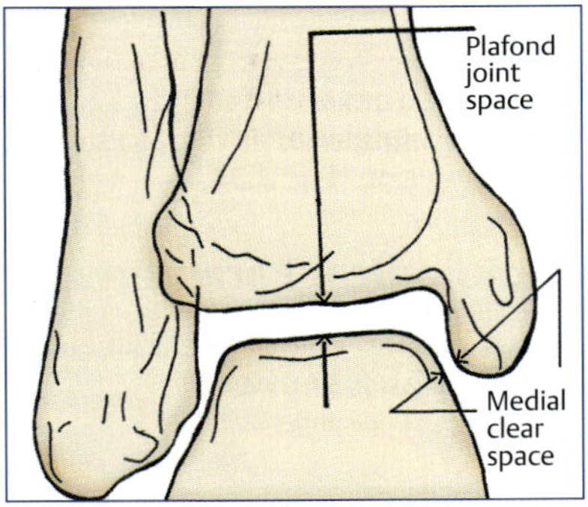

Fig. 2.34 Figure showing the evaluation of ankle instability sign.

Radiological Parameters for Calcaneus

Two angles are most commonly measured for evaluation of calcaneus morphology: Bohler's angle and Gissane's angle.

Bohler's Angle

This is the angle formed at the outer aspect between lines drawn tangentially to the anterior and posterior aspects of calcaneus. Normal value ranges between 20 and 40 degrees. It can be abnormal in both intra and extraarticular calcaneus fractures (**Fig. 2.35**).

Gissane's Angle

This angle is formed between the downward and upward slopes of superior surfaces of calcaneus. An angle of more than 130 degree suggests depression of the

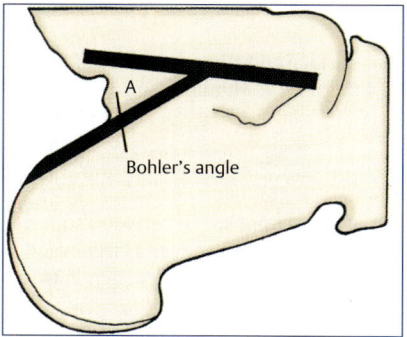

Fig. 2.35 Figure shows measurement of Bohler's angle.

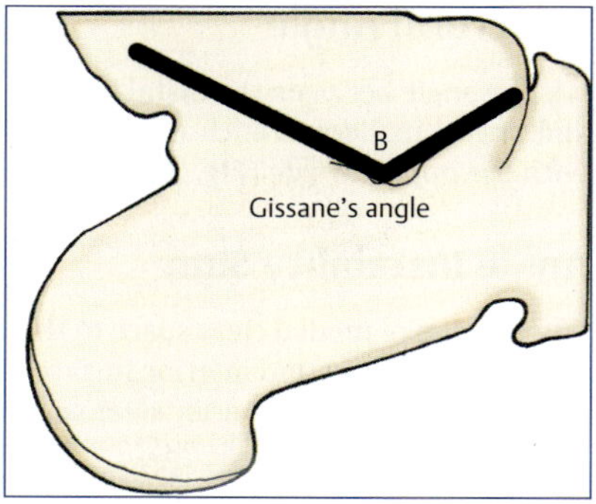

Fig. 2.36 Figure shows the measurement of Gissane's angle.

posterior subtalar articular facet. The parameter is used to analyze fracture calcaneus reduction (**Fig. 2.36**).

Radiological Parameters for Lisfranc Injuries

Six radiological analytical parameters for the diagnosis of Lisfranc injury are illustrated in **Figs. 2.37** to **2.42**.

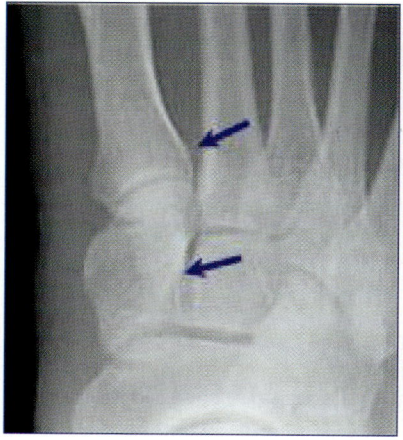

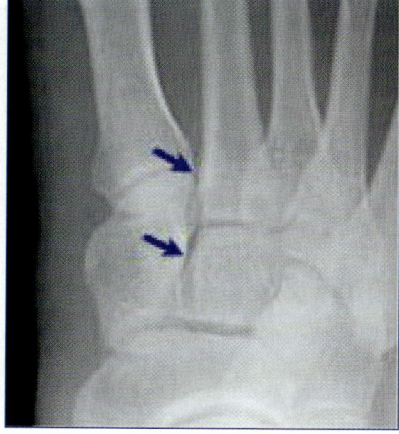

Fig. 2.37 Lateral border of first metatarsal is in line with the lateral border of first cuneiform. Any disruption is suggestive of Lisfranc injury.

Fig. 2. 38 Medial border of second metatarsal is in line with the medial border of second cuneiform. Any disruption is suggestive of Lisfranc injury.

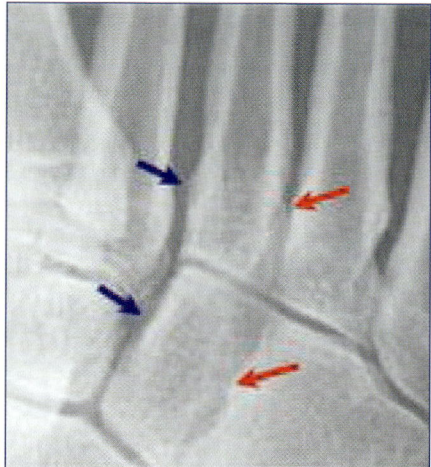

Fig. 2.39 Medial and lateral borders of third metatarsal are in line with medial and lateral border of third cuneiform. Any disruption is suggestive of Lisfranc injury.

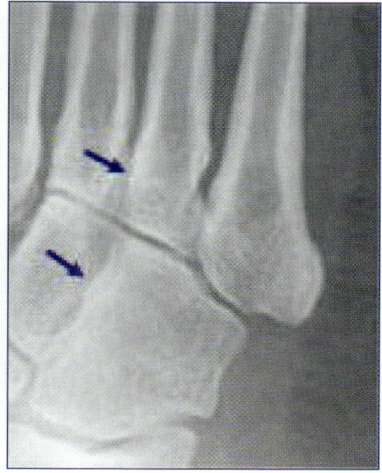

Fig. 2.40 In an oblique view, medial border of fourth metatarsal is in line with medial border of cuboid. Any disruption is suggestive of Lisfranc injury.

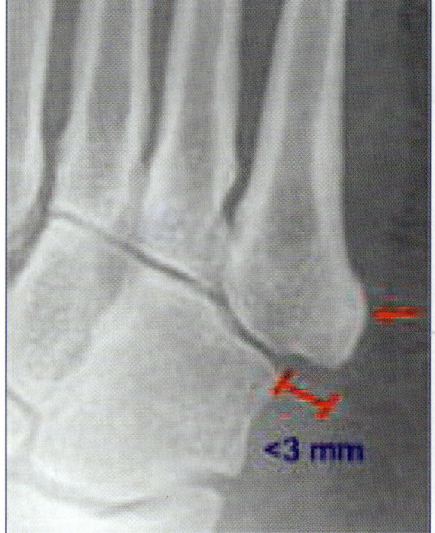

Fig. 2.41 In an oblique view, fifth metatarsal projects just 3 to 5 mm from lateral border of cuboid. Any deviation suggests Lisfranc injury.

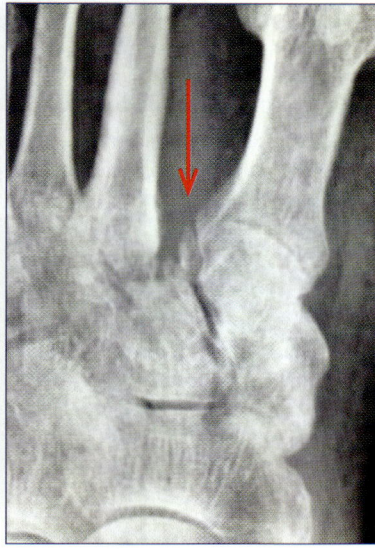

Fig. 2.42 Fleck sign: Presence of bony fleck in between intermetatarsal space is suggestive of Lisfranc injury.

Radiological Parameters for Acquired Flat Foot

♦ Talo-first metatarsal line is called *Meary's line*. This is straight in normal individuals. In cases of acquired flat feet, this line gets distorted on weight-bearing X-rays, suggesting diagnosis of flat feet (**Fig. 2.43**).
♦ Talo-navicular coverage angle is assessed to diagnose the forefoot abduction and thereby the severity of flat foot. Normal angle is less than 7 degree and any increase suggests presence of forefoot abduction (**Fig. 2.44**).

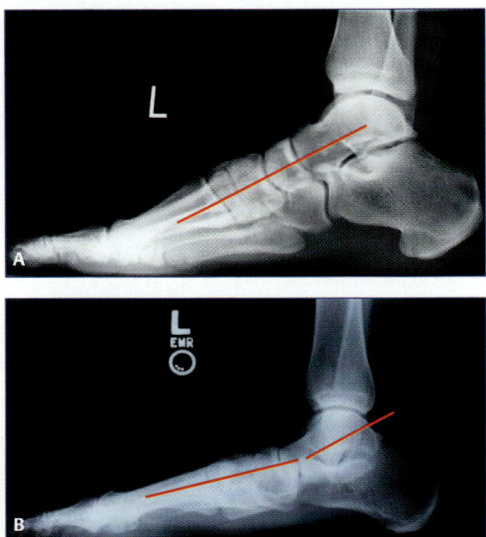

Fig. 2.43 (A and B) Comparative pictures of **(A)** normal and **(B)** abnormal Meary's line in a patient of flat foot in non–weight bearing and weight-bearing radiograph, respectively.

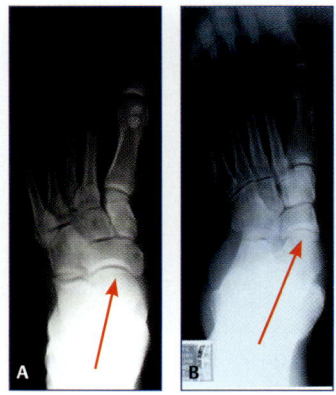

Fig. 2.44 (A and B) Comparative pictures of **(A)** normal and **(B)** abnormal talonavicular coverage angles.

Apart from radiographs, other investigative techniques that help in the diagnosis of foot and ankle diseases are listed in **Box 2.2**.

Box 2.2	Other investigative techniques
♦ Ultrasonography (USG)	
♦ Computed tomography (CT scan)	
♦ Magnetic resonance imaging (MRI)	

Ultrasonography

♦ This is a cheap, effective, and dynamic tool. Comparison with the opposite limb makes diagnosis simpler.
♦ High-frequency probe (8–16 Hz) needs to be used. Formal training for USG seems worth to advocate for foot and ankle surgeon.
♦ Disadvantage of USG is its user dependability.

Advantages and disadvantages of USG are described in **Table 2.2**.

Table 2.2 Advantages and disadvantages of USG

Advantages	Disadvantages
Inexpensive	Small field of view
Quick	Operator dependent
Allows high-resolution imaging of the periarticular soft tissues and tendons	Inability to completely visualize the joint cavity or the synovium
Dynamic imaging	Inability to evaluate the osseous structures due to inability of ultrasound to penetrate the cortex
Color and power Doppler allows assessment of vascularity of the involved region without having to inject any contrast medium	
Allows ultrasound-guided interventions	
Portable	
Imaging of postoperative ankle with metallic hardware	

Indications for Foot and Ankle USG

♦ Tendon pathology: tenosynovitis, tendinosis, tendon tears, subluxation, or dislocation.
♦ Joint and bursal pathology: joint effusion, intra-articular loose bodies, bursitis.

♦ Soft-tissue pathology: foreign bodies, plantar fasciitis, Morton neuroma, gangli-
   ons, cellulitis, or abscesses.
♦ Assessment when metallic artifact would limit imaging with MR imaging or CT.
♦ Guidance for intervention: joint aspiration, synovial or Soft-tissue biopsy, joint
   or tendon sheath injection.

Figs. 2.45 to 2.47 depict ultrasound images of ligaments and tendons of foot and
ankle.

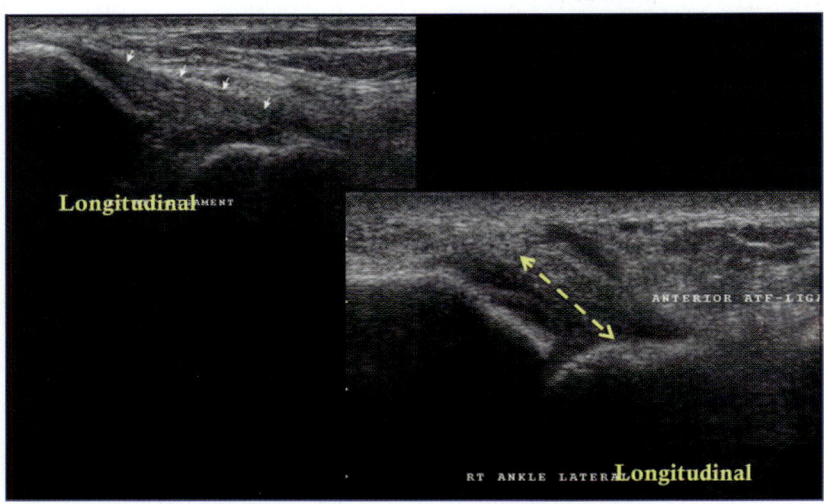

Fig. 2.45 Ultrasound image of anterior talofibular ligament.

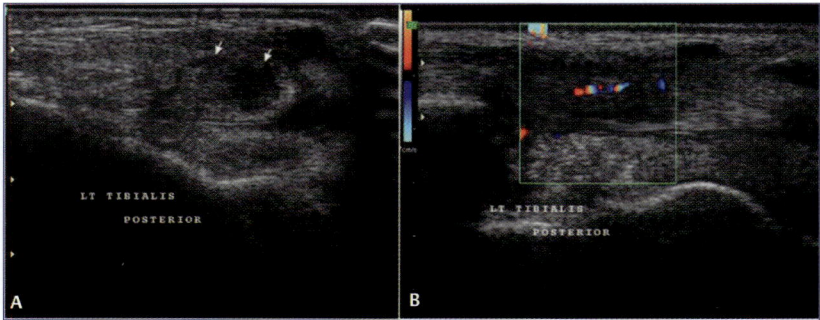

Fig. 2.46 (A and B) Ultrasound image of **(A)** normal and **(B)** inflamed tibialis posterior
tendon.

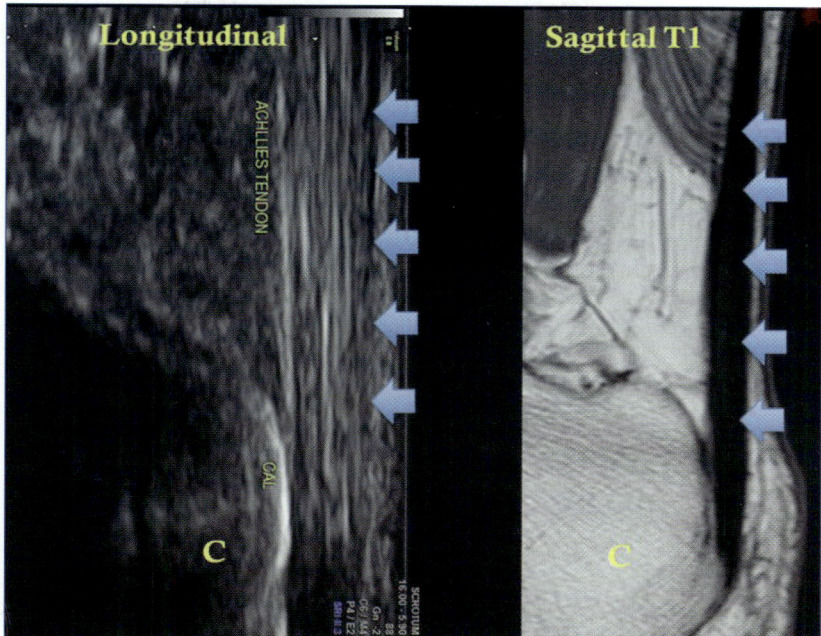

Fig. 2.47   Ultrasound image of normal Achilles tendon.

Computed Tomography

♦ CT scan is used for diagnosis and assessment of structural abnormalities, trauma, arthritides, infection, bony and soft-tissue tumors, and tendon injuries.
♦ CT scan has greater ability to discriminate low-contrast objects and shows tissue characters and cross-section display of tissues.
♦ Multiplanar reconstruction helps in obtaining three-dimensional views of structures.
♦ Because of extensive overlap of bony and joint surfaces seen on conventional radiographs, the cross-section capability of CT is most useful in foot and ankle.
♦ Image plane selection in foot and ankle is most important and is specific to given bone and joint examination.

Advantages and disadvantages of CT scan are listed in **Table 2.3**.

Table 2.3 Advantages and disadvantages of CT scan

Advantages	Disadvantages
Modality of choice in evaluation of osseous anatomy	Ionizing radiation
3D CT allows better visualization and surgical planning in complex fractures of the foot and ankle	Inability to demonstrate bone marrow
Allows CT-guided interventions such as bone biopsy and radio-frequency ablation	
Quick	
Modality of choice in detection of abnormal calcification	

Foot and ankle conditions-specific ordering of CT scan planes is listed in **Table 2.4**.

Table 2.4 Foot and ankle conditions–specific ordering of CT scan planes

Structure	Pathology	Optimal plane for scan
Ankle	Fracture, epiphyseal	Coronal, transverse
Ankle	Fracture, pilon	Transverse
Talus	Fracture, OCD	Coronal
Talus	Fracture neck	Transverse
Talus	Fracture body, neoplasm	Coronal, transverse
Calcaneus	Fracture: depression, tongue	Coronal
Calcaneus	Calcaneocuboid joint involving fracture, tumor	Coronal, transverse
Navicular bone	Fracture: acute or stress	Coronal
Talonavicular joint	Arthritis	Transverse
Calcaneocuboid joint	Arthritis	Transverse
Midfoot	Fracture, dislocation, diastasis	Coronal, transverse
Forefoot	Malalignment, metatarsal heads	Coronal
Sesamoids	Fracture, arthritis, AVN	Coronal, transverse

Abbreviations: OCD, osteochondral defect; AVN, avascular necrosis.

Magnetic Resonance Imaging

- MRI gives excellent soft-tissue visualization.
- MRI can differentiate soft-tissue structures and lesions from bony pathologies.
- MRI does not emit dangerous ionizing radiations to patient.

Limitations of MRI

♦ MRI has disadvantages of being time consuming and costly.
♦ USG gives scope of dynamic examination as well as comparative evaluation.
♦ Presence of metal would interfere with MRI imaging unlike CT scan or USG.
♦ At acute turning of tendons near bony ends, MRI gives magical effect thereby obscuring tendon tears unlike in USG.
♦ MRI is contraindicated in cases with aneurysm clips, electronic pumps, and cardiac pacemakers unlike CT scan or USG.
♦ Cortical bony outline is poorly defined by MRI unlike by CT scan and USG.
♦ Soft-tissue calcifications and small intra-articular loose bodies will produce same low-density signals in T1 and T2 imaging studies in MRI unlike in CT scan or plain radiographs.
♦ Following are the conditions where both USG and MRI should be ordered:
  • Os trigonum syndrome
  • Tarsal tunnel syndrome
  • *Haglund's* syndrome
  • Os peroneum syndrome
  • Anterolateral gutter syndrome
  • Sinus tarsi syndrome

Advantages and disadvantages of MRI are listed in **Table 2.5**.

Table 2.5 Advantages and disadvantages of MRI

Advantages	Disadvantages
No ionizing radiation involved	Expensive
Excellent depiction of the intra- and extra-articular soft-tissue anatomy, including the articular cartilage	Contraindicated in patients with pacemakers and cochlear implants
Allows visualization of bone marrow	Longer scanning time
Provides a global view of the evaluated area	Patients with claustrophobia
Newer imaging sequences allow functional imaging like cartilage mapping	Postoperative ankle with metallic hardware
	Inability to detect soft-tissue calcification

How to Read and Evaluate Foot and Ankle MRI?

♦ 30% of MRI is labelled normal with problems in patient!
♦ T1 and PD fat images are the best for evaluation.
♦ Identify structures in at least two planes.
♦ Correlate with clinical picture.
♦ If necessary, combine with USG examination.

♦ Observer must follow a strict motion path for reading MRI of foot and ankle (**Table 2.6**).

Table 2.6   Motion path for reading foot and ankle MRI

S. No.	Structures to be evaluated
1	Ankle joint
2	Subtalar joint
3	Midfoot joint and Lisfranc ligament
4	Interosseous membrane and syndesmosis
5	Ligaments: lateral, posterior, medial, and anterior
6	Tendons: Achilles, peroneus longus and brevis, tibialis posterior, flexor digitorum longus, flexor hallucis longus, and tibialis anterior
7	Sinus tarsi
8	Plantar fascia
9	Bones, accessory bones, stress fractures
10	Nervous tissues: tarsal tunnel and Morton neuroma

♦ Observer must know which sequence is best for the evaluation of a specific structure (**Table 2.7**).

Table 2.7   Structures versus MRI sequence to be selected for reading foot and ankle MRI

Structure	Sequence of MRI to be preferred
Joints	Coronal and sagittal T1 and T2, PD fat sat
Tendons	Axial and coronal
Ligaments	Axial and coronal
Plantar fascia	Combined with USG

♦ Observer must know the signal pattern of various tissues in T1 and T2 MRI images (**Table 2.8**).

Table 2.8 Signal patterns of various tissues in T1 and T2 MRI images

Tissue	T1	T2
Cortex	Low	Low
Ligaments	Low	Low
Articular cart	Intermediate	Intermediate
Red marrow	Intermediate	Intermediate
Old blood	High	High
Osteomyelitis	Low	High
Sarcoma	Low	High
Marrow edema	Low	High
Fat	High	Intermediate
Pus	Intermediate	High

MRI images of tendons and ligaments of ankle are shown in **Figs. 2.48 to 2.52**.

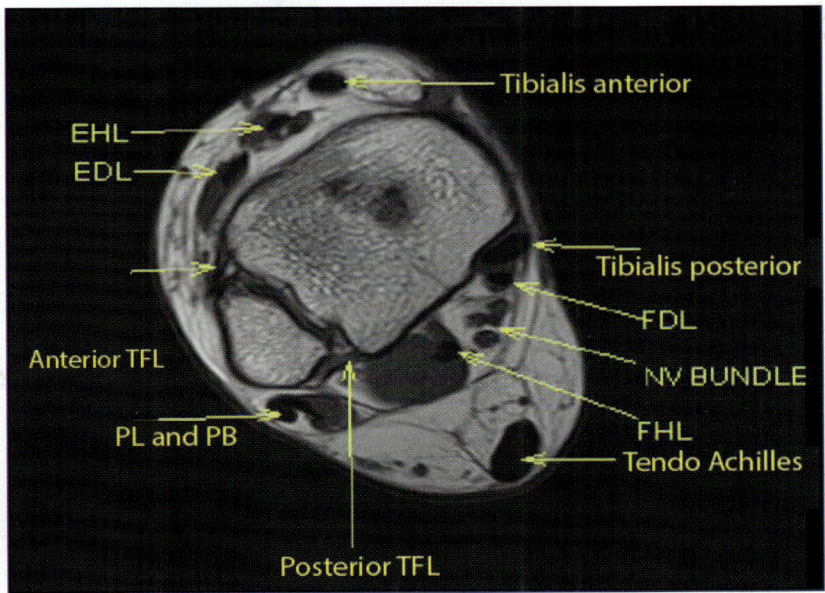

Fig. 2.48 MRI picture of tendons around ankle joint. EHL, exterior hallucis longus; EDL, exterior digitorum longus; TFL, talofibular ligament; PL, peroneus longus; PB, peroneus brevis; FDL, flexor digitorum longus; FHL, flexor hallucis longus; NV bundle, neurovascular bundle.

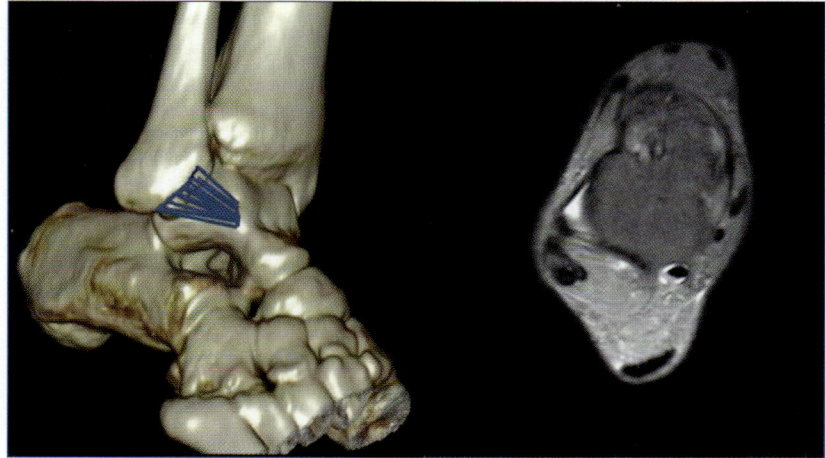

Fig. 2.49 MRI picture of anterior talo-fibular ligament.

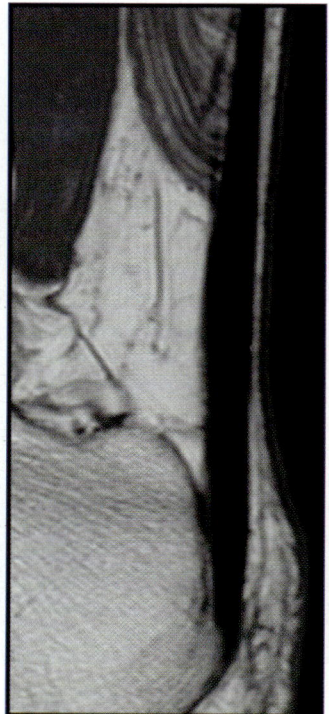

Fig. 2.50 MRI picture of normal Achilles tendon.

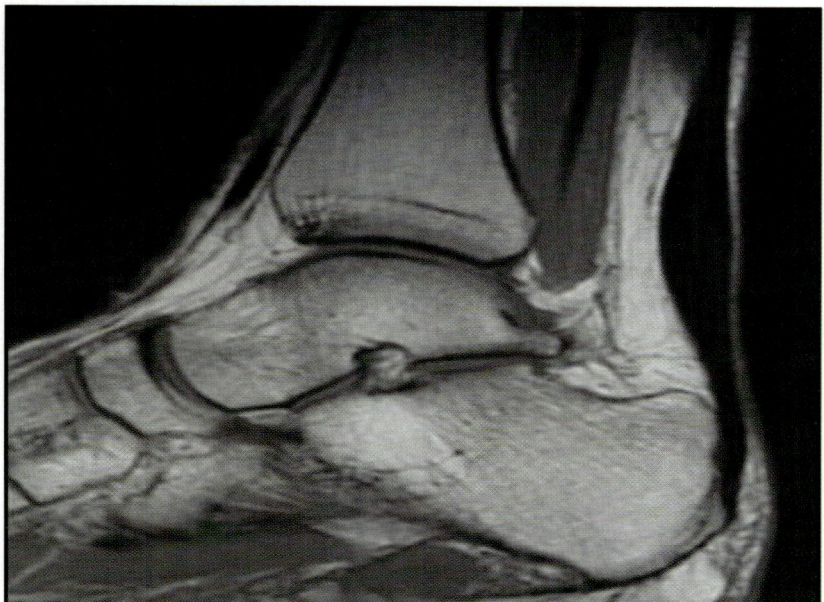

Fig. 2.51   MRI picture of Achilles tendinosis.

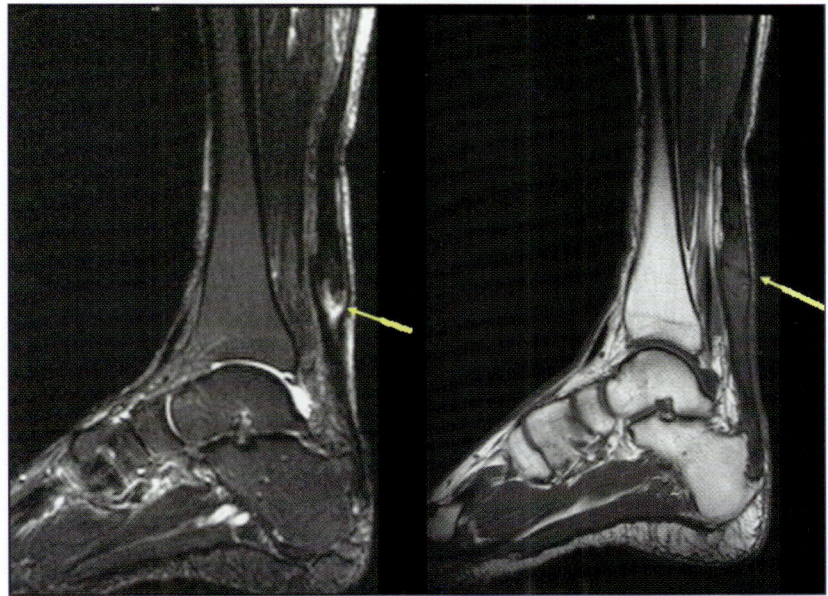

Fig. 2.52   MRI picture of Achilles tear.

Rational Prescription of Foot and Ankle Orthotics

Orthotic prescription mirrors expertise of a specialist!

Orthotic prescription should have logic and rationale. Consideration of a few simple points will make a prescription perfect.

Criteria for Prescribing Orthotic or Shoe Modification

Criteria for orthotic prescription are listed in **Box 3.1**.

♦ *Age of the patient*: A young and active patient would need stronger and durable material. These orthotics need to be slim in order to be easily accommodated in the shoe. Orthotics for female patients must take care of cosmetic aspects. In the older age group, associated comorbid conditions, poor vision, presence of arthritis, and issues of balance are of prime consideration.

Box 3.1	Criteria for orthotic prescription

♦ Age of the patient
♦ Activity level of the patient
♦ Type and location of deformity
♦ Status of sensations in foot
♦ Bony prominences and ulcers
♦ Study and analysis of existing orthotics

♦ *Activity level of the patient*: Activity level has a direct bearing on the wear and tear of orthotics, which needs repetitive check-ups, changes, and replacements.
♦ *Type and location of deformity? Is the deformity rigid or flexible?* Complete description of deformity is needed. Flexible deformity needs corrective orthotics, while a rigid deformity needs accommodative orthotics.
♦ *Status of sensations in foot*: An impaired sensation in the foot requires special care to make sure that there is no pressure from orthotics. Repetitive examination by patient, consultant, and orthotist is required to ensure proper fit of orthotics and lack of any pressure on an insensate foot by orthotics.
♦ *Bony prominences and ulcers with its location and details*: Drawing of bony prominences or ulcers on a paper is advisable. Locations with depth or prominence are noted. Amount of discharge from ulcer is specified to judge the need for space for dressing material.
♦ *Study and analysis of existing orthotics or shoe modifications*: Wear and tear of existing orthotic/shoe would give an idea about usage, habits, and hygiene of the patient. It is advisable to send all previous orthotics/shoes to an orthotist for study before preparing a new one.

Formulation of an Orthotic/Shoe Modification

The key is to get answers to the following questions:

♦ Why do I want orthotic or footwear modification in this patient? What objectives should it fulfil? Objectives could be any one of the following:
  • Reduce the impact and improve shock absorption
  • Relieve the pressure over sensitive structures
  • Correct the flexible deformity
  • Accommodate the fixed deformity and compensate for reduced movements
  • Provide support and maintain the neutral position
  • Limit abnormal or excessive movements
♦ Does this patient need custom-molded orthotics or would a prefabricated orthotics work?
♦ Presence of deformity and abnormal shape and size of foot would mandate the use of custom-molded orthotics.
♦ Any other specific factors to be considered? Age, activity level, cosmesis, and sensations are the factors to be considered.

Table 3.1 gives details of various foot and ankle conditions and commonly prescribed orthotics or shoe modifications for them.

Table 3.1 Conditions and common orthotic prescriptions

Foot and ankle problems	Goal	Prescribed orthotics/shoe modifications
Hallux valgus	Align first ray Offload first metatar-sophalangeal (MTP) joint	Night splint Toe spreader Gel pad inside shoe/insole Rocker bottom shoe/insole Carbon fiber insole
Hallux rigidus	Total plantar surface contact to reduce load over first MTP	Silicone gel sleeve Low heel, high toe crest footwear Rocker bottom shoe Carbon fiber insole
Hammer, claw, and mallet toes	Total surface bearing Stress-free toe tip Stretching of shortened extensors	Flexible: Metatarsal bar Night splints Rigid custom-molded total contact orthosis Toe crest pad
Morton neuroma	Offload painful neuroma site	Silicone gel pad Metatarsal pad Carbon fiber foot plate
Metatarsalgia	Maintain parabolic arch of foot	Metatarsal arch pad Carbon fiber foot plate insert Total contact orthosis
Plantar corn/callosity	Take pressure off the painful area	Offloading pads Scalloping inside insole Silicone gel pad
Flat foot—stages 1 and 2	Arch correction Deformity prevention	Valgus pads with C and E heel UCBL Supramalleolar orthosis
Flat foot stage 3	Accommodation of deformity	Total contact foot orthosis/insole Foot mold orthosis
Heel varus	Maintaining subtalar joint to neutral	Lateral/outer heel wedge Reverse C and E heel High wall UCBL
Pes cavus	Minimizing foot fatigue with total surface contact	Custom-molded total contact foot orthotic
Midfoot arthritis	Arrest progression of deformity Take load off painful site	Supramalleolar orthosis Short ankle–foot orthosis (AFO) Longitudinal firm arch support
Plantar fasciitis	Relieve load over inflamed fascia	Silicone heel cushion Scooped heel Arch support

Table 3.1 Conditions and common orthotic prescriptions (Contd.)

Foot and ankle problems	Goal	Prescribed orthotics/shoe modifications
Retrocalcaneal bursitis, insertional tendinitis	Release tension on tendo Achilles	Heel raise/lift (minimum 3 cm) Silicone heel (donut shape)
Foot drop	Prevent gravitational dropping of foot Assist in gait	Toe-raising splints Dynamic AFO Static AFO
Charcot neuroarthropathy	Stabilization of foot	Charcot restraint orthotic walker (CROW)

Model for Orthotic/Footwear Alteration Prescription

An exemplary model for orthotic prescription is explained in **Fig. 3.1.**

Name of the patient:

Age: Occupation:

Diagnosis:

Sensations:

Deformity/Ulcer:

Foot drawing:

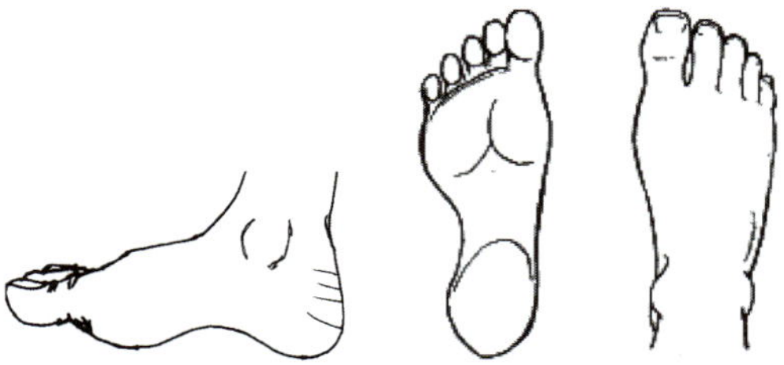

Aim of orthotic/footwear modification:

Shock absorption/ Pressure relief/ Deformity correction/

Deformity Accommodation/ Position maintenance / Motion limitation

Description of orthotic:

Instructions, if any:

Signature:

Fig. 3.1   Exemplary model for orthotic prescription.

Points to be checked once orthosis/footwear modifications are done are listed in **Box 3.2.**

Box 3.2	Postorthosis checks

♦ Comfort of patient
♦ Pressure areas
♦ Gait with orthotics
♦ X-ray with orthotics

In the Foot and Ankle Operation Theater

*Time taken in planning the operation is the time
reduced in carrying the operation!*

Regional Anesthesia and Blocks

Tips and Tricks

- Done at least 30 minutes prior to the procedure for allowing some time for the anesthesia to take effect.
- Long-acting molecules take longer time to give effect.
- Take 30 mL of total solution with 10 mL of xylocaine and 20 mL of Marcaine and use a 22-gauge needle.
- Never use epinephrine.
- Use of sodium bicarbonate may speed up the onset of effect.
- Use of nerve stimulator or ultrasound would make procedure precise.
- Always aspirate before injecting.
- Be careful with the volume-tourniquet effect.
- Be cautious in cases with peripheral vascular diseases and diabetes.
- Take care in cases with infection where local anesthetic may not work due to acidotic effect, and there is a risk of infection spreading to healthy tissues.

Ankle Block

Surface anatomy of nerves in foot and ankle is depicted in **Figs. 4.1 and 4.2**. Important points to consider for ankle block are listed as follows:

♦ Used for procedures at or distal to ankle.
♦ Five nerves are blocked:
  • Tibial nerve
  • Sural nerve
  • Deep peroneal nerve
  • Superficial peroneal nerve
  • Saphenous nerve

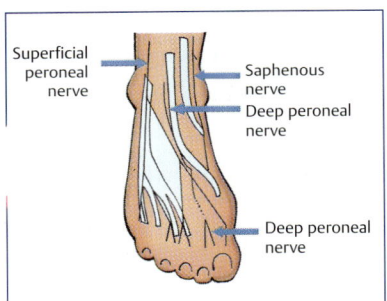

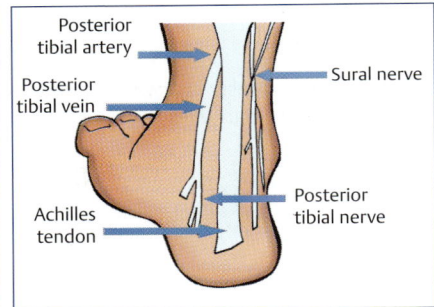

Fig. 4.1 Surface anatomy of nerves in foot.

Fig. 4.2 Surface anatomy of nerves in ankle.

Tibial nerve

Hold ankle dorsiflexed and put needle next to Achilles tendon at the level of ankle joint; direct it from posterior to anterior, advance to the bone, and withdraw 5 mm and inject 10 mL (**Fig. 4.3**).

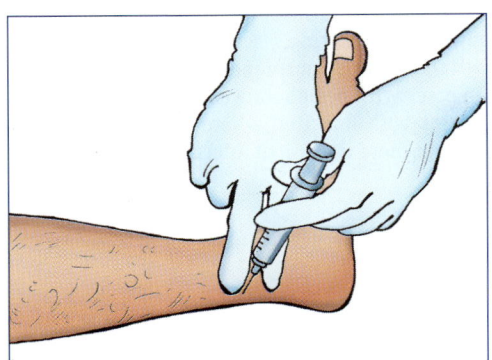

Fig. 4.3 Method of blocking of tibial nerve.

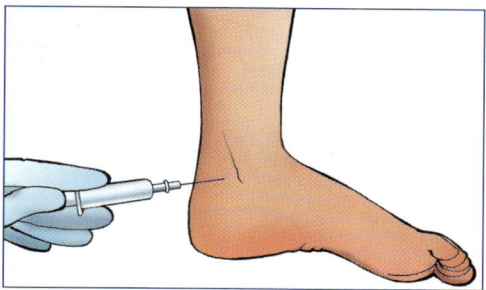

Fig. 4.4   Method of blocking of sural nerve.

Sural nerve

Inject subcutaneously halfway between the tendo Achilles and peroneal tendons and inject 5 mL (**Fig. 4.4**).

Deep peroneal nerve/Superficial peroneal nerve/Saphenous nerve

Inject subcutaneously in the form of bolus, starting from the medial malleolus going up to the fibula proximal to the ankle joint in superficial plane. About 10 to 12 mL is injected (**Figs. 4.5–4.7**).

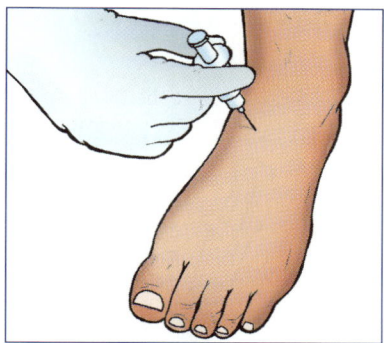

Fig. 4.5   Method of blocking of deep peroneal nerve.

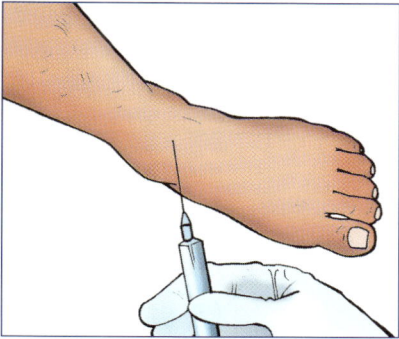

Fig. 4.6   Method of blocking of superficial peroneal nerve.

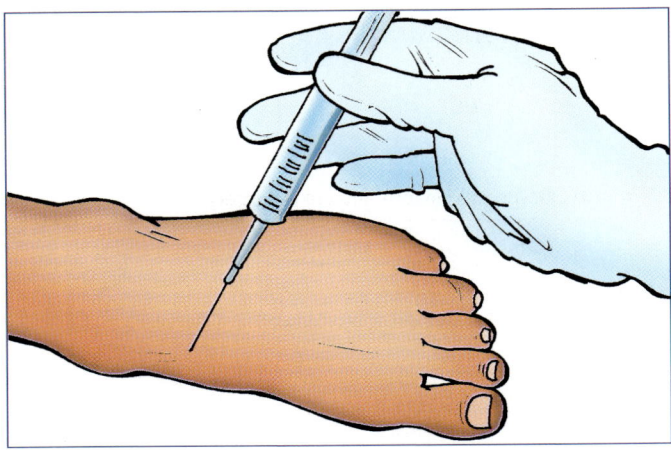

Fig. 4.7 Method of blocking of saphenous nerve.

Forefoot Block

Important points to consider for forefoot block are listed as follows:

♦ Used for forefoot and toe surgeries
♦ Nerves blocked are digital nerves (**Fig. 4.8**)
♦ Usually injected in the web space and around the bases of metatarsals. Once the needle is inside the web space, it is advanced dorsal to plantar. Skin is tented and injectioning is done simultaneously with withdrawal of needle

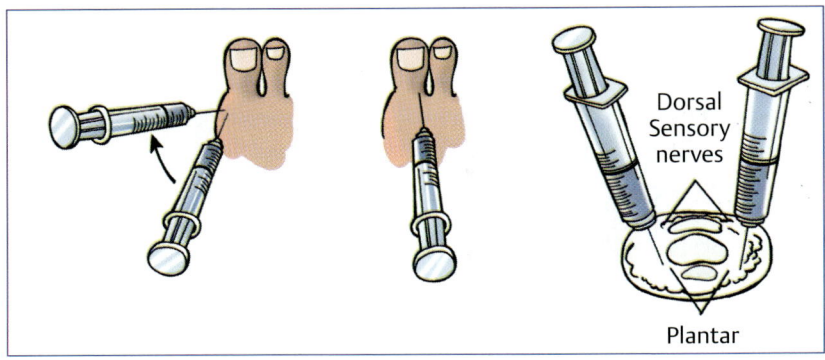

Fig. 4.8 Relationship of nerves in digit and method of blocking them.

Special Instruments for Foot and Ankle Surgery

Some special instruments used in the foot and ankle surgery are listed in **Box 4.1** and are shown in **Figs. 4.9 to 4.15**.

Box 4.1	Instruments used in foot and ankle surgery

- ◆ Weitlaner retractor
- ◆ Gelpi retractor
- ◆ Cobb elevator
- ◆ Key elevator
- ◆ Freer elevator
- ◆ Lamina spreader
- ◆ Hintermann distractor

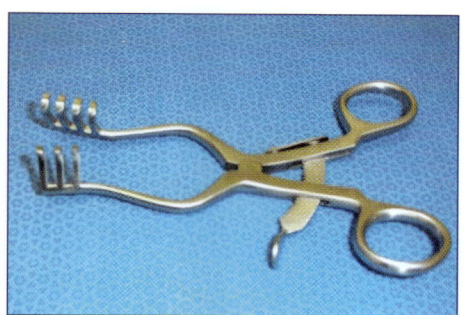

Fig. 4.9 Weitlaner retractor.

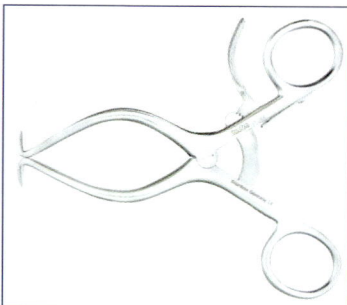

Fig. 4.10 Gelpi retractor.

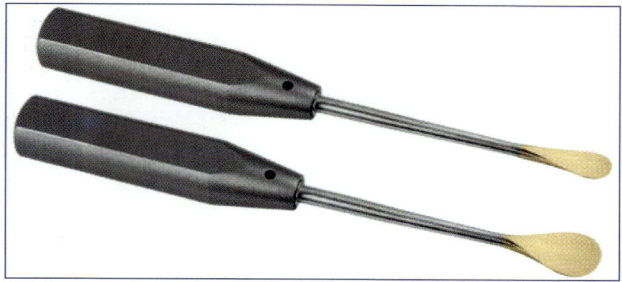

Fig. 4.11 Cobb elevators.

Fig. 4.12   Key elevator.

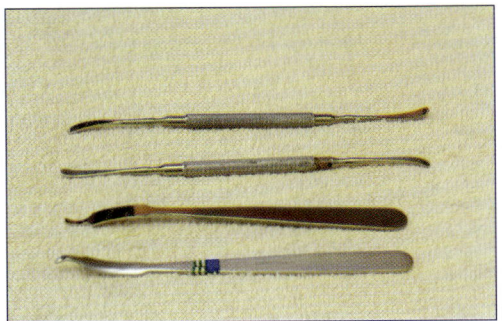

Fig. 4.13   Freer elevators.

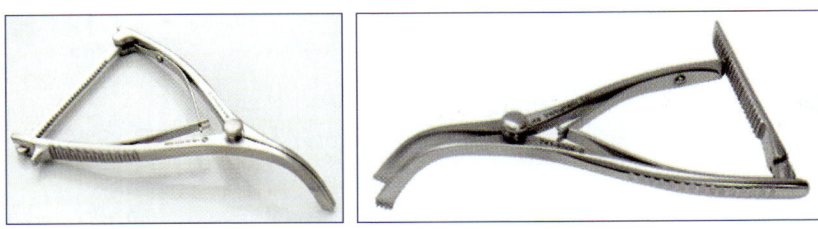

Fig. 4.14   Smooth and toothed lamina spreaders.

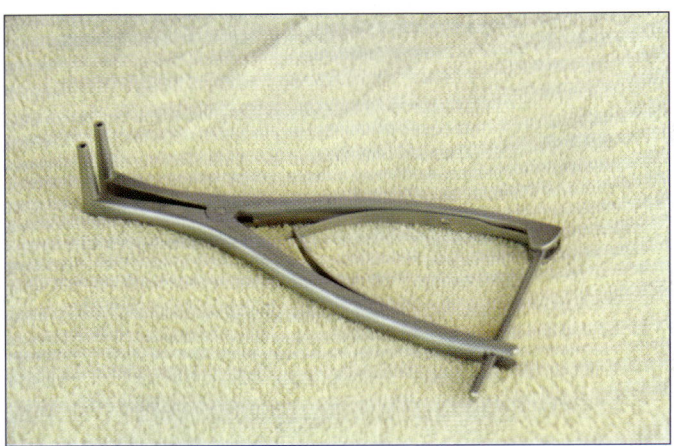

Fig. 4.15   Hintermann distractor.

Patient Positioning for Foot and Ankle Surgeries

Foot and ankle surgeries are done with six different positions, which are mentioned in **Box 4.2**.

Box 4.2	Positioning for foot and ankle surgeries

♦ Supine
- Supine with bump under gluteal region
- Supine position with pillow under knee and leg above ankle keeping ankle off the table (**Fig. 4.16**)
- Reverse Trendelenburg position

♦ Lateral

♦ Prone

♦ Foot is positioned flat on table (**Fig. 4.17**)

♦ Foot over C-arm machine with camera reversed and foot resting on it (**Fig. 4.18**)

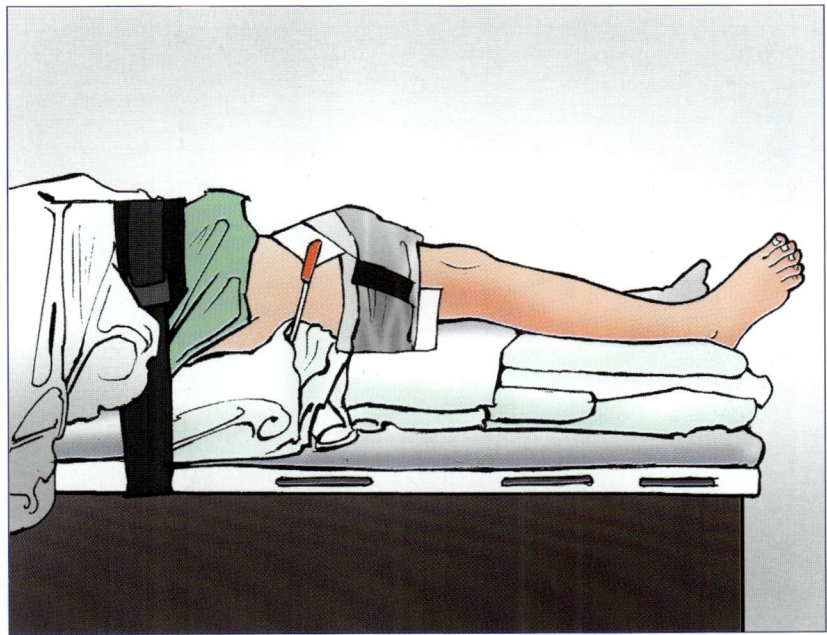

Fig. 4.16   Supine position with pillow under knee and leg ending above ankle, keeping ankle off the table.

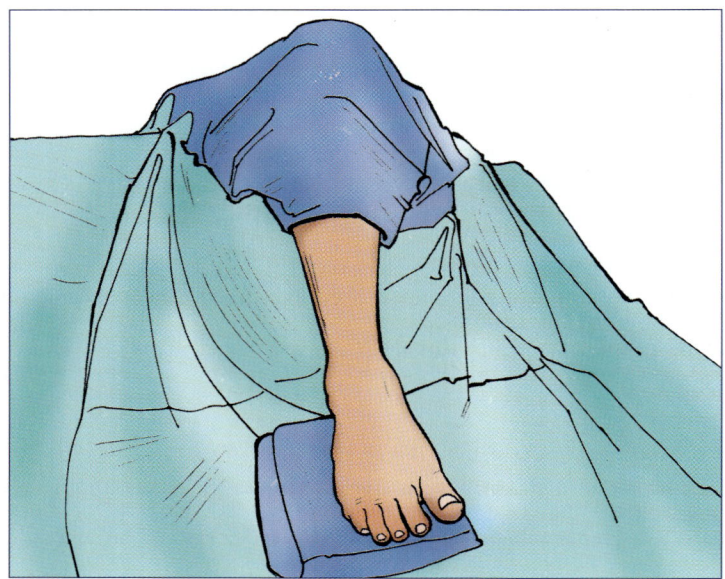

Fig. 4.17   Foot is positioned flat on table.

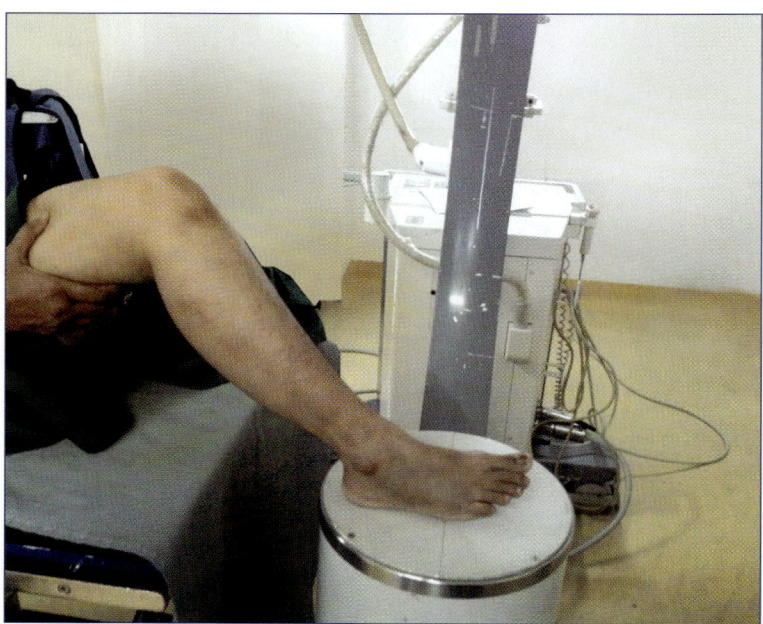

Fig. 4.18   Foot is positioned on C-arm, which is reversed in such a form that the foot rests over the camera side.

Flowchart 4.1 displays the supine positions for foot and ankle surgeries with their respective indications.

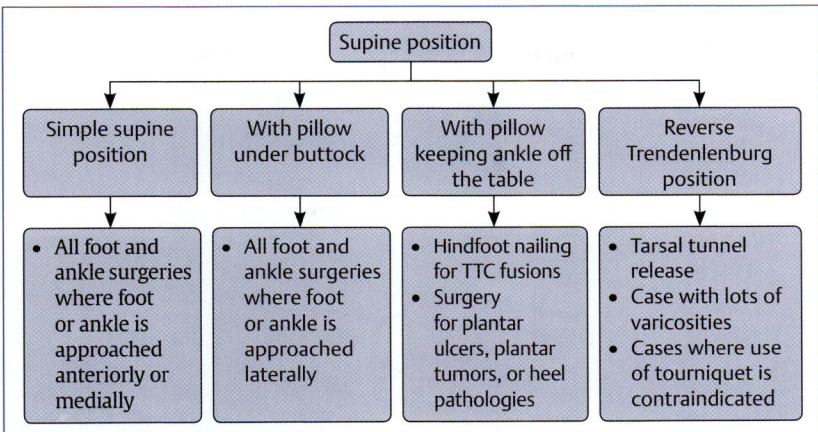

Flowchart 4.1 Supine positions with their respective indications. TTC, tibiotalocalcaneal fusion.

Flowchart 4.2 displays other positions for foot and ankle surgeries with their respective indications.

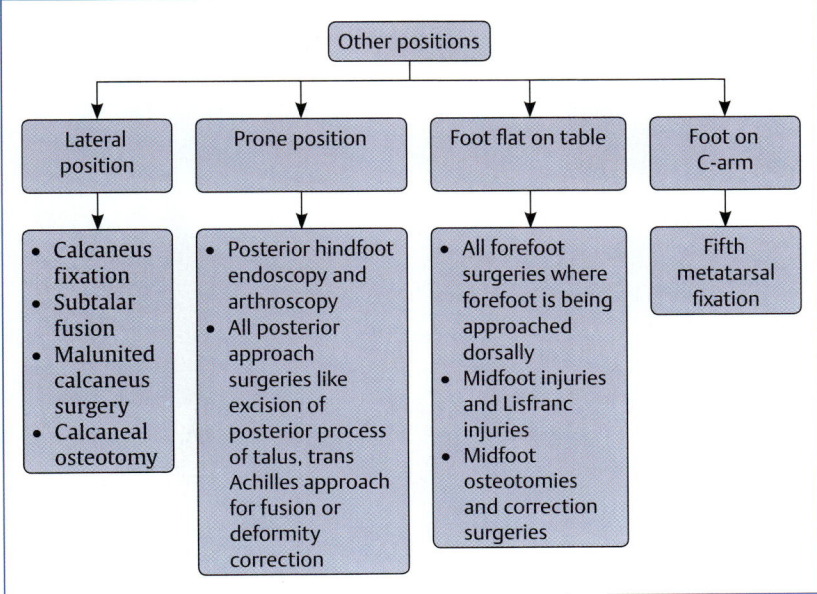

Flowchart 4.2 Other positions for foot and ankle surgeries with their respective indications.

There are three basic C-arm positions as listed in **Box 4.3**.

Box 4.3	C-arm positions

♦ C-arm on the opposite side of surgeon
♦ C-arm on the side of surgeon
♦ C-arm diagonal to table (**Fig. 4.19**)

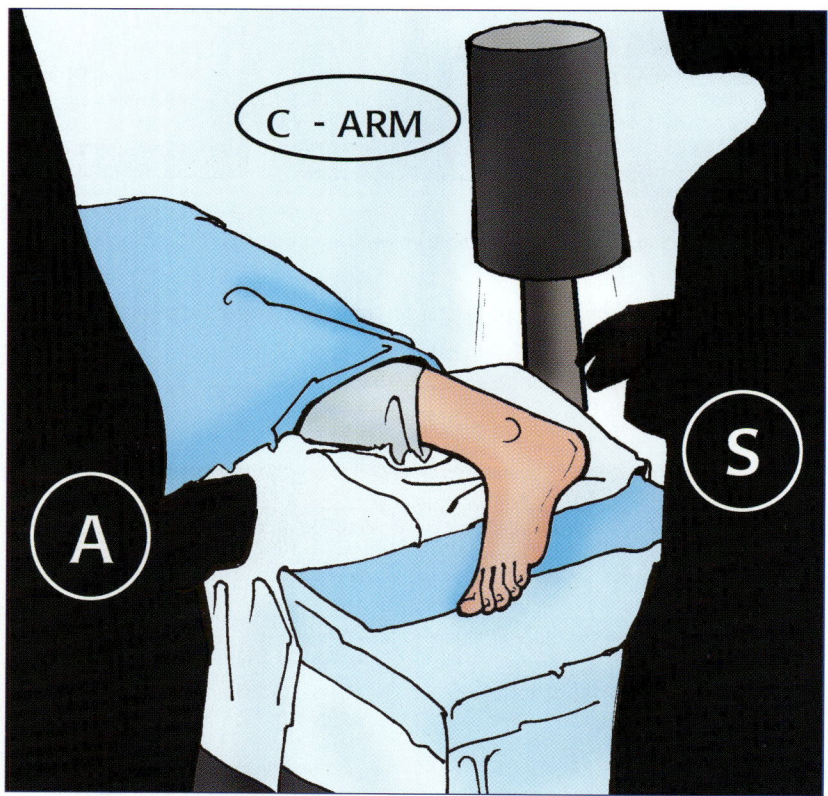

Fig. 4.19 C-arm positioned diagonally. A, position of the assistant; S, position of the surgeon.

Flowchart 4.3 displays the C-arm positions with indications.

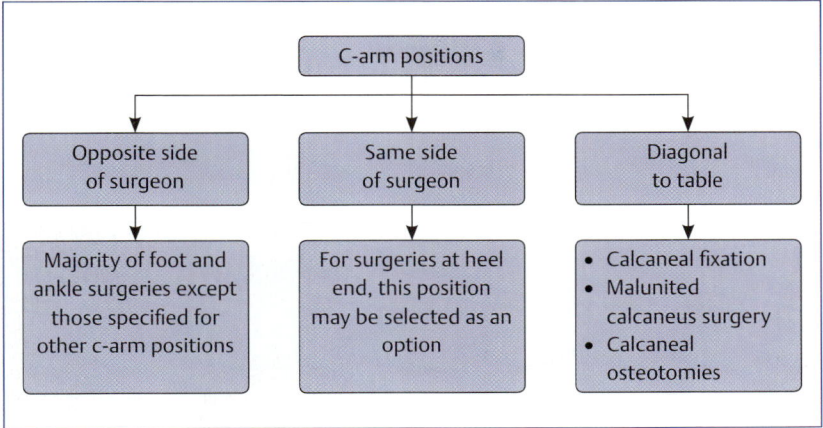

Flowchart 4.3   C-arm positions with indications.

There is another special C-arm position for fifth metatarsal fracture screw fixation. In this, the knee is flexed and C-arm is turned so that foot rests on camera of C-arm over a bump of folded towel sheets (**Fig. 4.20**).

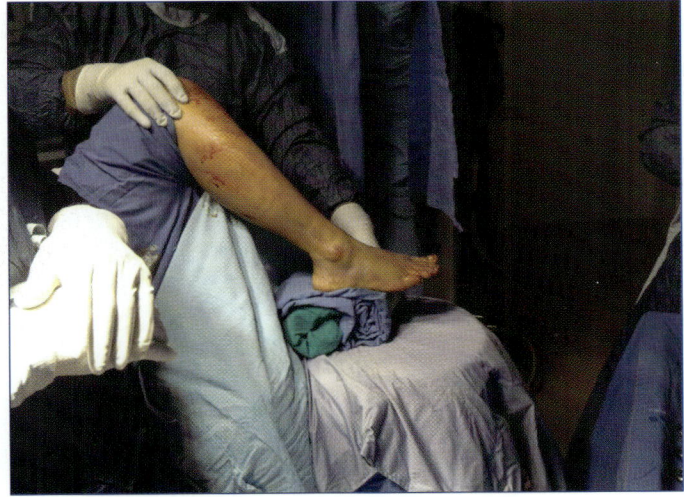

Fig. 4.20   Foot position with respect to C-arm position for fifth metatarsal surgery.

5

Ten Commandments of Foot and Ankle Trauma Management

Foot and ankle trauma is different!

For good outcome of foot and ankle trauma, it is mandatory to strictly adhere to specific management principles. They are best described as the "Ten commandments of foot and ankle trauma management." and are illustrated in **Fig. 5.1**.

Commandment No. 1: High Index of Suspicion!

Many of the foot and ankle fractures can be easily missed, if not suspected! Quality of high index of suspicion would rescue a surgeon in many situations because, if missed, these injuries would lead to long-term disability.
Commonly missed or misdiagnosed foot and ankle injuries are as follows:

- ◆ Syndesmotic ankle sprain
- ◆ Subtalar joint sprain
- ◆ Anterior process of calcaneus fracture
- ◆ Lateral talar process fracture
- ◆ Posterior process talus fracture
- ◆ Osteochondral fractures of talus
- ◆ Fifth metatarsal base fracture
- ◆ Tendo Achilles rupture

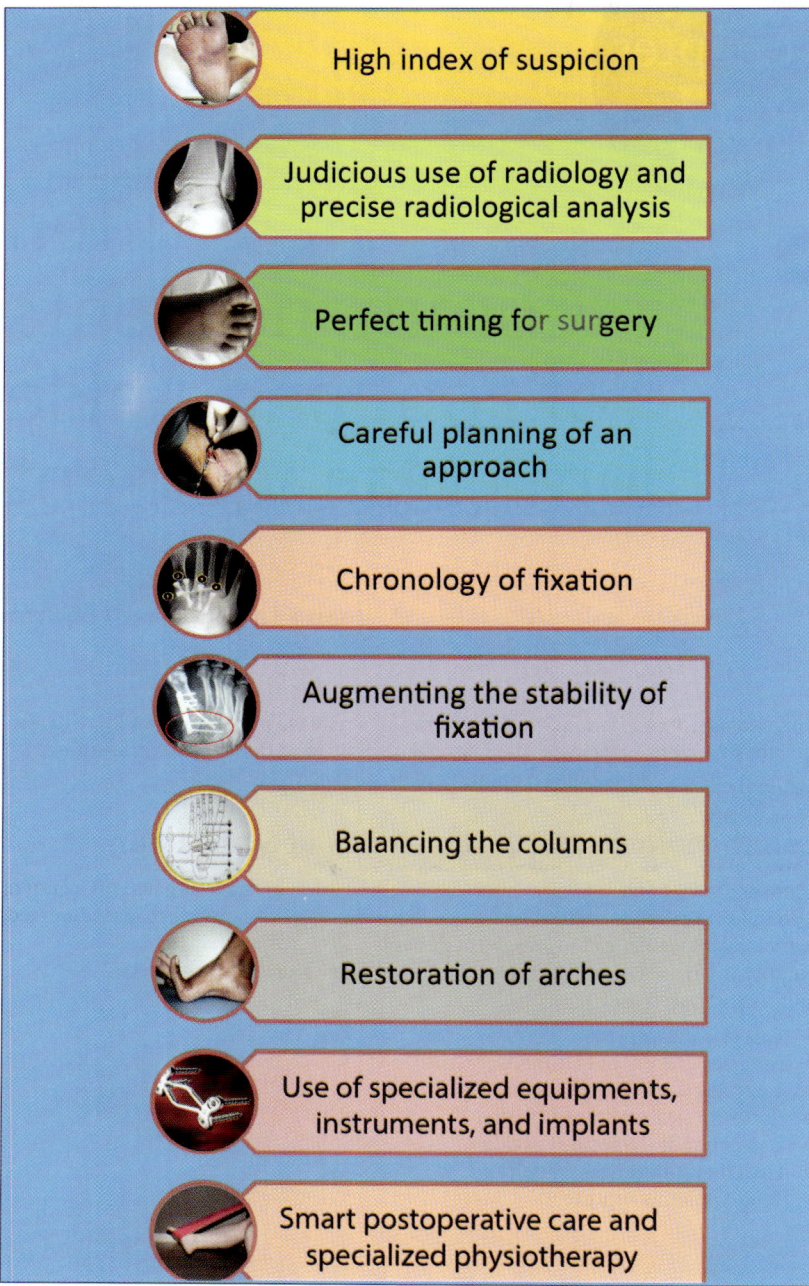

Fig. 5.1 Ten commandments of foot and ankle trauma.

◆ Peroneal tendon injury (all the aforementioned conditions can be mistaken for ankle sprain)
◆ Ankle and midfoot fractures associated with neuropathy (careful history taking, clinical examination, and monofilament testing would differentiate neuropathic fracture)
◆ Lisfranc injury (it could be misdiagnosed as midfoot sprain. Plantar ecchymosis, clinical examination, weight-bearing X-rays, and stress tests would lead to precise diagnosis)
◆ Cuboid fracture (midfoot bones are like forearm bones where isolated injury of one is rare and will almost always be associated with radiologically undetectable subtle injury of others. Specialized as well as comparative X-rays together with careful clinical examination would lead to diagnosis)
◆ Sesamoid injuries (mode of trauma, careful clinical examination, and specialized radiology would support suspicion)
◆ Stress fractures (specialized investigations such as CT scan, bone scan, and MRI shall follow suspicion of stress fractures, more so in athletes and weekend warriors)

Commandment No. 2: Judicious Use of Radiology and Precise Radiological Analysis

Radiology plays a vital role in the diagnosis as well as management of foot and ankle trauma. Familiarity to specialized radiological views is mandatory. Careful analysis of radiology is equally important.

Importance of weight-bearing radiology cannot be overemphasized in foot and ankle trauma care. Reader is referred to Chapter 2 of this book for further reading.

Table 5.1 summarizes about the pivotal role radiography plays in diagnosing and managing different traumatic conditions in foot and ankle.

Table 5.1 Injury-specific radiology

Condition	Specific radiology	Remarks
Ankle fractures	AP, LAT, and OBL ankle views	Look for nine ankle radiology signs
Calcaneus fractures	Axial view Broden's view	Useful for intraoperative subtalar joint reduction assessment
Talus fractures	Canale and Kelly's view	Pre- and intraoperative use to look for medial comminution
Midfoot fractures	Medial oblique view Lateral oblique view Traction view Comparative view	To look for both the columns of foot and subtle compression injuries of cuboid
Lisfranc injuries	AP, OBL, and LAT foot views weight-bearing views Stress views	Look for five Lisfranc signs and Fleck sign
Sesamoid injuries	Sesamoid views	

Abbreviations: AP, anteroposterior; LAT, lateral; OBL, oblique

Commandment No. 3: Perfect Timing for Surgery, a Must!

Bones in foot and ankle are subcutaneous and are contained in a closed compartment with poor soft-tissue envelope. Injury would lead to extensive edema and formation of blisters. Timing of surgery is crucial to avoid skin problems such as wound break-down, inability to close incisions, and delayed healing. Following are some important points of consideration:

♦ Presence of wrinkles is a good sign to move in for surgery. The sign is religiously followed for pilon, ankle, calcaneus, and midfoot injuries
♦ Waiting for 5 to 7 days is justified for many foot and ankle injuries such as midfoot trauma, Lisfranc injuries, and forefoot trauma. Waiting up to 3 weeks is recommended for hindfoot trauma
♦ While surgeon is waiting for edema to subside, a spanning external fixator may be utilized to keep tissues in tension and maintain the ligamentotaxis
♦ Span, scan, and plan are the philosophies for foot and trauma, more so for high-velocity trauma

Commandment No. 4: Careful Planning of an Approach

Approach must be meticulously planned for foot and ankle trauma.

♦ Avoid incising through the blisters
♦ In case of a double approach, proper spacing between two approaches is impor-tant to avoid wound healing issues
♦ To target a specific bone for a surgery in midfoot, approach may be taken with the assistance of radiology
♦ Involvement of rays in Lisfranc injury may vary the placement of incision
♦ While placing incision over the midfoot, an initial soft incision is made, followed by hemostat-guided deep dissection to avoid injuring cutaneous nerves and for-mation of painful postoperative neuroma
♦ While planning approach for fracture talus, need for its probable extension for doing osteotomy must be thought

Commandment No. 5: Chronology of Fixation Must Be Followed

Fixation in foot and ankle trauma follows a set chronology to avoid issues of malpo-sitioning.

♦ In most of the pilon fractures, fibula fixation precedes application of external fixator over tibia because the maintenance of fibular length is of paramount significance
♦ Medial wall and sustentacular reduction is achieved first before building articular reduction in fracture calcaneus
♦ Lateral screw is put first in fracture neck talus because the lateral bone is denser and the lateral side comminution is rare. This helps in prevention of varus malunion
♦ In cuboid reconstruction, fixation ladder starts with reconstruction from intact joint side toward more damaged joint side and from inside out
♦ Second metatarsal is the key stone for midfoot injuries and needs to be reduced and stabilized first

♦ Mobile medial column is always rigidly fixed first, followed by rigid lateral column that is fixed by soft fixation
♦ Metatarsal parabola maintenance mandates surgeon to start his fixation from second metatarsal and proceed to fifth metatarsal

Commandment No. 6: Art of Augmenting Stability of Fixation

Fixation stability augmentation is required for all midfoot and forefoot fractures and all neuropathic fractures.

♦ Crossing and spanning of joints is advisable. This may necessitate planned removal of implant. Joint spanning plates that do not violate articular cartilage are best used for forefoot and midfoot trauma
♦ Stability may also be augmented with spanning external fixator, which may be kept for 4 to 6 weeks, depending on the need
♦ Multiple fixations and longer and stronger fixations are required for neuropathic joints

Commandment No. 7: Balance the Columns!

Length of both medial and lateral columns is the most vital for restoration of foot biomechanics. If the length is not restored, then adduction or abduction may result at the forefoot, leading to pain, stiffness, difficult ambulation, and later on arthritis. Temporary spanning external fixators or plates are used for this purpose in midfoot and forefoot trauma.

Commandment No. 8: Restore the Arches!

Longitudinal as well as transverse parabolic arch of foot needs perfect restoration while dealing with posttrauma reconstruction. Resultant flat arch would pose its own set of problems such as gait and pressure issues, and later on arthritis.

♦ In foot and ankle trauma management, preservation of attachment of tibialis posterior at navicular or reattachment of its insertion is most important
♦ If parabolic arch of metatarsals is not restored, it would lead to metatarsalgia and formation of corns and callosities due to abnormal plantar pressures
♦ Every metatarsal fracture needs accurate length restoration, which is the sole reason for pendulum shift in its management toward operative care

Commandment No. 9: Use Specialized Instruments, Equipments and Implants

Specialized instruments such as lamina spreaders, Hintermann retractors, motorized wire and burr drivers, and reduction clamps are always needed for seamless foot and ankle trauma management.

♦ Fragment-specific anatomically shaped implants are implants of choice
♦ Screws have given a way to wires
♦ Headless screws are required for articular fixation

Commandments No. 10: Smart Postoperative Care and Specialized Physiotherapy

In foot and ankle trauma, postoperative protocols are never generalized as elsewhere.

♦ Postoperative arch support is required for 6 for 8 weeks following midfoot fixations
♦ Removal of screws, external fixators, distractors, spanning plates must be planned in advance and communicated to patients
♦ Breakage of these implants is very common
♦ Physiotherapy is more focused toward eccentric strengthening and proprioception.
♦ Theraband plays an important role in physiotherapy
♦ Long-lasting venous edema is the rule and must be informed to patients well in advance

Chapter 6

Tips, Tricks, and Management Algorithm for Foot and Ankle Injuries

Success mantra for foot and ankle trauma management:
Ten commandments of foot and ankle trauma management!

Ankle Fractures

Till date, ankle fractures are one of the most controversial fractures in foot and ankle! Algorithm of management with respect to timing of patient presentation is described in **Flowchart 6.1**.

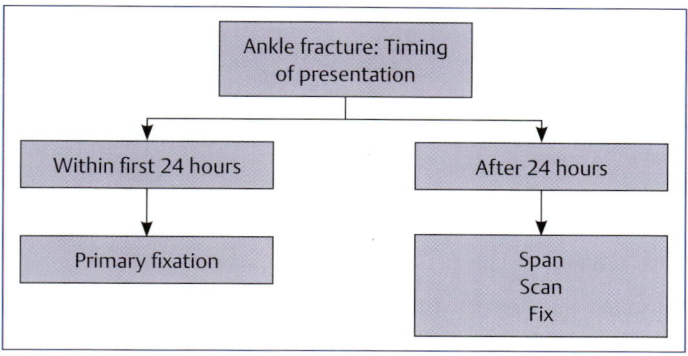

Flowchart 6.1   Algorithm of management as per the timing of presentation of ankle fractures.

Ankle fractures are treated with typical ladder of fixation. **Flowchart 6.2** enumerates that ladder.

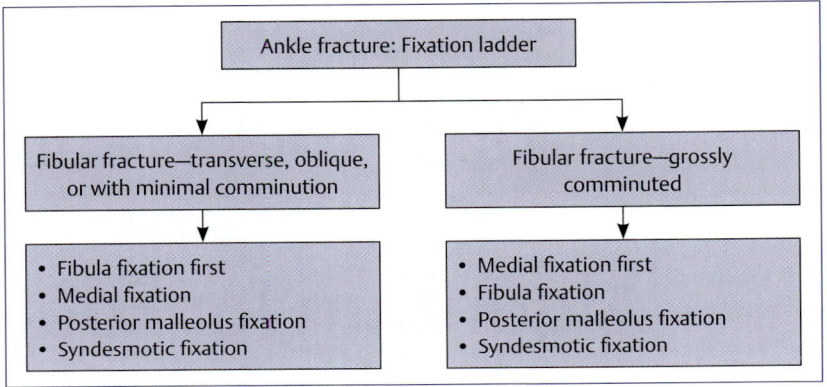

Flowchart 6.2   Ankle fracture fixation ladder.

Ankle fractures associated with deltoid ligament injury are treated differently (**Flowchart 6.3**).

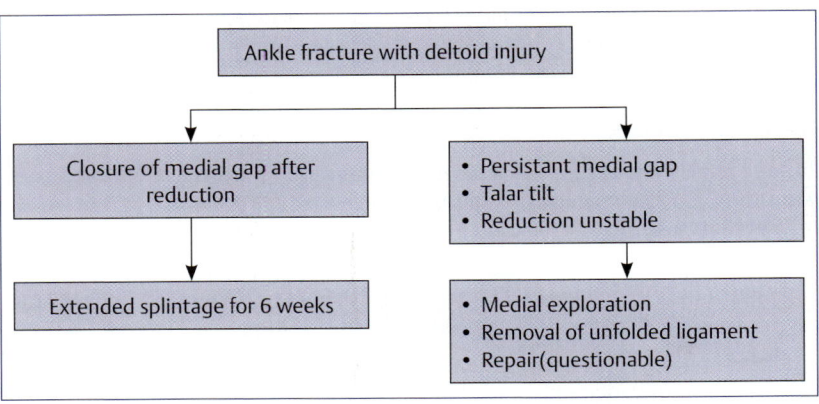

Flowchart 6.3   Treatment of ankle fracture with associated deltoid injury.

Tips and Tricks

♦ Early fixation of fractures (within 24 hours of injury) gives better outcome.
♦ Late-presenting injuries need protocol of span, scan, and plan with waiting up to 1 week.
♦ For late presentations, temporary joint spanning external fixator is used for a few days.
♦ Presence of wrinkles on the skin is a sign for safe intervention.

- ◆ Early surgical intervention prevents blister formation.
- ◆ If blisters are already present, wait for it to heal and avoid incising through it.
- ◆ Avoid use of tourniquet in cases with diabetes mellitus and peripheral vascular disease.
- ◆ Use of tourniquet is associated with increased postoperative pain and swelling and delayed achievement of range of motion. As far as possible, avoid tourniquet in most of the cases!
- ◆ Steps of fixation shall be fibular length restoration, medial exploration and fixation, posterior malleolus fixation, followed by syndesmotic assessment and fixation except in cases with gross comminution of fibula.
- ◆ Fibular length achievement and perfect rotational alignment of fibula are the most important factors for successful end result.
- ◆ Fixation chronology may be altered depending upon fracture geometry. In cases with fibular comminution, medial exploration and stabilization shall be done first.
  - • Infrasyndesmotic fibular fractures—screw or tension band wiring
  - • Transsyndesmotic fibular fractures—plate, screw, or tension band wiring
  - • Suprasyndesmotic fibular fractures—plate
- ◆ For all isolated fibular fractures, gravity stress X-ray is a must to assess syndesmotic integrity and need for syndesmotic fixation (**Fig. 6.1**).

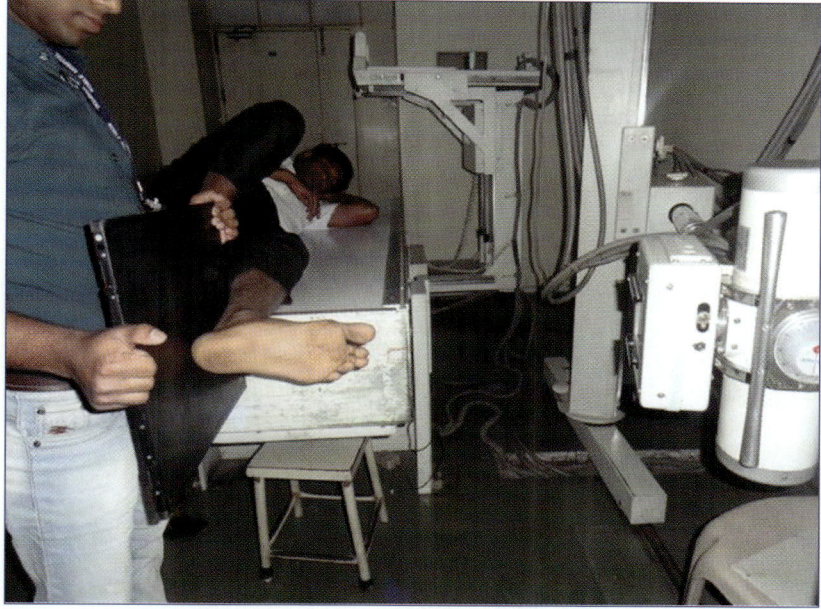

Fig. 6.1   Positioning of patient for taking gravity stress view.

- ◆ Antiglide plate (plate put on the posterior surface of the fibula) gives strongest fixation and is preferred in osteoporotic situations.
- ◆ Use of intramedullary nailing should be reserved for selected transverse, suprasyndesmotic fibula fractures only.

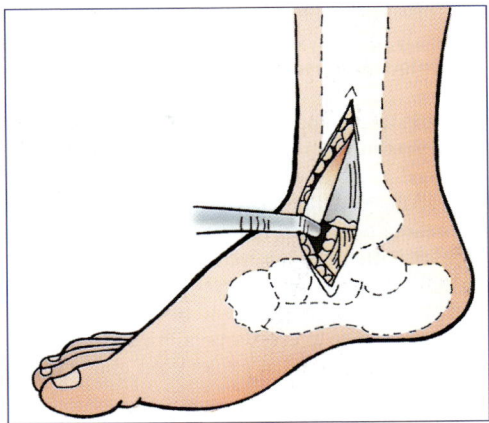

Fig. 6.2 Anteriorly placed medial incision helps in visualizing ankle joint.

- Anteriorly taken medial incision provides the opportunity of looking inside the ankle joint to identify osteochondral lesion and is a must **(Fig. 6.2)**.
- Routine repair of deltoid ligament is not indicated.
- Explore deltoid ligament to remove its unfolding in cases where either after fibular reduction medial clear joint space remains wide or fibular reduction is difficult to maintain.
- Large medial malleolar fragment should be buttressed with a plate **(Fig. 6.3)**.
- Always fix posterior malleolar fragment irrespective of its size for better reconstruction of incisura. Such a fixation often obviates the need for syndesmotic screw fixation **(Fig. 6.4)**.

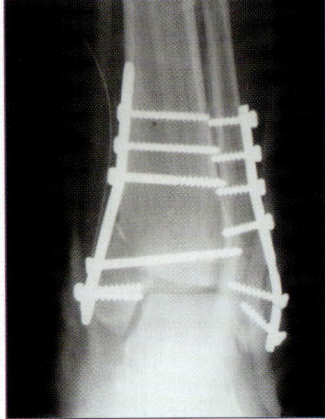

Fig. 6.3 Postoperative X-ray image of a case where large medial fragment was fixed up with buttress plate.

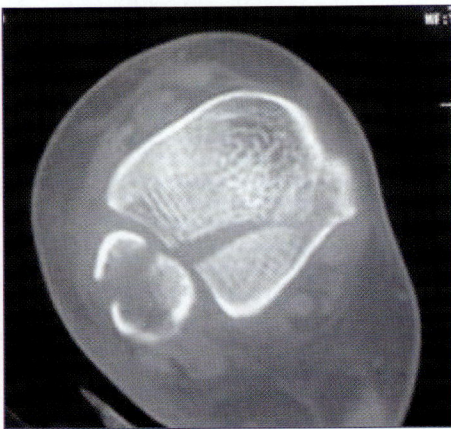

Fig. 6.4 Axial CT image of ankle showing the posterior malleolar fracture extending up to incisura of fibula.

♦ Posterior malleolar fractures are better stabilized by a biomechanically strong screw put from posterior to anterior.
♦ For a large posterior malleolar fragment, use of buttress plate is a must (**Fig. 6.5**).

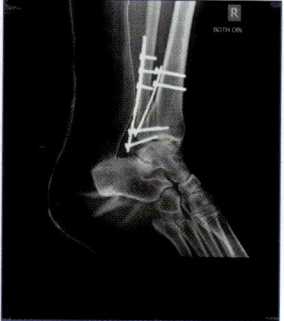

Fig. 6.5   Postoperative radiograph of a case where large posterior malleolus fracture was stabilized with buttress plate.

♦ Ankle fracture protocols:
  Preoperative: prepare and drape both the limbs.

  Intraoperative: Follow six-step ankle protocol.

  • Comparative image-assisted mortise view to look for medial clear space, dime sign, and ankle instability sign
  • *Hook test*: It is done by putting a bone hook in the interosseous membrane of the fibula and the fibula is pulled outward to look for instability at syndesmosis (**Fig. 6.6**)
  • *Tap test*: It is performed by pushing tap through one of the screw holes of the fibular plate and separation of fibula from tibia is noted, which is suggestive of syndesmotic instability (**Fig. 6.7**)

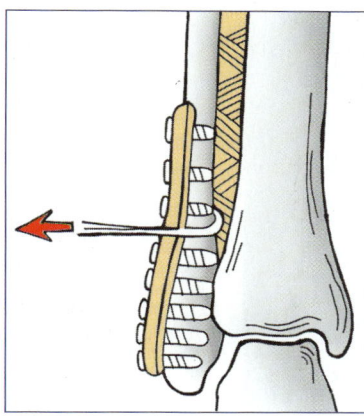

Fig. 6.6   Hook test.

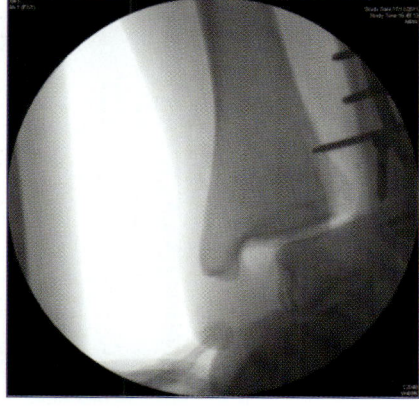

Fig. 6.7   Tap test.

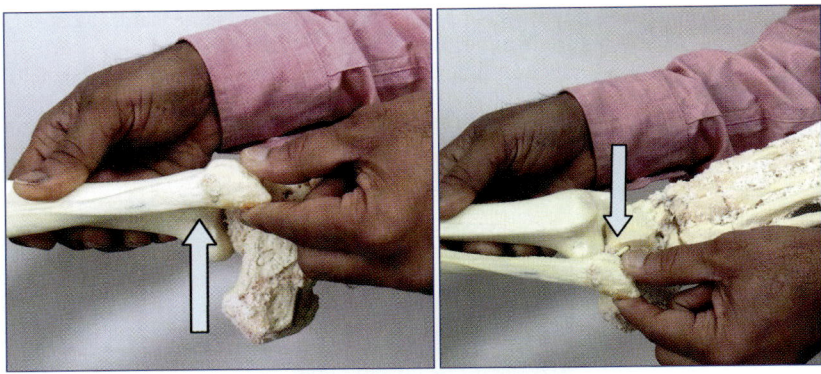

Fig. 6.8 Anteroposterior ballottement test.

- Anteroposterior ballottement test (**Fig. 6.8**). In this test fibula is rolled anteroposteriorly over tibia and amount of instability at syndesmosis is noted.
- Gravity stress test
◆ When in doubt, it is better to fix syndesmosis.
◆ Author's preference is use of two 3.5 mm syndesmotic screws with purchase of four cotices and removal only if at the end of three post-operative months ankle dorsiflexion is limited.
◆ Use two screws with four cortices for syndesmotic fixation in unstable situations, diabetics, revision fixation, and osteoporosis for better stability.
◆ Foot should be in neutral position during syndesmotic screw fixation.
◆ In osteoporotic ankle fractures, use of antiglide fibula plate, bicortical screw fixation, and combination fixations are preferred.
◆ Use intramedullary K-wires supported with plate, locking plate, bone substitutes, and cement augmentation for osteoporotic cases.
◆ In neuropathic fractures, stronger, longer, combination, and spanning fixations are preferred. Use of fibula pro tibia screws is advised (**Fig. 6.9**).

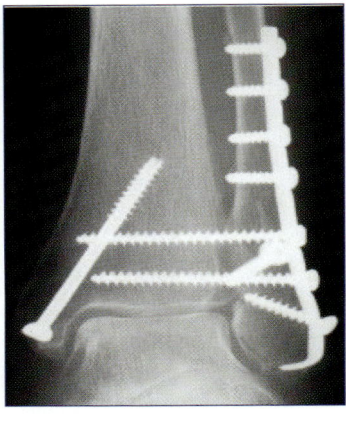

Fig. 6.9 Radiograph showing fibula pro tibia screws.

Ankle Sprain

Every ankle injury is not ankle sprain!
Unresolved ankle sprain is the deadliest enemy of orthopedic surgeon!
Flowcharts 6.4 and **6.5** demonstrate the management of acute and chronic lateral ligament injury.

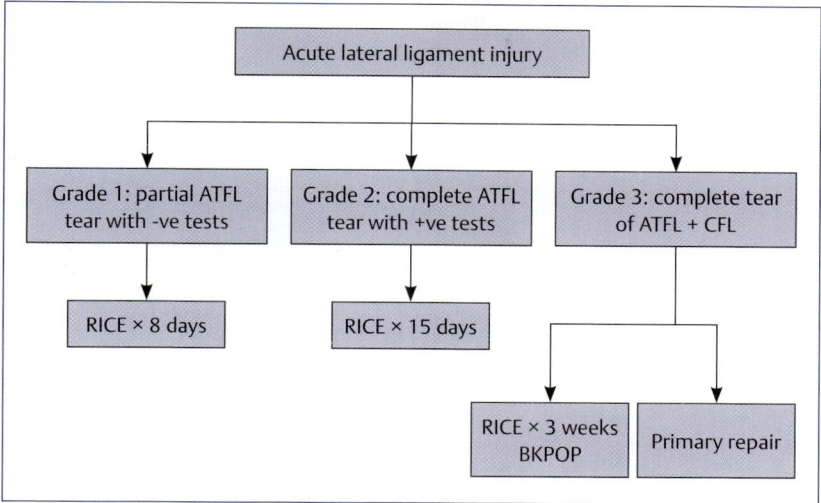

Flowchart 6.4 Management of acute lateral ligament injury. ATFL, anterior talofibular ligament; CFL, calcaneofibular ligament, RICE, rest, ice, compression and elevation; BKPOP, below knee plaster.

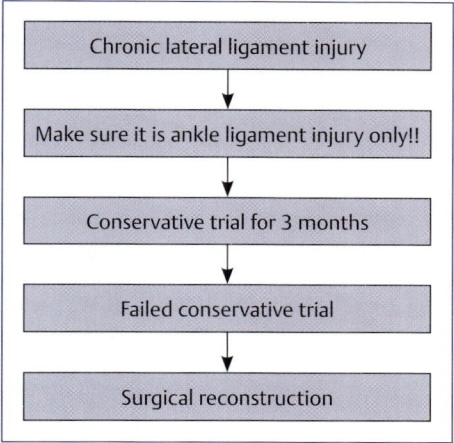

Flowchart 6.5 Management of chronic lateral ligament injury.

Tips and Tricks

♦ Always rule out conditions that can mimic ankle sprain. The following conditions can mimic ankle sprain:
  • Fracture of anterior process of calcaneus
  • Fracture of lateral process of talus
  • Fracture of posterior process of talus
  • Osteochondral lesion of talus
  • Fracture base fifth metatarsal
  • Tendo-Achilles rupture
  • Peroneal tendon injuries
  • Syndesmotic injury with high fibular fracture
♦ Follow five-phase protocols for ankle sprain management (**Flowchart 6.6**).

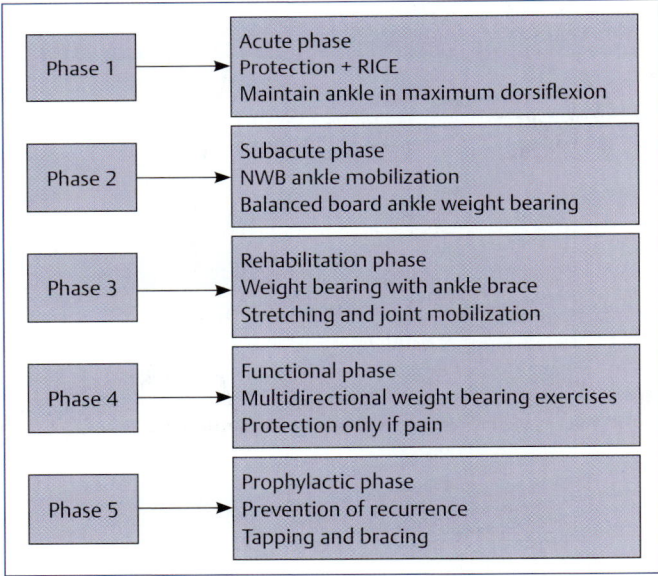

Flowchart 6.6 Protocols for ankle sprain management. RICE, rest, ice, compression and elevation.

Fully activated and strong peronei are the best protection against instability!

♦ Use balanced board, proprioception exercises, and theraband judiciously for rehabilitation of ankle sprain cases.
♦ Reassess every ankle sprain case at the end of 6 weeks because 20% of properly treated ankle sprain cases progress to functional ankle instability.
♦ Get MRI images if symptoms persist beyond 10 weeks.
♦ Anatomical reconstruction of lateral ligament should always be preferred over nonanatomical reconstruction.
♦ At reconstructive lateral ligament surgery, correct bony malalignments like hindfoot varus or forefoot varus.

Syndesmotic Injuries

Syndesmotic injuries are one of the most controversial injuries in foot and ankle!
The following facts have emerged in the present era with respect to management of syndesmotic injuries.

Screws Used in Syndesmotic Injuries

◆ Material: Steel, titanium, and bioabsorbable, all showed comparable results.
◆ Where: Between 2 and 5 cm above plafond **(Fig. 6.10)**.
◆ Number and size: 2 × 3.5 vs. 1 × 4.5 screws. Early results are good with 3.5 screws, but no difference visible at 1 year.

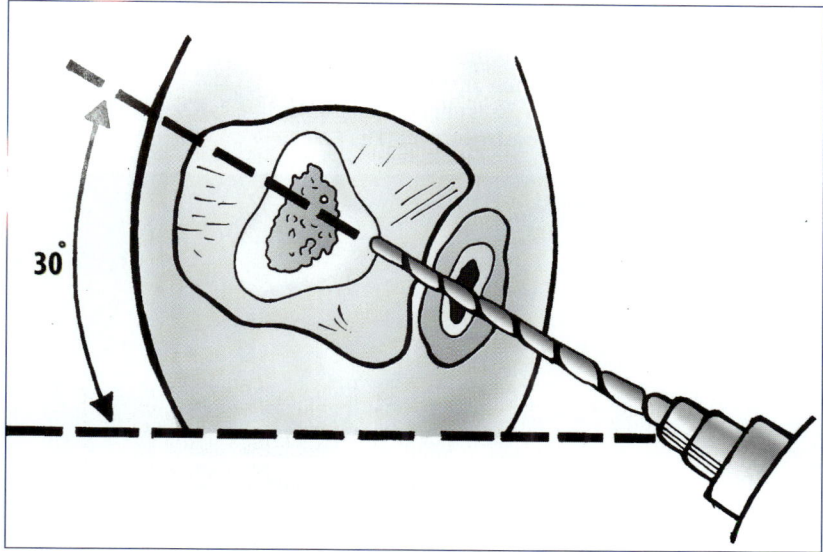

Fig. 6.10 Direction of syndesmotic screw.

◆ No difference in outcomes between tricortical or quadricortical screws, but quadricortical screws can be removed easily if they break and are symptomatic.

Diagnosis of Syndesmotic Injury

◆ Four clinical tests:
  • Direct palpation causing pain on syndesmosis
  • External rotation of foot causing pain
  • Calf squeeze causing pain
  • Dorsiflexion with syndesmotic squeeze/taping relieving pain after taping than before
◆ External rotation test is most sensitive.

No single test is reliable to demonstrate syndesmotic instability. In case of clinical suspicion in symptomatic patient, MRI scan with high sensitivity and high specificity is recommended.

◆ X-rays: AP and mortise views.
◆ Tibiofibular overlap between the lateral border of posterior tibia and the medial border of fibula if it is more than 6 mm on AP and more than 1 mm on mortise views.
◆ Tibiofibular clear space at the medial border of fibula and anterior tibial tubercle if it is more than 6 mm on both views.
◆ Medial clear space in mortise view is less than 4 mm or equal to talotibial plafond space.
◆ Intraoperative tests:
  • Cotton test (Hook test): Pull fibula laterally and take AP X-ray
  • External rotation test: Hold leg straight and externally rotate the foot and take AP X-ray
  • Modified cotton test: Pull fibula posteriorly and take a lateral X-ray
  • Ballotment test: Roll fibula antero-posteriorly
◆ Latest method of CT-based assessment: Tibiofibular line can be checked preoperatively/postoperatively/posttreatment (**Fig. 6.11**).

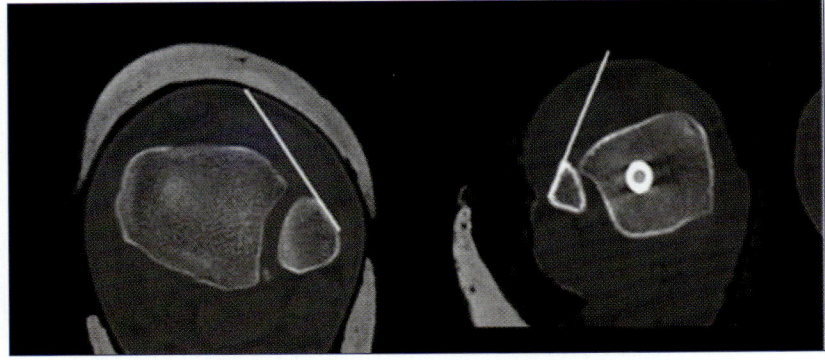

Fig. 6.11 CT image showing the tibiofibular line for diagnosis of syndesmotic injuries.

◆ Line from flat anterolateral surface of fibula to anterior tubercle of tibia measured 1 cm above tibial plafond on axial cut of CT scan. Must be within 2 mm from the anterior surface of tibia.

Tips and Tricks for Syndesmotic Screws

◆ Put a clamp at the same horizontal level. If the clamp is put obliquely, it can pull the fibula out of its anatomical groove
◆ Aim the drill posterior to anterior from the fibula, otherwise one may miss the tibia
◆ Position of the foot is immaterial. Let it stay in the resting position
◆ May allow the syndesmosis to fall back into its original position and allow for the natural movement of distal fibula during ankle movement

♦ Recent studies show no difference in symptoms and functional scores at 1 year between removal of screws or not
♦ Syndesmosis may not be healed by 3 months and removal of screws may lead to loss of position

Pilon Fractures

Flowcharts 6.7 and **6.8** demonstrate various types of closed pilon fractures and their respective treatment options.

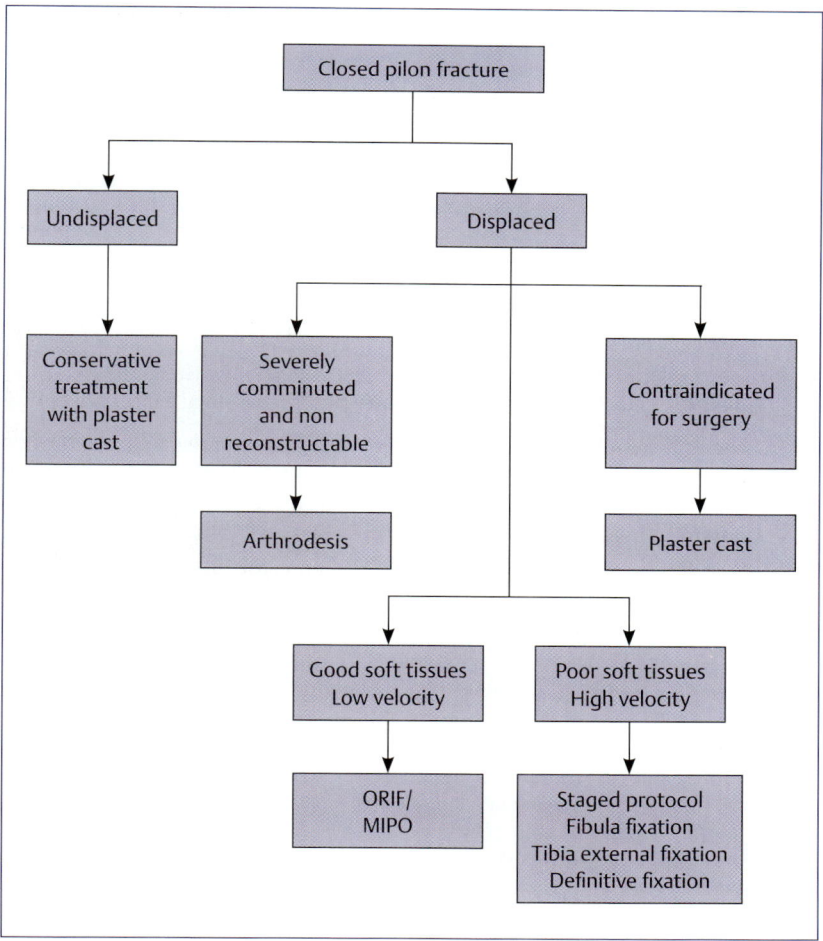

Flowchart 6.7   Types of closed pilon fractures and their respective treatment options. ORIF, open reduction internal fixation; MIPO, minimally invasive plate osteosynthesis

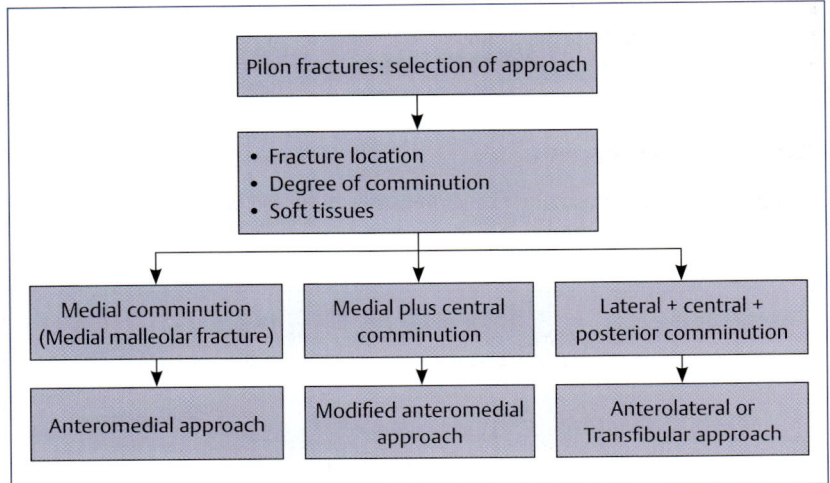

Flowchart 6.8   Approach selection in the case of pilon fractures.

Tips and Tricks

♦ Plan your treatment based on the answers to the following five questions:
  • **Question 1:** Is this a low-velocity injury or a high-velocity injury?

  History of mode of injury and presence of associated injuries will answer this question. By and large, sagittal fracture line suggests high-velocity trauma, while coronal fracture line suggests low-velocity trauma

  • **Question 2:** What is the status of soft tissues?
  • **Question 3:** Is this injury reconstructible?

  Amount of comminution and bone loss would guide.

  • **Question 4:** Is it displaced injury or undisplaced injury?
  • **Question 5:** Are there any comorbid conditions?
♦ Best fixation for fibula is a plate that maintains the length and rotation. Nail should only be used in short oblique or transverse fibular fractures
♦ Use joint spanning external fixator with a delta frame to give optimum stability. Sometimes soft tissues may not permit definitive internal fixation and continuing the same fixator may be needed and will work as well
♦ Follow the principle of span, scan, and plan
♦ The more minimally invasive you wish to be, the more preoperative planning you need to do
♦ Read, reread, and reread CT scan
♦ Do keep CT scan in operation room
♦ CT scan guides about the direction and placement of screws to build articular block
♦ Always use a direct approach
♦ Always mark future incision sites before putting an external fixator
♦ Placement of plate is always on the unstable side

◆ At least one stiff implant is a must
◆ Use talus as a template for building the reduction
◆ Restoration of articular surface by open reduction, followed by metaphyseal block fixation mostly by minimally invasive biological fixation is the today's tune

Calcaneus Fractures

Flowchart 6.9 shows the management of extra-articular calcaneal fractures.
Flowchart 6.10 shows the method of fixation in different classes of intra-articular calcaneus fractures according to Sander's classification.

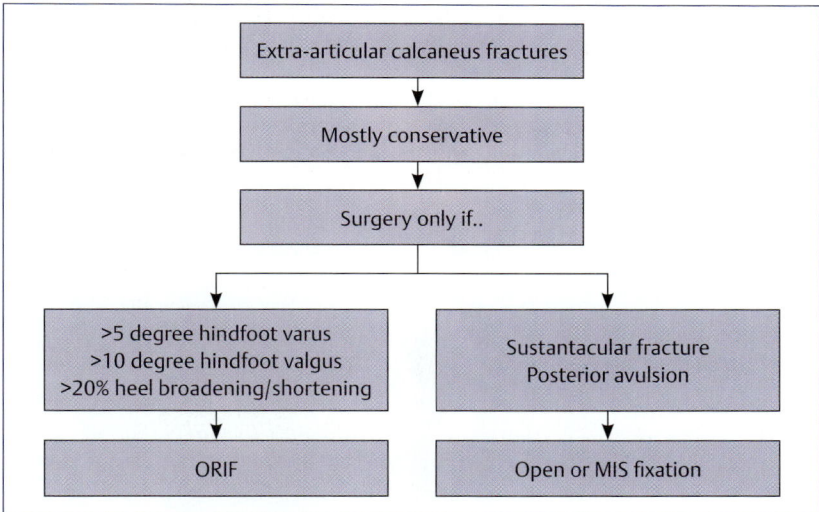

Flowchart 6.9   Management of extra-calcaneal fractures. ORIF, open reduction internal fixation; MIS, minimal invasive surgery.

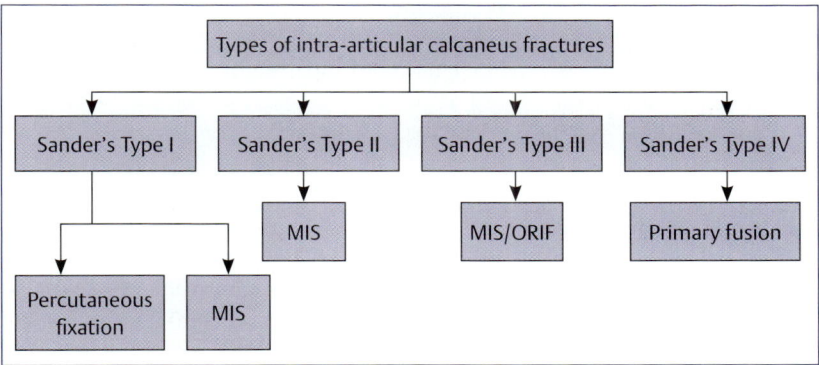

Flowchart 6.10   Fixation in case of Sander's Type I to IV. MIS, minimal invasive surgery; ORIF, open reduction internal fixation.

Tips and Tricks

♦ A periodic X-ray check for 3 weeks is a must while treating calcaneus fractures conservatively
♦ Before proceeding to surgery based on either X-rays or CT scan, assess the following parameters and then plan your surgery
  • Medial comminution
  • Medial wall blast
  • Involvement of calcaneocuboid joint
  • Comminution of posterior articular facet
  • Heel position
  • Heel shortening
  • Heel broadening
♦ Avoid incising through the blisters
♦ Serous blisters shall be aspirated and are not much of an issue, while blood-filled blisters necessitate delaying of surgical intervention
♦ *Wrinkle test*: If dorsiflexion and eversion of foot show the presence of wrinkles at the junction of dorsal and plantar skin then that is the surest sign to safe surgical intervention **(Fig. 6.12)**

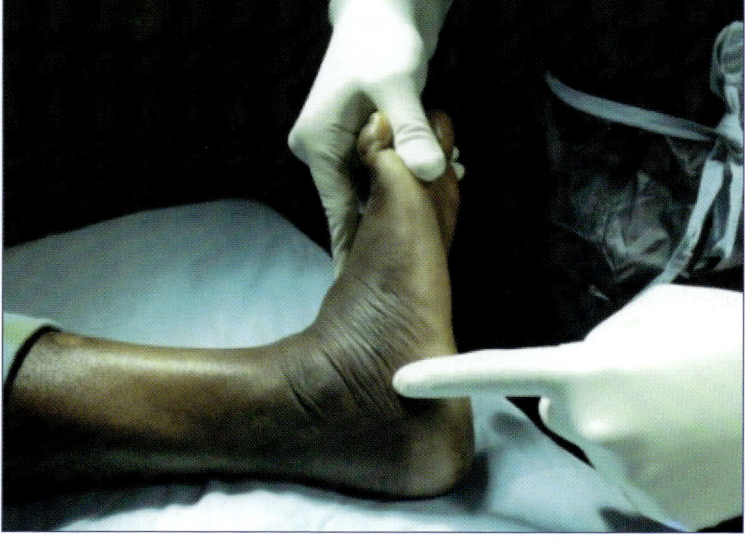

Fig. 6.12   Wrinkle test is being demonstrated by dorsiflexion and eversion of foot showing presence of wrinkles at heel.

♦ Beyond 3 weeks, treat calcaneus fracture on lines with malunited calcaneus fracture.
♦ Before surgery ensure about the need for reduction of sustentacular fragment or medial wall. Plan separate medial incision for the same, if needed.
♦ At surgery, surgeon stands at the heel end and assistant stands at the forefoot end, while the image intensifier is positioned diagonally opposite in a manner that AP

projection shows lateral heel image and lateral projection shows axial heel image (**Fig. 6.13**).

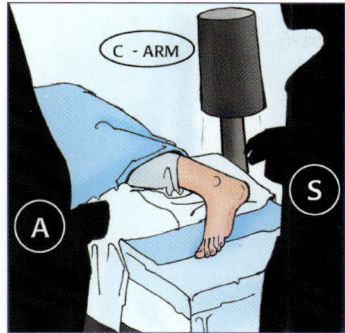

Fig. 6.13 Patient position at surgery for calcaneus fracture. A, position of assistant; S, position of surgeon.

♦ To have a clear axial image, assistant must always dorsiflex the forefoot.
♦ Vertical limb of incision needs to be taken more posteriorly to avoid seeing the sural nerve (**Fig. 6.14**).
♦ In a case with involvement of calcaneocuboid joint, horizontal limb of incision should be taken more distal and should be curved upward (**Fig. 6.15**).

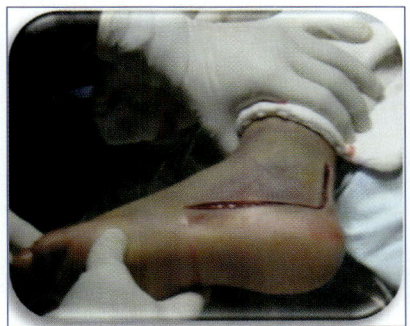 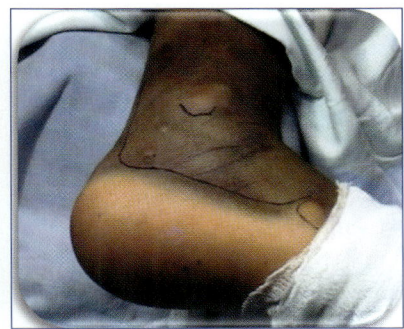

Fig. 6.14 Incision for extended lateral approach for calcaneus fracture surgery.

Fig. 6.15 Modification of incision for involvement of calcaneocuboid joint.

♦ Flap should be handled with plain forceps and is retracted with blunt skin hooks.
♦ While putting talar wire for flap retraction, heel inversion should be done, and for putting cuboid wire for flap retraction, heel eversion should be done.
♦ Reduction is built from inside out, starting from medial wall and sustentacular fragment and coming out laterally.
♦ A use of freer, hemostat, or bone spike from the lateral side for manipulation will facilitate medial-sided reduction.

♦ For two fragments of posterior articular facet principle of compression is adopted, while for more than two fragments of posterior articular facet principle of position screw is adopted.
♦ For multiple fragments of posterior articular surface, temporary K-wire is threaded in a retrograde manner (**Fig. 6.16**).

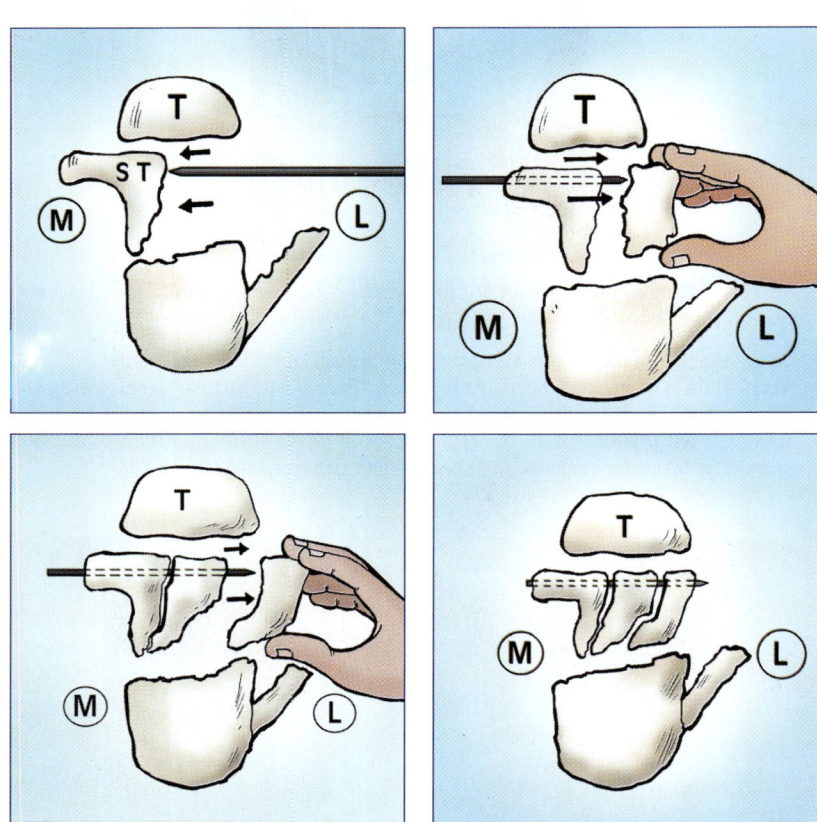

Fig. 6.16 Diagrammatic demonstration of threading of posterior articular fragments with K-wire. M, medial side; L, lateral side; T, talus; ST, sustantacum tali.

♦ In severely comminuted situations, temporary stabilization wires may be pushed further into the talus or cuboid.
♦ Putting compression or position screws outside the plate for posterior articular facet reduction makes surgery easy.
♦ Always suture inadvertently incised peroneal tendon sheath before closure.
♦ Never suture back calcaneofibular ligament.

♦ All knots must come outside the flap (**Fig. 6.17**).

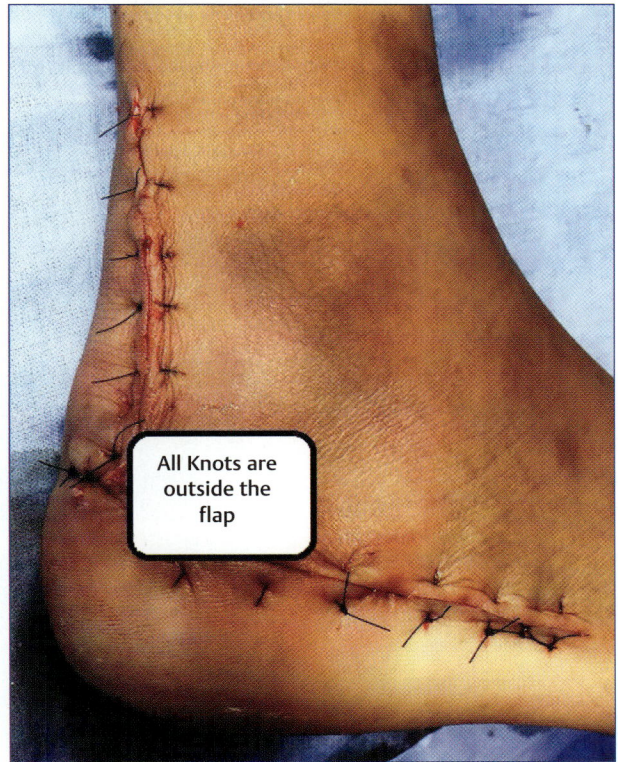

Fig. 6.17   Picture showing position of knots at closure of incision.

♦ Start closure from ends and go toward apex.
♦ For MIS fixations, use of joysticks and image assistance are two most important prerequisites.
♦ Use either external fixator or JESS fixator as aid to reduction during minimally invasive surgery.
♦ Peroneal tendon sheath is dissected free from bone to slide subperoneal low-profile plate through the sinus tarsi approach.
♦ Achieving perfect reduction is the first step for primary fusion as fusion is never done *in situ* without correcting heel height, heel broadening, and various bony protrusions.
♦ Both the iliac crests must be prepared while contemplating primary fusion of calcaneus.

Talus Fractures

Flowchart 6.11 shows the management of talar process fractures. **Flowcharts 6.12** to **6.14** cover the management of the fracture of various regions of talus, head body, and neck, respectively. **Flowchart 6.15** shows the closed reduction of the fractures with dislocation.

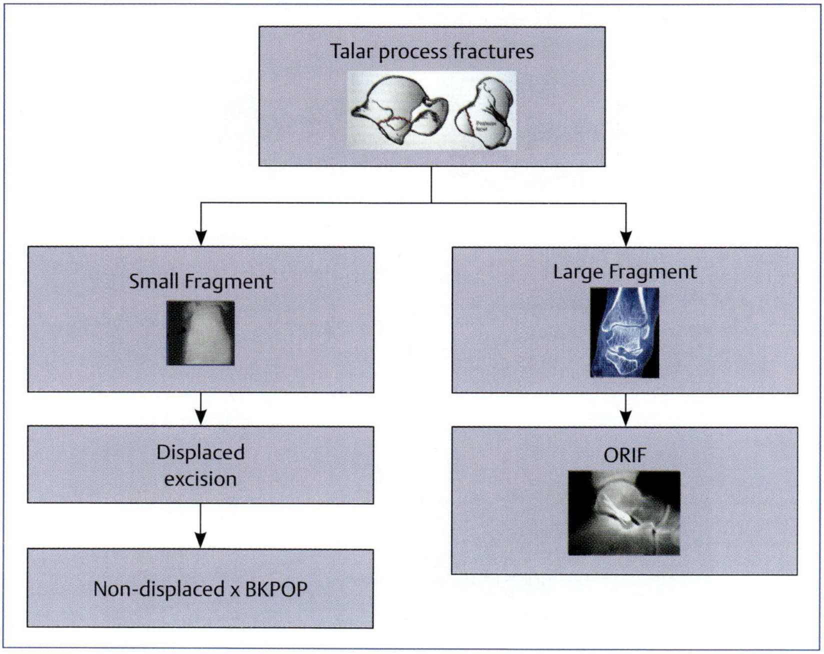

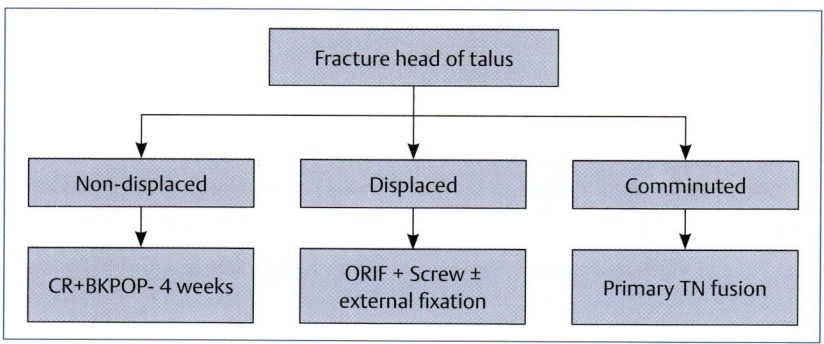

Flowchart 6.11 Management of talar process fractures. BKPOP, below knee plaster; ORIF, open reduction internal fixation.

Flowchart 6.12 Management of the fracture of head of talus. BKPOP, below knee plaster; CR, closed reduction; TN, talo-navicular.

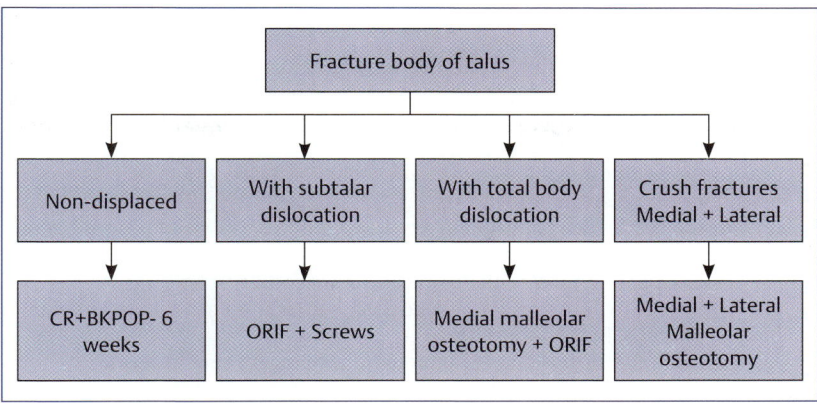

Flowchart 6.13 Management of the fracture of body of talus. BKPOP, below knee plaster; CR, closed reduction; ORIF, open reduction internal fixation.

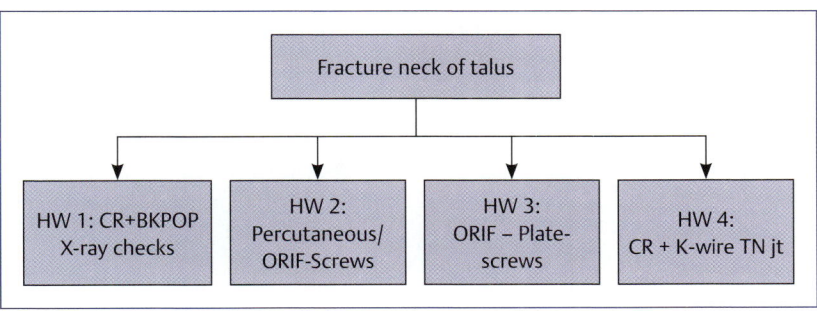

Flowchart 6.14 Management of the fracture of neck of talus. CR, closed reduction; ORIF, open reduction internal fixation; TN, talo-navicular; HW, hawkin.

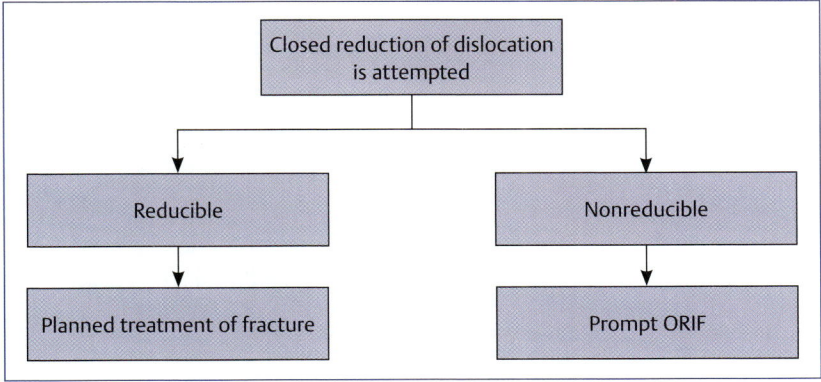

Flowchart 6.15 Management of the fracture of talus with dislocation.

Tips and Tricks

♦ *Be suspicious, be aggressive*
♦ Suspect fracture talus in every hindfoot trauma and every polytrauma case
♦ Suspect displacement and comminution and get Canale and Kelly view as well as CT scan before treating these injuries
♦ Any unresolved post–ankle trauma pain should be suspected to be a case of osteochondral fracture of talus
♦ Any unresolved ankle sprain should be suspected to be a case of missed fracture lateral or posterior process of talus
♦ Serial radiology is a must while treating fracture conservatively
♦ Clinician needs to be aggressive to reduce any dislocation or subluxation of talus before advising CT scan
♦ Aggression in the form of emergent reduction or surgery should be shown in cases with vascular jeopardy, compartment syndromes, and protruding fragments underneath skin **(Fig. 6.18)**
♦ Whenever in doubt, take double approach **(Fig. 6.19A** and **B)**

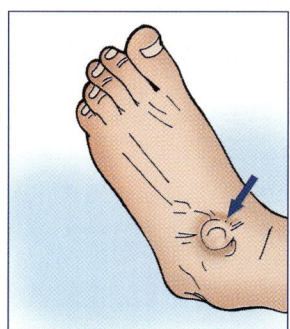

Fig. 6.18 Fragment of fracture talus just beneath the skin.

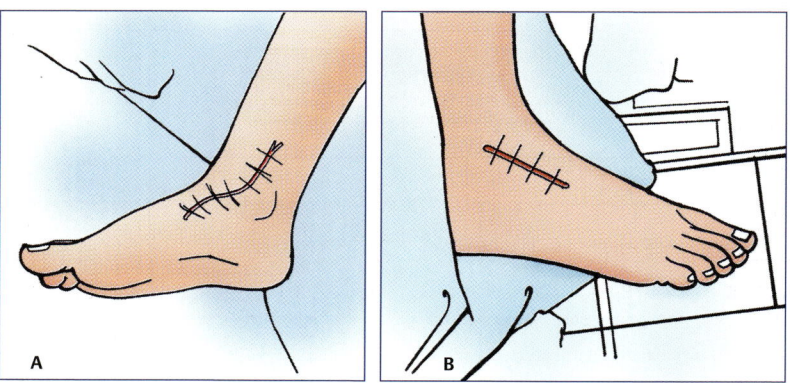

Fig. 6.19 (A and B) Double approach (anteromedial and anterolateral) for treating fracture talus.

♦ Anterior approach gives great visualization but these are disadvantages such as delayed healing, wound issues, and inability to visualize subtalar joint
♦ Always be prepared to add either medial or lateral malleolar osteotomy for facilitation of reduction **(Fig. 6.20)**
♦ Use a hemostat as a cartilage protector during medial malleolar osteotomy **(Fig. 6.21A** and **B)**

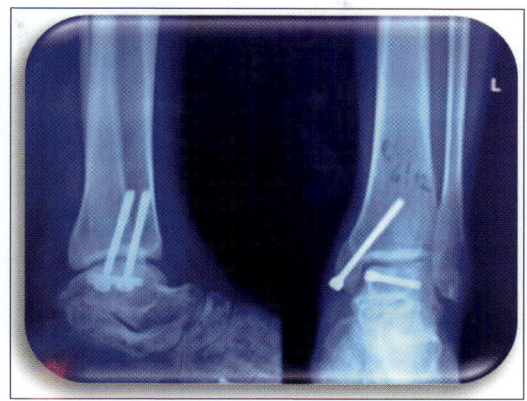

Fig. 6.20   Radiograph of a case of fracture talus treated with medial malleolar osteotomy.

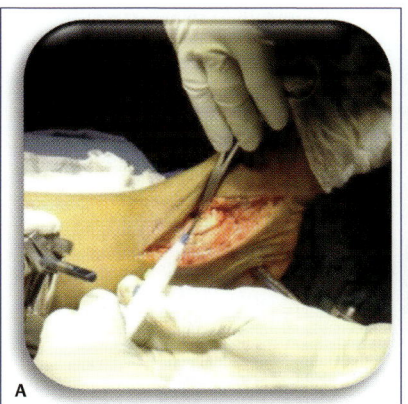
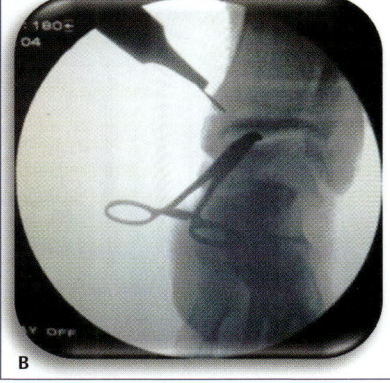

Fig. 6.21   (A and B) Pictures show the use of hemostat inside the ankle joint to serve not only as cartilage protector but also as a guide to osteotomy.

♦ Do not pull medial malleolar fragment vigorously down, otherwise it would damage the only source of blood supply to the head and neck of talus

♦ It would be advisable to put suture threads through the osteotomized medial malleolar fragment and use these sutures as retractors **(Fig. 6.22)**
♦ Always suture ligaments back while repositioning lateral malleolar osteotomy.
♦ Predrill and tap osteotomy
♦ Osteotomy should be directed over the talus dome and should not damage the talar articular surface **(Fig. 6.23)**

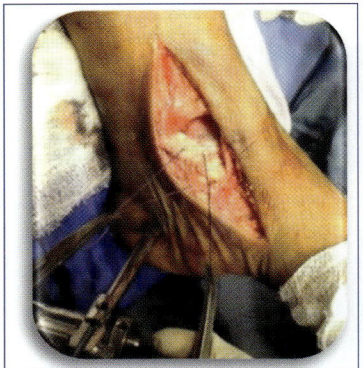

Fig 6.22   Use of sutures as retractor for medial malleolar osteotomy.

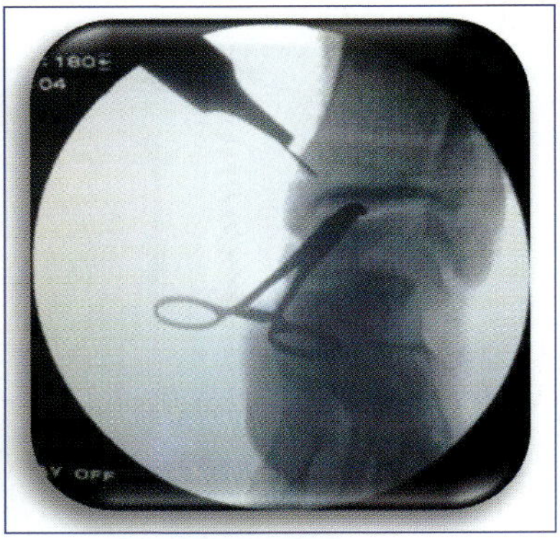

Fig. 6.23   Intraoperative image showing the direction of osteotomy.

♦ Posterior-to-anterior screws are biomechanically strong, but posterior approach has a very narrow window of opportunity to push screws
♦ Size and location of fragment would dictate the placement of screws, anterior to posterior or vice versa **(Fig. 6.24)**

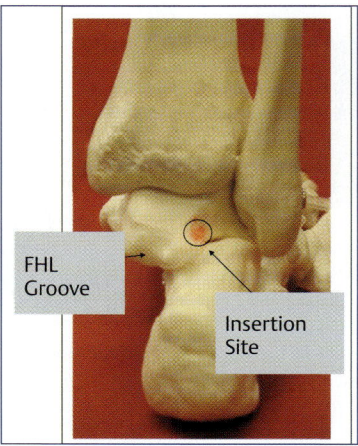

FHL
Groove

Insertion
Site

Fig. 6.24   Diagrammatic picture of area available for placement of posterior screws. Insertion site is lateral to grove for passage of tendon of flexor hallucis longus (FHL).

♦ Joysticks are put parallel in both the planes to make sure not to open up fracture either in coronal or in sagittal planes (**Fig. 6.25**)
♦ Superficial peroneal nerve, saphenous nerve, and sural nerve need special care while taking talar approaches

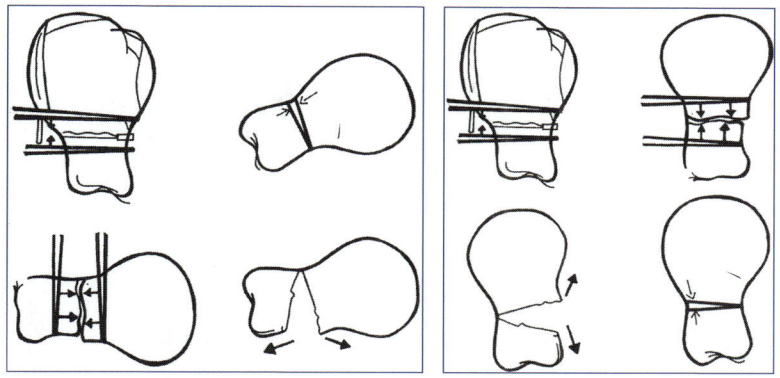

Fig. 6.25   Figures show the placement of joysticks and problems related to its placement.

Midfoot Injuries

Flowcharts 6.16 to **6.18** show the chronology for reconstruction of midfoot injury, reconstruction of cuboid injury, and management of cuboid void.

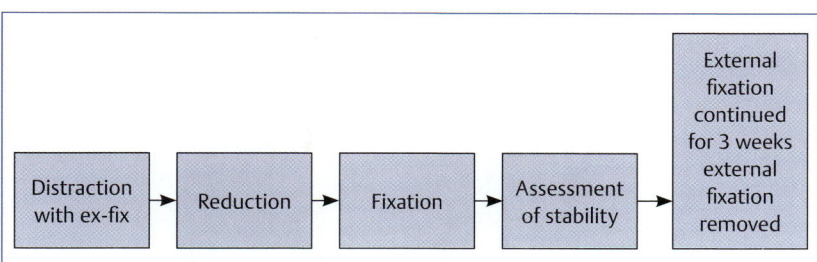

Flowchart 6.16   Chronology of midfoot injury reconstruction.

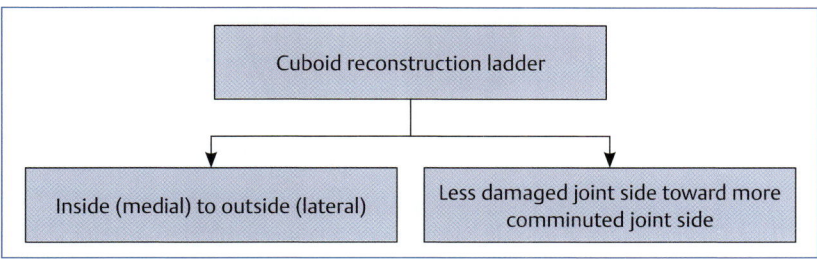

Flowchart 6.17   Chronology of cuboid reconstruction.

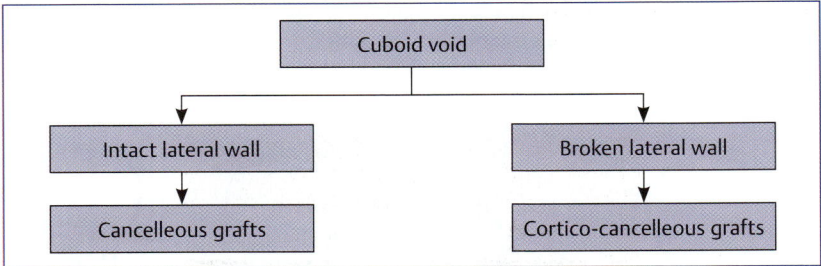

Flowchart 6.18   Management of cuboid void.

Tips and Tricks

♦ Midfoot injuries need highest degree of suspicion. Suspect these injuries in all high-velocity traumas. It should also be suspected in low-velocity traumas such as sprains, strains, falls, and twisting injuries

♦ Suspect for stress midfoot injuries in sports population **(Fig. 6.26)**

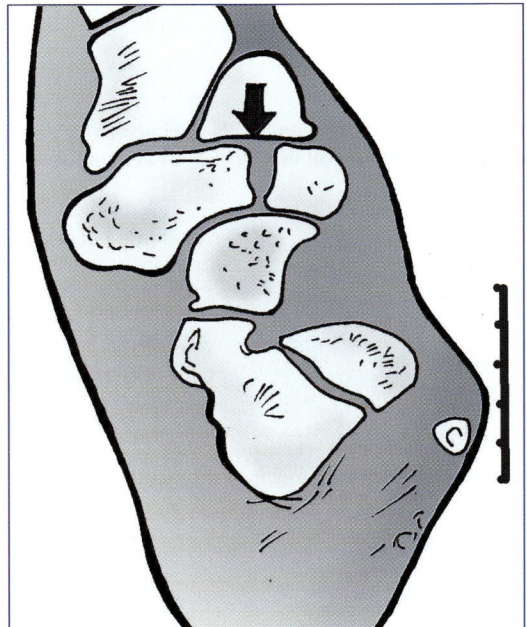

Fig. 6.26   CT image showing stress fracture of navicular in a sportsman.

♦ Always suspect and look for injuries of other bones and joints

♦ There can be injury to dorsalis pedis artery, tendons of tibialis posterior, extensors, and also compartment syndrome associated with midfoot injuries. All need high index of suspicion

♦ Midfoot bones are like both forearm bones and isolated injuries of one are rare. Always suspect and look for radiologically undetectable injury of the other bone (**Fig. 6.27**)

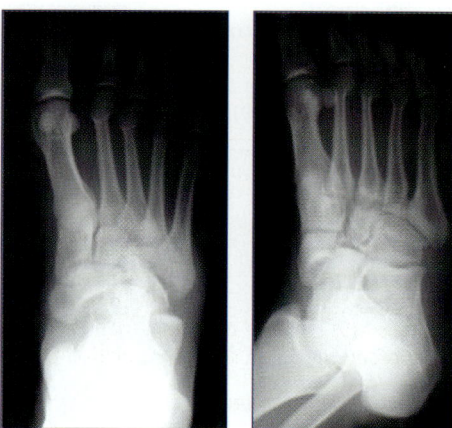

Fig. 6.27   X-rays showing injury of navicular with subtle injury of cuboid bone.

♦ Specialized X-rays such as medial oblique views, traction views, and comparative views may be needed for precise diagnosis of these injuries.
♦ A CT scan is a must
♦ Stress views and weight bearing views would help whenever possible
♦ Midfoot neuropathic fractures are with trivial trauma in diabetics and may mimic infection. Precise history taking, monofilament testing, and weight bearing radiology over and above high index of suspicion would rescue clinician (**Fig. 6.28**)

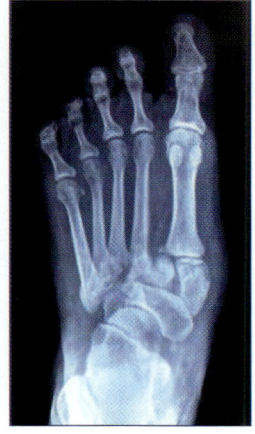

Fig. 6.28   X-ray of a midfoot neuropathic fracture.

◆ At conservative care of midfoot trauma, weekly X-ray check for 3 weeks is mandatory
◆ Talonavicular and fourth and fifth TMT joints should always be salvaged
◆ Naviculocuneiform joints, calcaneocuboid joint, and first, second, and third TMT joints can be sacrificed
◆ Always reattach navicular tuberosity or tibialis posterior tendon back to preserve medial arch
◆ Presence of wrinkle is a good sign for safe surgical intervention and waiting for a few days is always justified **(Fig. 6.29)**

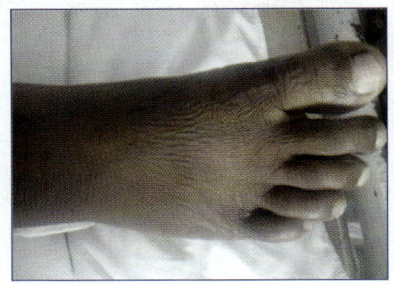

Fig. 6.29   Wrinkle sign at midfoot injury.

◆ While waiting for soft tissue to be conducive for surgery, span the midfoot and reduce subcutaneous bony fragments to prevent skin necrosis
◆ Care of vessels and superficial nerves is a must while approaching the midfoot
◆ Use of power equipment, pointed reduction forceps, distractors, lamina spreaders, and Hintermann retractors are must to treat midfoot injuries
◆ K-wires have given way to screws and fragment-specific low-profile plates
◆ Midfoot fixation follows typical fixation pattern of distraction, reduction, assessment, and decision making whether to continue distractor or to remove the same.
◆ Spanning or crossing of joints is advisable and preferred in midfoot injuries **(Fig. 6.30)**

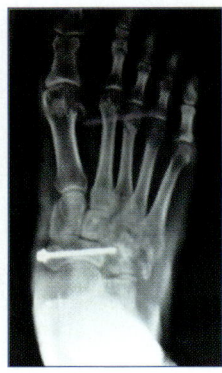

Fig. 6.30   X-ray showing crossing of joints for fixation of navicular bone.

♦ For a comminuted navicular fracture, screws are put as position screws or as lag screws otherwise
♦ Spanning plate not violating joint may work well in comminuted situations **(Fig. 6.31)**

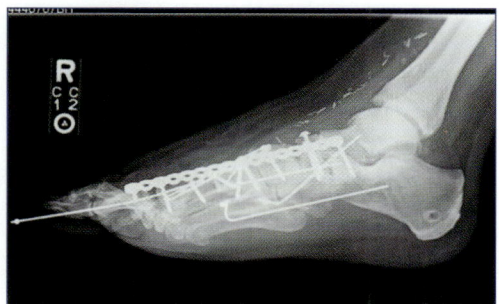

Fig. 6.31   X-ray showing use of spanning plate at midfoot fixation.

♦ Cuboid reconstruction is started from inside out and from less comminuted side to more comminuted side
♦ Always feel the void in cuboid
♦ With intact lateral wall cuboid void should be filled with cancellous bone grafts, while with damaged lateral wall void needs to be filled up with cortico-cancellous bone grafts
♦ Accessory navicular fracture should be treated with excision and reattachment of tibialis posterior insertion. There may be need for adjuvant flat foot reconstruction procedures
♦ Non-reconstructible injuries are subjected to primary fusion
♦ At surgery of midfoot, always restore lengths of both the columns **(Fig. 6.32)**
♦ At midfoot surgery, reconstruction must take care of restoration of medial longitudinal arch

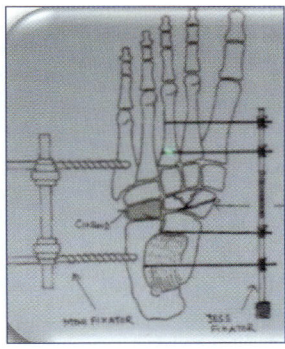

Fig. 6.32   Column length restoration by use of spanning external fixator.

Lisfranc Injuries

Plan of treatment of Lisfranc injuries is demonstrated in **Flowchart 6.19**. Different methods of treatment of Lisfranc injuries are shown in **Flowchart 6.20**. Treatment depending on the displacement of bone is explained in **Flowchart 6.21**.

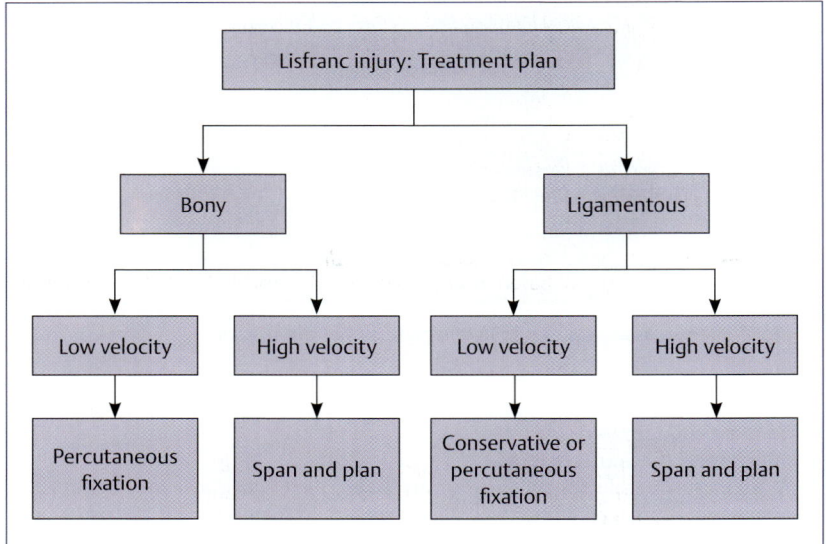

Flowchart 6.19 Plan of treatment of Lisfranc injuries.

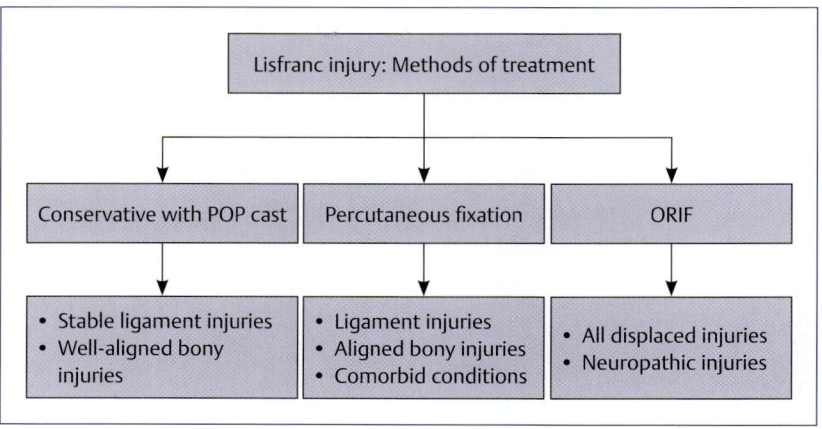

Flowchart 6.20 Methods of treatment of Lisfranc injuries. ORIF, open reduction internal fiixation; POP, plaster.

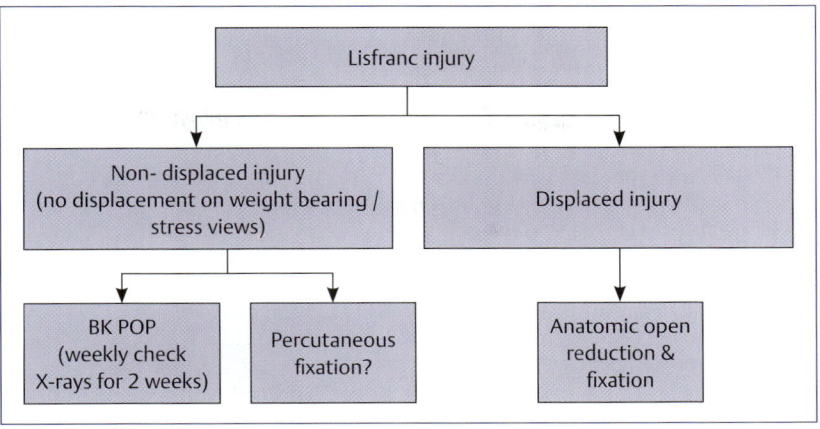

Flowchart 6.21   Treatment based on displacement of bones. BKPOP, below knee plaster.

Tips and Tricks

♦ Diagnosis needs high index of suspicion.
♦ Look for plantar ecchymosis, weight bearing views, and stress views for precise diagnosis **(Fig. 6.33)**.
♦ On plain radiology, look for typical Lisfranc injury signs plus fleck sign.
♦ For weight bearing radiology, X-ray tube must be kept parallel to foot and not to the floor **(Fig. 6.34)**.

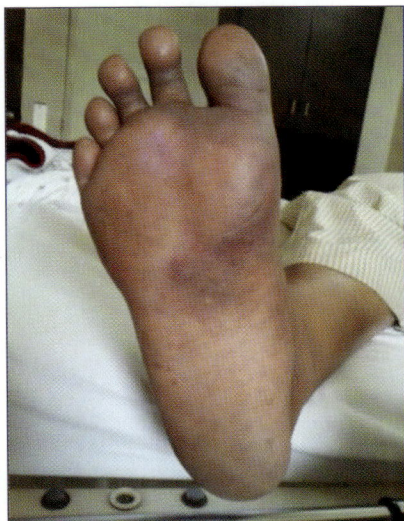

Fig. 6.33   Clinical picture showing plantar ecchymosis.

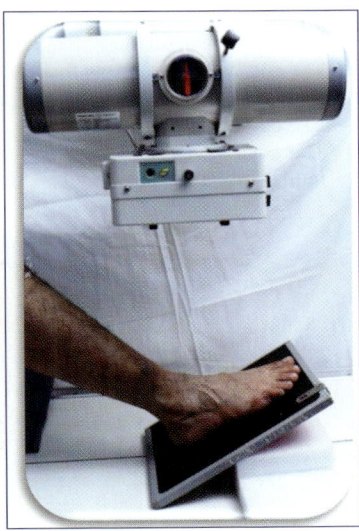

Fig. 6.34   Position of X-ray beam for imaging Lisfranc injury.

♦ CT scan is a must for evaluation before management.
♦ Diagnostic local injections under image assistance may be needed for diagnosis of subtle Lisfranc injury.
♦ Surgery may need to be delayed up to 10 to 20 days depending on local conditions.
♦ Placements of incisions may vary according to injury patterns.
  • Only first—medial to EHL
  • First and second—lateral to EHL, medial to vessels
  • Second—Lateral to vessels
  • Second and third—far lateral to vessels
  • Fourth and fifth—over forth
♦ Keep good distance between two incisions to prevent skin damage.
♦ Lengthening of extensor digitorum brevis is needed.
♦ Vessels and cutaneous nerves must be taken care of.
♦ Always make a pocket-starting hole for screw placement to prevent a crack running from screw hole to articular surface (**Fig. 6.35**).

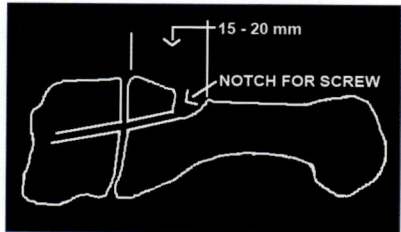

Fig. 6.35   Pocket hole for placement of lisfranc screw.

♦ Second metatarsal must be reduced first and rest of the reduction is built around it.
♦ The chronology of screw fixation is second metatarsal to medial cuneiform, first metatarsal to medial cuneiform, and then individual metatarsal bases to respective cuneiform bones.
♦ The advantages of passing screw from the base of second metatarsal to medial cuneiform are shown in **Fig. 6.36**.

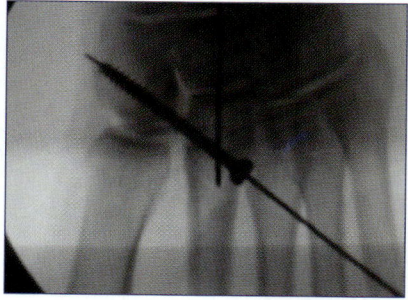

Fig. 6.36   X-ray picture showing passage of screw from base of second metatarsal to medial cuneiform.

- Aiming from smaller to bigger target is easy.
- Longer threaded portion in medial cuneiform bone gives better fixation.
- Screw goes into a denser plantar medial part of medial cuneiform.
- If the screw breaks, then it is easier to remove.
- Fourth and fifth rays are fixed with soft fixation like K-wires, while medial rays are fixed with rigid fixation with screws (**Fig. 6.37**).

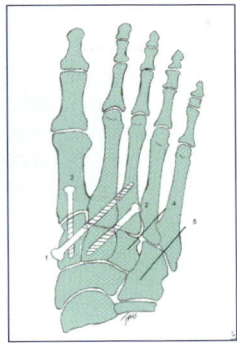

Fig. 6.37   Picture showing Lisfranc fixation.

- Secondary closure may be needed in many cases.
- Screws are put as position screws.
- All toes are dorsiflexed while tightening screws (**Fig. 6.38**).

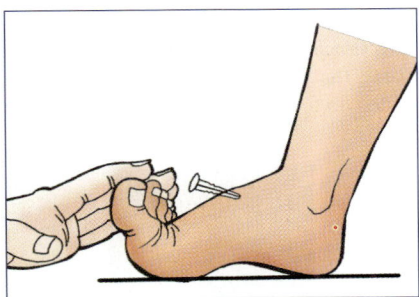

Fig. 6.38   Picture showing dorsiflexion of toes while tightening of screws.

♦ Spanning plate for comminuted situations serves best as it gives no articular damage and adds stability and removal may not be necessary (**Fig. 6.39**).

♦ For neuropathic fractures, the principles of fixation are as follows (**Fig. 6.40**):

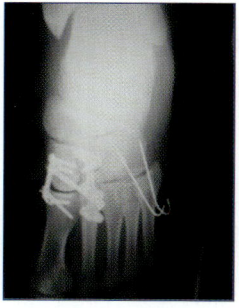

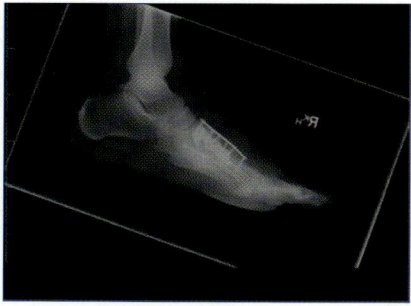

Fig. 6.39 X-ray showing use of spanning plate for lisfranc fixation.

Fig. 6.40 X-ray showing fixation of midfoot neuropathic fracture.

- Longer fixations
- Stronger fixations
- Combination fixations
- Spanning fixations
- Double protection
- Delayed weight bearing
- Long bracing

♦ Bone grafting from calcaneus, lower-end tibia, or from proximal tibia may be required for primary fusions.

♦ Removal of implants is planned as removal of K-wires by 6 to 8 weeks and screw removal by 4 to 6 months.

♦ Screws may be left *in situ* provided they are nonsymptomatic, but patient must be informed in advance that screws may break (**Fig. 6.41**).

♦ Postoperatively molded arch support or shoe inserts are a must for 6 to 8 weeks.

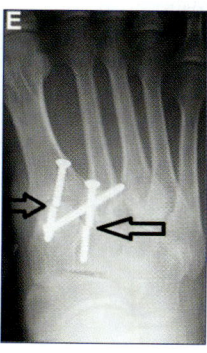

Fig. 6.41 X-ray showing broken screws after lisfranc fixation.

Metatarsal Fractures

Management of fractures of neck, shaft, and bases of first and fifth metatarsals are explained in **Flowcharts 6.22** to **6.25**, respectively.

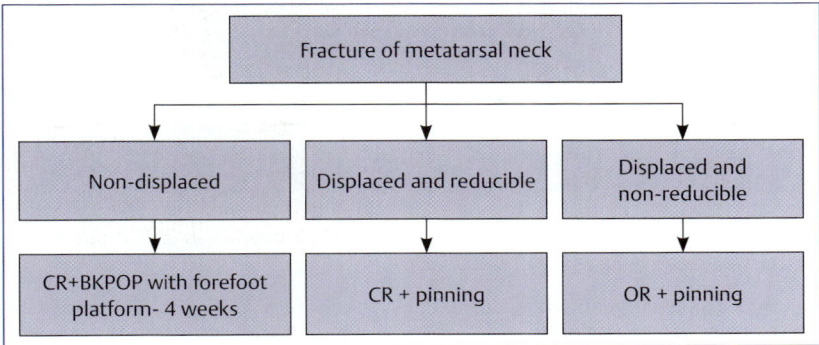

Flowchart 6.22 Management of fracture of neck of metatarsal. BKPOP, below knee plaster; CR, closed reduction; OR, open reduction.

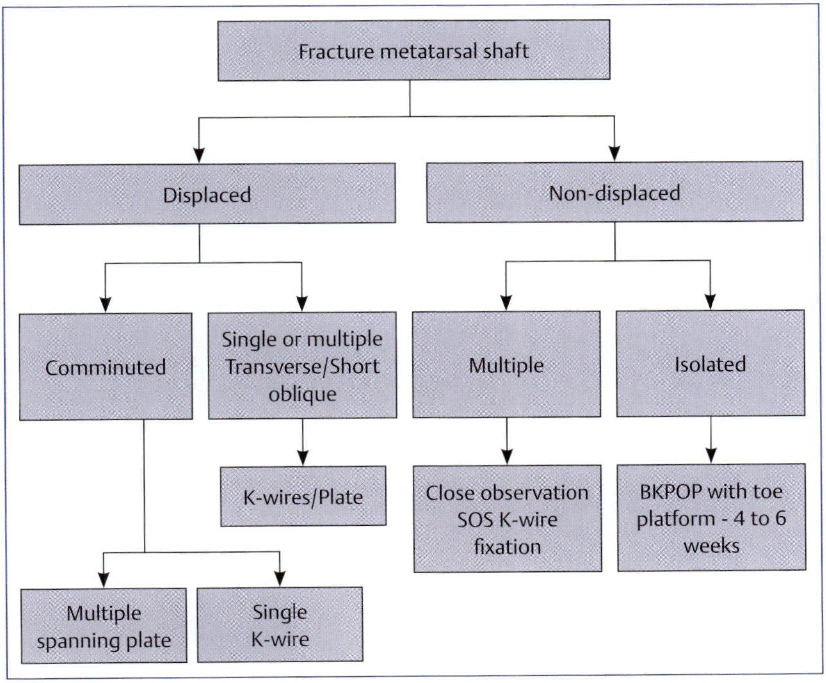

Flowchart 6.23 Management of fracture of shaft of metatarsal. BKPOP, below knee plaster.

Fracture of first metatarsal
Non-displaced, isolated
Non-displaced with comminution or other MT fractures
Displaced, comminuted
CR+BKPOP- 4 to 6 weeks
CR + Pin fixation ± External fixation
Spanning plate/K-wire + External fixation

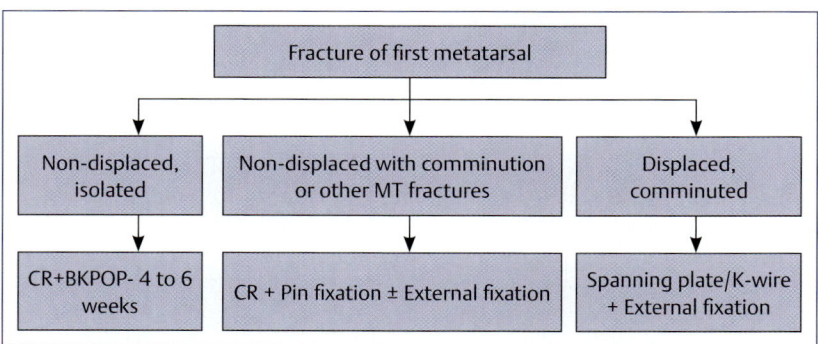

Flowchart 6.24 Management of fracture of base of first metatarsal. BKPOP, below knee plaster; CR, closed reduction; MT, metatarsal.

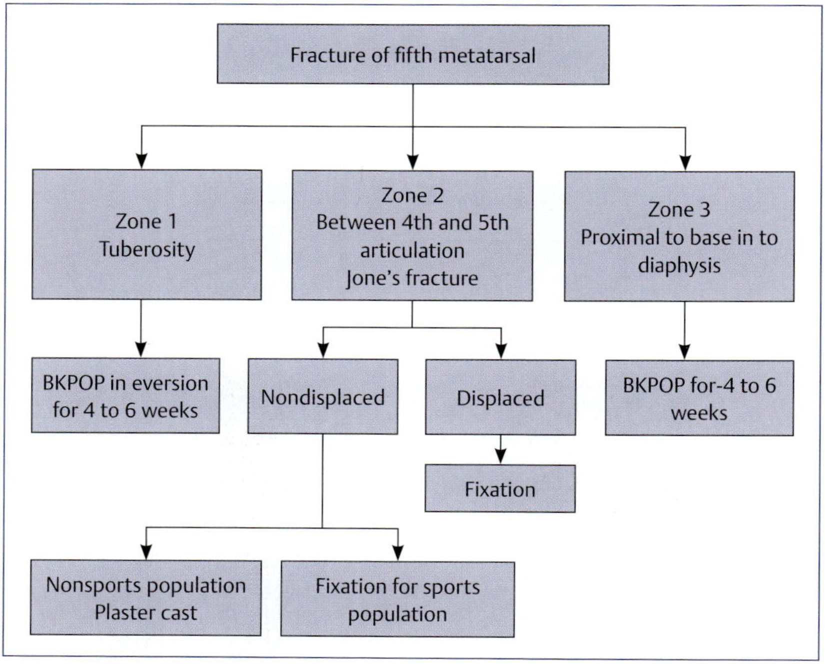

Fracture of fifth metatarsal
Zone 1 Tuberosity
Zone 2 Between 4th and 5th articulation Jone's fracture
Zone 3 Proximal to base in to diaphysis
BKPOP in eversion for 4 to 6 weeks
Nondisplaced
Displaced
BKPOP for-4 to 6 weeks
Fixation
Nonsports population Plaster cast
Fixation for sports population

Flowchart 6.25 Management of fracture of base of fifth metatarsal.

Tips and Tricks

- Tangential view for metatarsal head fractures, sesamoid views for sesamoid injuries, and oblique views for shaft and base fractures are important
- Contralateral limb radiology gives an idea about the metatarsal length

◆ Maintenance of length of the first metatarsal is most important and may need spanning external fixator **(Fig. 6.42)**
◆ Defining Jones fracture and having a suspicious look at its union is mandatory

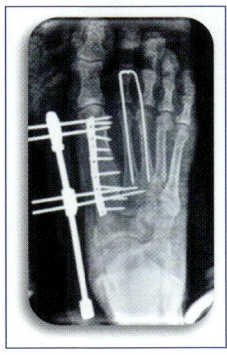

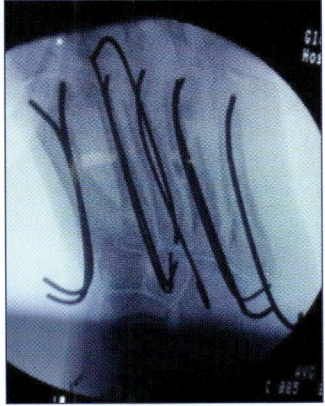

Head fractures

Shaft fractures

Stress fractures

"True Jones" fractures

Tuberosity fractures

Fig. 6.42   X-ray showing first metatarsal fixation stabilized with external fixator.

Fig. 6.43   Fracture base fifth metatarsal zones.

◆ In obese patients and in patients with hind foot varus, Jones fracture is treated with surgery in form of intramedullary screw fixation **(Fig. 6.44)**
◆ Fracture of head, neck, and shaft of metatarsal needs fixation to restore length and to maintain parabolic arch of forefoot **(Fig. 6.45)**

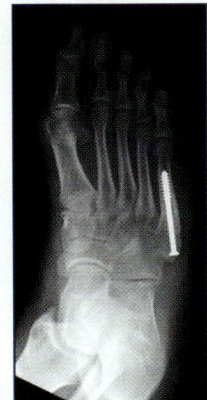

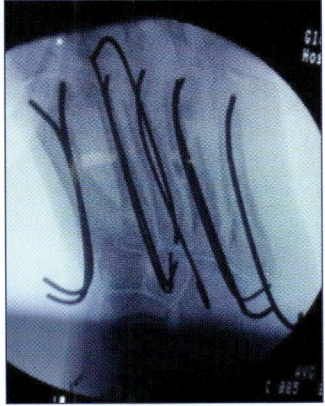

Fig. 6.44   X-ray showing fixation of fifth metatarsal fracture with intramedullary screw.

Fig. 6.45   X-ray showing fixation of multiple metatarsal fractures to maintain length and parabolic arch of forefoot.

♦ Angulated fractures of head and neck of metatarsals need to be corrected to prevent plantar pressure due to malunion **(Fig. 6.46)**

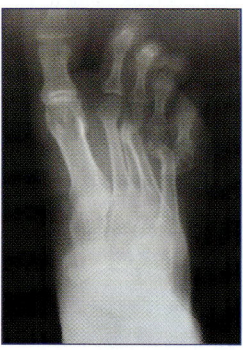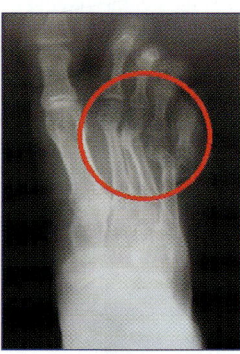

Fig. 6.46   X-ray showing malunion of metatarsal neck.

♦ Spanning and crossing the joints in distal and proximal metatarsal fractures adds stability to fixation and is advisable
♦ Intramedullary K-wires used to stabilize metatarsal should be pushed as far as possible upto subchondral level and are not passed through the joint
♦ Intramedullary K-wires passed to stabilize metatarsal fractures must not violate articular cartilage, and hence tips of these K-wires must be cut flat
♦ Intramedullary K-wires passed to stabilize metatarsal shaft fractures must fan out at the opposite end to get better purchase and better stability **(Fig. 6.47)**
♦ Use of spanning plates to stabilize comminuted metatarsal fractures is the better option **(Fig. 6.48)**

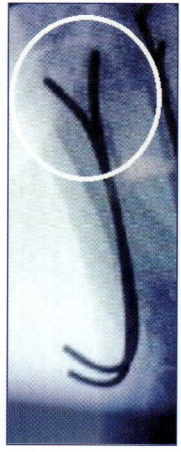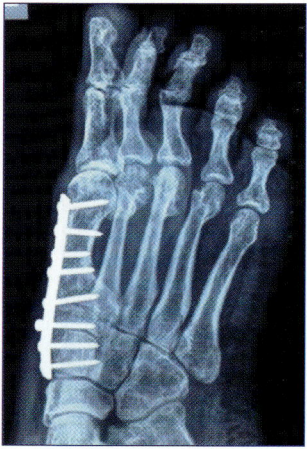

Fig. 6.47   Picture showing preferred position and fanning of intramedullary K-wires for fixation of metatarsals.

Fig. 6.48   X-ray showing use of spanning plate for fixation of unstable and comminuted fracture of base of first metatarsal.

Chapter 7

Foot and Ankle Malunions

Foot and ankle malunions are unique!

Three major differences are seen in foot and ankle malunion in comparison to malunion elsewhere.

1. *Secondary arthritis of adjoining joints is quick and inevitable*:
   Structurally, foot and ankle have multiple small bones having many articulations with each other. Movements are coupled and interlocked. Malposition of one bone thereby would affect many joints located proximally, distally, and sideward, leading to fast and inevitable arthritis of these joints (**Figs. 7.1** and **7.2**).

2. *Pressure effects over surrounding muscles, tendons, fascia, and nerves*:
   Malunion of calcaneus may give pressure effect on plantar fascia, peronei, calcaneofibular ligament, tendon of tendo-Achilles and flexor hallucis longus,

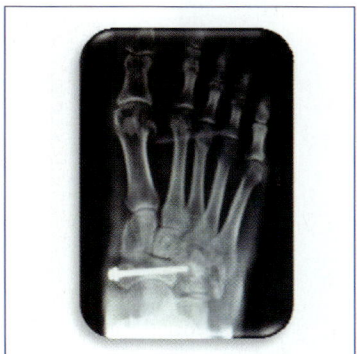

Fig. 7.1 X-ray picture showing malunion of cuboid while navicular fracture was only treated.

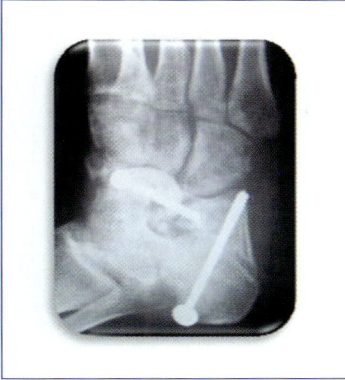

Fig. 7.2 Malunion of navicular leading to arthritis of adjoining joints.

sural and posterior tibial nerves. Lisfranc and midfoot bone malunions can give pressure over dorsal cutaneous nerves and tendon of tibialis anterior and long extensors (**Figs. 7.3** and **7.4**). Forefoot malunion will give pressure effect on plantar skin, leading to formation of corns and callosities (**Fig. 7.5**).

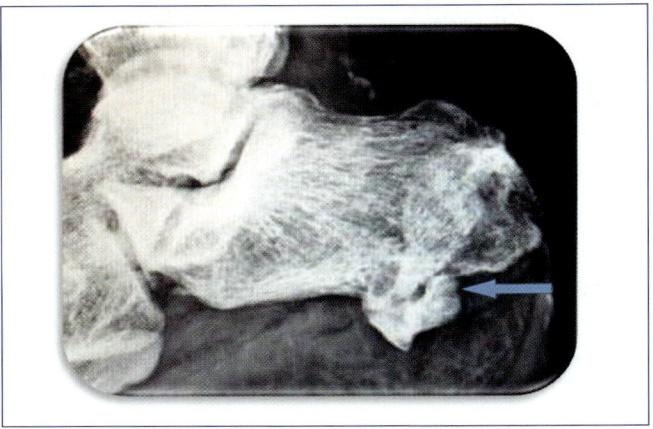

Fig. 7.3   Malunited calcaneal fracture giving plantar pressure and pain.

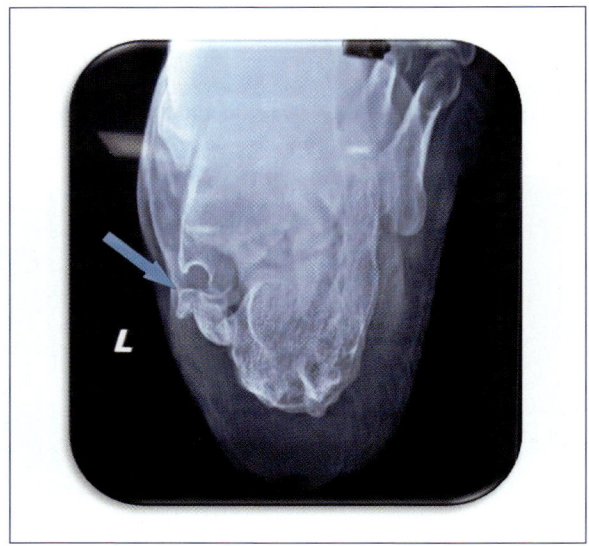

Fig. 7.4   Malunited calcaneus giving pressure medially on flexor hallucis longus tendon and posterior tibial nerve, leading to tendinitis of flexor hallucis longus tendon and secondary tarsal tunnel syndrome.

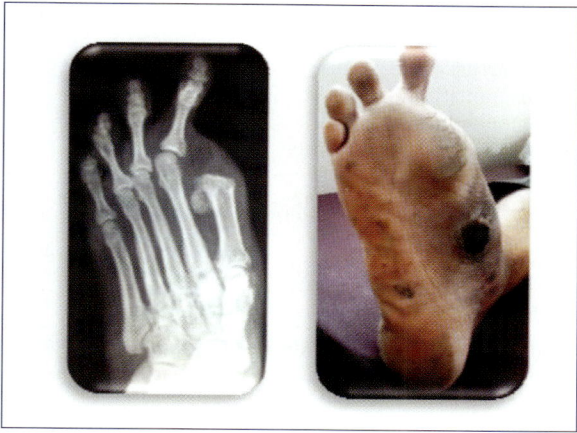

Fig. 7.5   Malunited forefoot and midfoot injury giving rise to plantar pressure effect.

3. *Difficulty in gait and footwear utilization*:
   Increased foot size following malunion poses difficulty in wearing standard footwear. Gait would be altered due to secondary deformities and pain due to the same (**Fig. 7.6**).

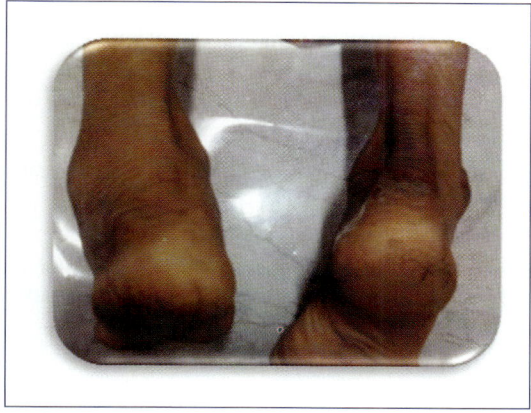

Fig. 7.6   Calcaneus malunion on right side giving rise to broadening and shortening of heel making it difficult for the standard shoe to fit.

Assessment of Delayed Presentation and Malunion

Malunion could be assessed by taking into account the following points:
- Chief complaints and duration of the same
- Treatment taken

- Swelling and deformities
- Shape of foot
- Examination of arches
- Neurological examination
- Assessment of individual muscles
- Assessment of movements of all joints
- Gait examination
- Footwear evaluation
- Foot and ankle series X-rays
- Standing radiography
- Comparative radiographic evaluation
- CT scan and MRI, if needed

Differential injectioning technique to diagnose various pain generators forms the most important part of examination.

Management

Management of malunions varies from that of the original fractures. The points of difference are enumerated in **Box 7.1**.

Box 7.1   How does management differ?

- Revision fixation works well even for malunion of longer duration.
- Oftentimes, fusion has to be preceded by fixation to avoid pressure effects as well as to restore biomechanics. Combinations of both work well.
- Excision of exostosis or bony bumps forms the mainstay of treatment to decompress pressure effects over tendons, muscles, and nerves.
- Replacement arthroplasty has yet to establish its place.
- External fixation is required more often than elsewhere because of poor soft tissue envelope.
- Fusion overplays replacement in comorbid conditions.
- Excision arthroplasty is most commonly used for malunion affecting metatarsophalangeal, proximal interphalangeal, distal interphalangeal, and fourth and fifth tarsometatarsal joints.

Tips and Tricks

- Two basic sets of procedures are adopted: joint salvage and joint sacrificing (**Flowcharts 7.1–7.3**).
- For young active patients with good bone stock, joint salvage procedures are reserved.
- For old sedentary patients with comorbid conditions and poor bone stock, joint sacrificing procedures are undertaken.
- Joint salvage procedures are correction with revision fixation provided arthritis has not set in.

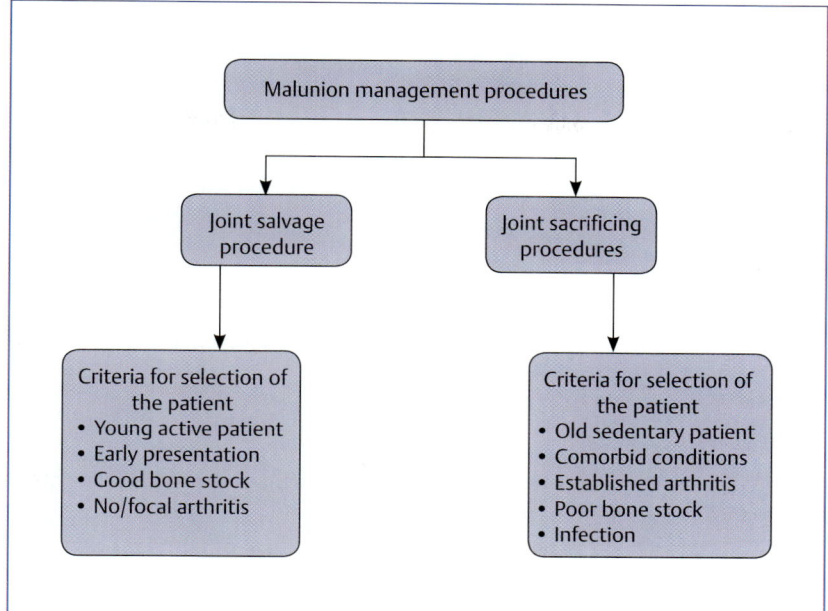

Flowchart 7.1   Management procedures for malunion.

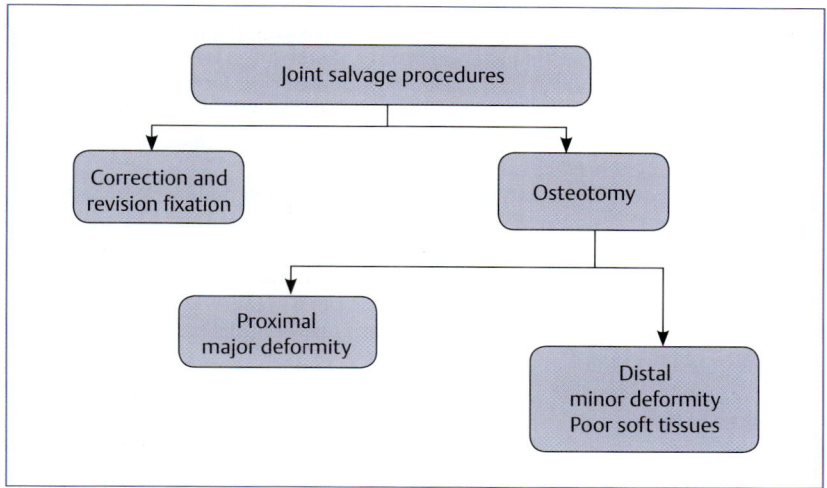

Flowchart 7.2   Treatment plan of joint salvage procedures.

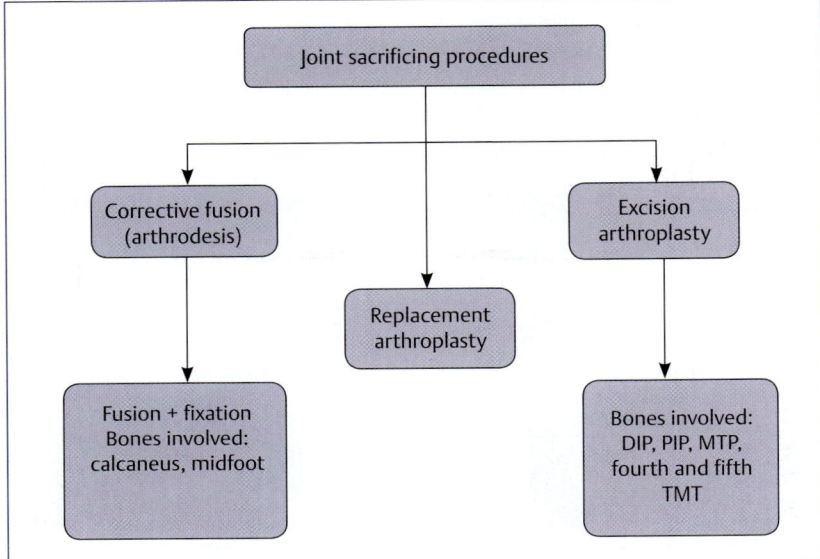

Flowchart 7.3   Treatment plan of joint sacrificing procedures. DIP, distal interphalangeal joints; PIP, proximal interphalangeal joints; MTP, metatarsophalangeal joints; TMT, tarsometatarsal joints.

◆ With focal or no arthritis in the presence of a deformity, osteotomy to correct the deformity is done. For a smaller deformity, distal corrective osteotomy would work, while proximal corrective osteotomy is preferred for better correction of axis in a case with major deformity.

◆ Arthrodesis, excision arthroplasty, and replacement arthroplasty are options for joint sacrificing procedures.

◆ Arthrodesis with fixation is carried out in calcaneal and midfoot malunions.

◆ Arthrodesis is the most preferred method, except for fourth and fifth tarsometatarsal joints, distal and proximal interphalangeal joints, and lesser metatarsophalangeal joints where excision arthroplasty is preferred.

◆ Arthroplasty is in consideration for ankle joint in patients with minimal deformity and good bone stock with good vascularity without the presence of any neuropathy or infection.

Decision Making

Decision making depends on various factors as shown in **Fig. 7.7**.

◆ *Duration of malunion*: Longer the duration, the more difficult is to do revision fixation through the original fracture site. Also, there are more chances of setting of arthritis in the adjoining joints making revision fixation more difficult.

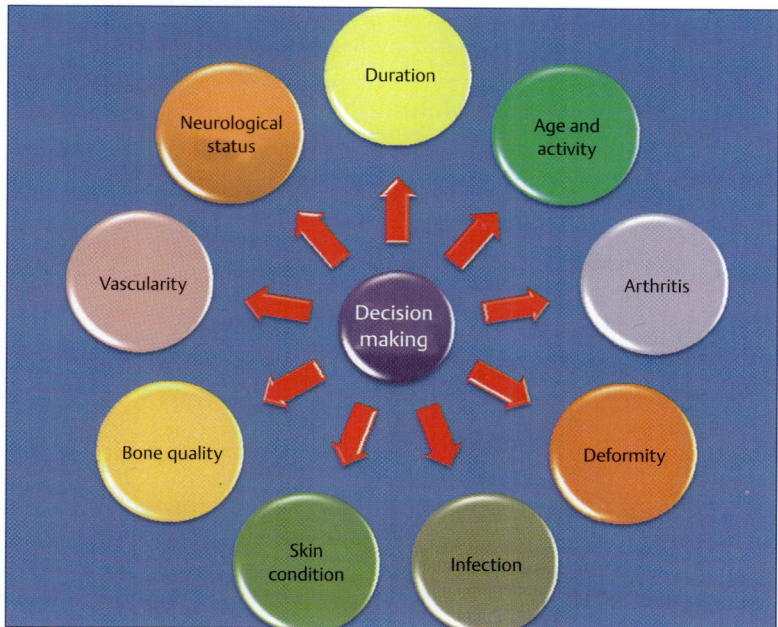

Fig. 7.7   Factors leading to the selection of management procedures for malunion.

♦ *Age and activity level of patient*: Arthrodesis may be reserved for old sedentary patients with comorbid conditions as a single-stage gold standard procedure. Heavy laborers may as well be treated with arthrodesis. Corrective revision fixation would be a procedure of choice in most others.

♦ *Presence of arthritis*: Arthritis warrants fusion over fixation. Cases with focal arthritis may be treated with corrective osteotomy in major joints like ankle.

♦ *Presence of deformity*: Deformity must be minimal for replacement surgery to be carried out and it must be corrected before final surgery. At arthrodesis also *in situ* fusion is avoided. Corrective osteotomy must precede removal of articular cartilage.

♦ *Presence of infection*: Infected cases are best fused than revised. Cases with active infection would favor use of external fixation devices for fusion.

♦ *Vascular status of the limb*: Evaluation of the vascular status of the limb plays most important role in decision making. With poor vascularity, healing is doubtful. Amputation may be a choice in such vascularity-deficient limbs.

♦ *Neurological status of the limb*: Neuropathy would dictate longer, stronger, and combination of implants for arthrodesis where adjoining joints are also spanned to get better stability. Failure rates are high.

♦ *Condition of skin at operative site*: Skin condition or scarring would force a surgeon to modify surgical approach and use of implants.

♦ *Quality of bone*: Osteoporotic situations demand stronger combination fixations, which spans bones to get better stability. Augmentation procedures are needed.

Management of Specific Malunions

Various specific malunions are listed in **Box 7.2**. Tips and tricks for the management of these specific malunions are explained as follows.

Box 7.2	Specific malunions

♦ Pilon malunion
♦ Ankle malunion
♦ Calcaneal malunion
♦ Talar malunion
♦ Midfoot malunion
♦ Forefoot malunion

Pilon Malunion

♦ Supramalleolar corrective osteotomies are good options for malalignment without arthritis (**Fig. 7.8**).
♦ Cases with significant articular cartilage damage need ankle fusion (**Fig. 7.9**).
♦ Open-wedge osteotomy gains length but needs bone grafting and it heals slowly, while closed-wedge osteotomy heals faster but it leads to shortening.

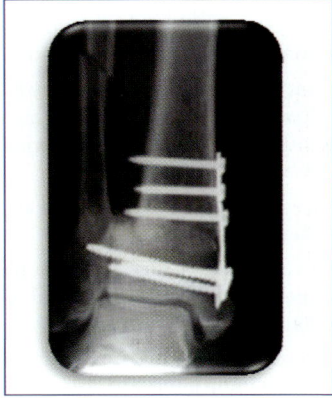

Fig. 7.8 X-ray showing correction of pilon malunion with supramalleolar osteotomy.

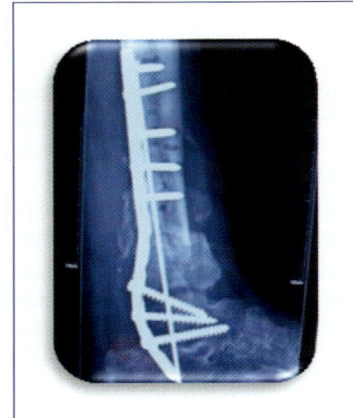

Fig. 7.9 X-ray showing ankle fusion post pilon malunion.

♦ Fibular osteotomy is always needed. Fibula is shortened for open wedge osteotomy and is cut either proximally or at the level of tibia for closed-wedge osteotomy.

Ankle Malunion

♦ There is no limit to revise fixation in ankle malunion provided arthritis has not set in.
♦ Ankle malunions with varus need to be revised, while those with mild valgus may be well tolerated by patients.
♦ Sagittal plane malunions are notorious and need immediate attention. Coronal plane malunions and medial malleolar malunions may not be revised.
♦ Revision fixation may warrant other procedures such as ankle arthroscopy and ligament balancing.
♦ Fibular shortening and rotational malunions are least tolerated and need to be revised and so are the posterior malleolar malunions that need early revisions.
♦ Syndesmotic malunions are revised.
♦ Procedure of revision is by fibular osteotomy, fibular lengthening, syndesmotic and fibular fixation, and bone grafting (**Figs. 7.10** and **7.11**).

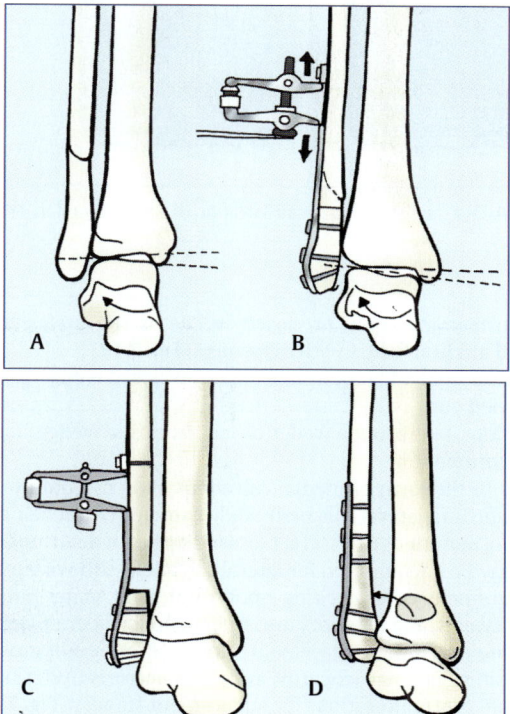

Fig. 7.10   (A-D) Schematic diagram of revision of fibular malunion in ankle fracture.

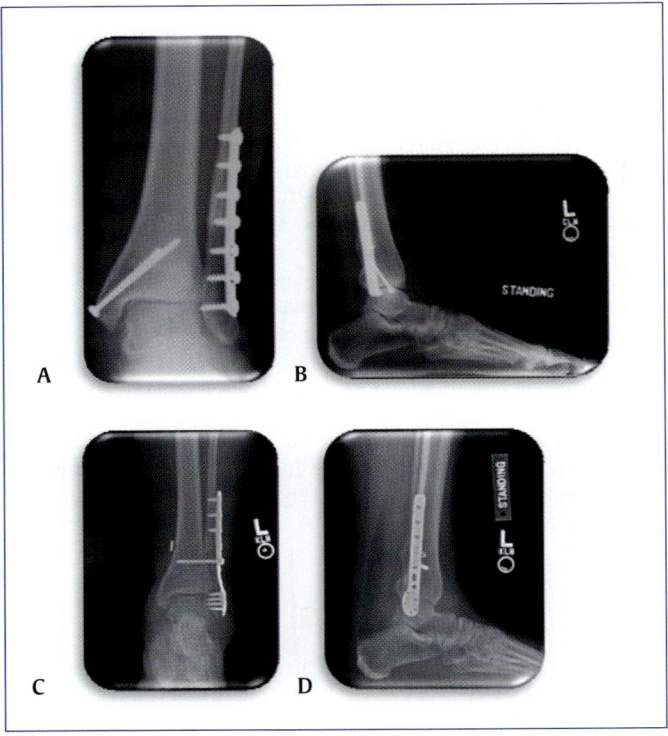

A

B

C

D

Fig. 7.11 **(A-D)** X-rays showing revised fixation of ankle malunion 3 months postsurgery.

♦ Supramalleolar osteotomy, open or closed wedge, is the preferred correction modality for focal ankle arthritis with deformity (**Fig. 7.12**).

♦ For varus malunions, medial open wedge or lateral closed wedge supramalleolar osteotomy is carried out.

♦ For valgus malunions, lateral open wedge or medial closed wedge supramalleolar osteotomy is performed.

♦ Distal osteotomy in the form of medial calcaneus slide osteotomy can be used for valgus malunion and lateral calcaneus slide osteotomy can be used for varus malunion. These osteotomies can correct lesser degrees of deformities and issues of skin closure may be encountered for lateral calcaneus slide osteotomy.

♦ Total ankle replacement is an exciting option but with many limitations. The implant availability, cost, and longevity are issues to be considered. Deformity must be corrected before executing replacement surgery. Presence of gross deformity, infection, neuropathy, vascular jeopardy, avascular necrosis (AVN), and poor soft tissues are absolute contraindications for replacement surgery (**Fig. 7.13**).

♦ Arthrodesis is the gold standard procedure for ankle malunions. Position of fusion is 0 to 5 degrees of valgus and 0 degree of dorsiflexion (**Fig. 7.14**).

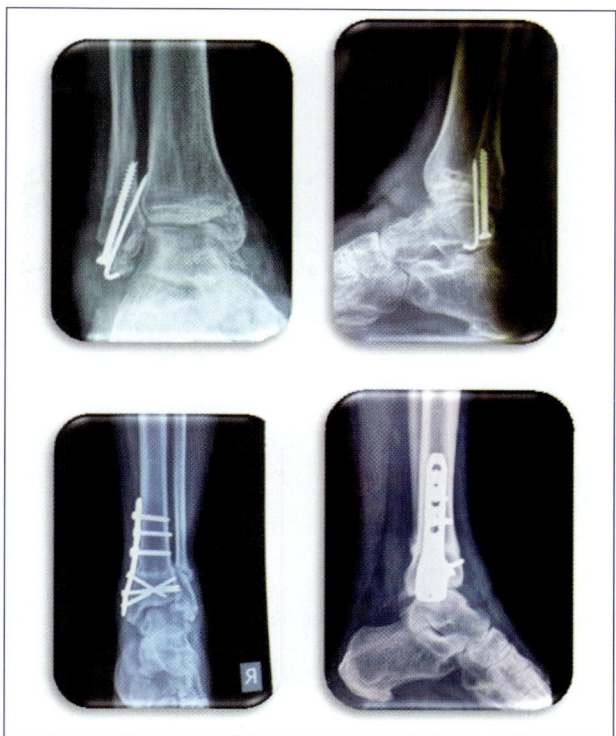

Fig. 7.12 Preoperative and postoperative X-rays of operated case of supramalleolar osteotomy in case of focal ankle malunion.

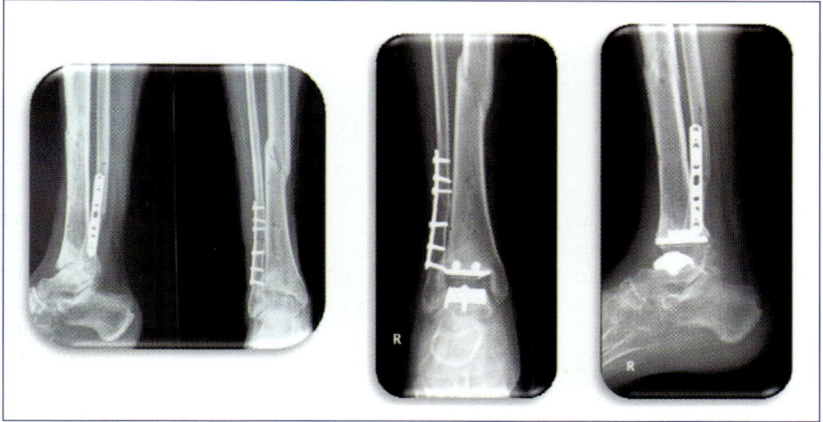

Fig. 7.13 X-rays showing total ankle replacement done in a case of ankle malunion.

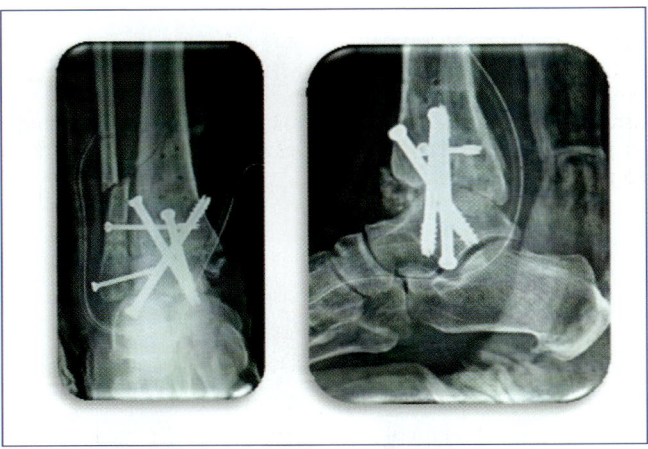

Fig. 7.14 X-rays showing ankle arthrodesis with screws through transfibular approach.

Calcaneal Malunion

Calcaneal malunion needs to be approached like a case of back pain where one tries to find out every pain generator!

Treatment is then directed to every pain generator for best outcome!

♦ Early malunion without subtalar arthritis but with heel deformation can be treated with joint-preserving osteotomy (**Fig. 7.15**).

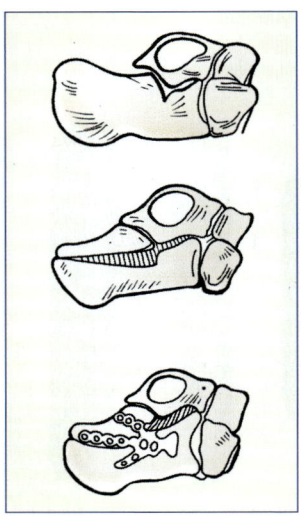

Fig. 7.15 Schematic representation of joint preserving osteotomy for calcaneal malunion.

- Many malunited bony exostoses in calcaneal malunion generate pressure effects over surrounding tendons, ligaments, muscles, and nerves. These exostosis need to be excised to relieve pressure effects.
- Such pressure effects medially could be on the tendon of flexor hallucis longus and posterior tibial nerve, laterally over calcaneofibular ligament and tendon of peronei, posteriorly over the tendo-Achilles and plantarward toward the heel fat pad and plantar fascia (**Figs. 7.16–7.18**).

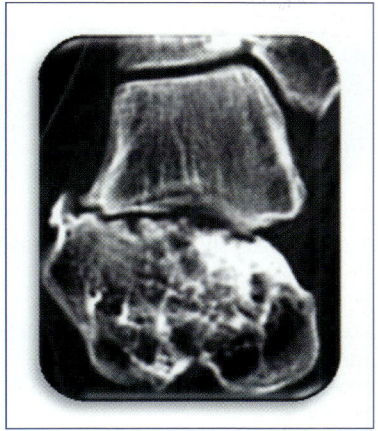

Fig. 7.16 Axial CT scan of calcaneus malunion showing lateral exostosis and pressure effect over tendon of peronei and calcaneofibular ligament.

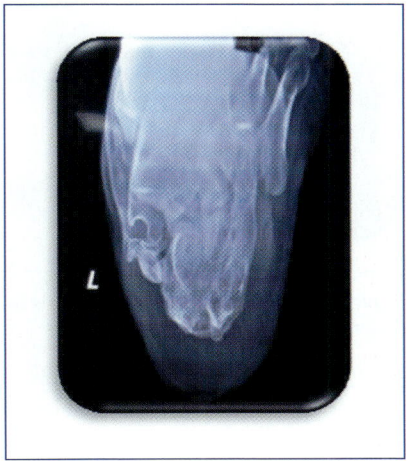

Fig. 7.17 X-ray of calcaneus malunion showing medial exostosis and pressure effect over posterior tibial nerve and tendon of flexor hallucis longus.

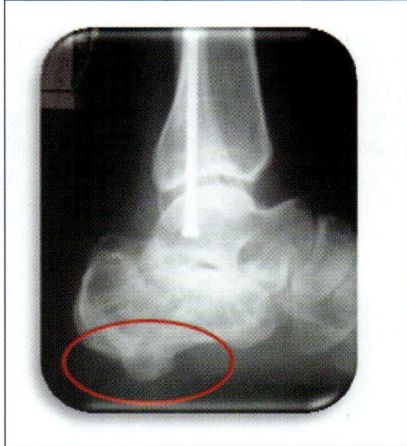

Fig. 7.18   X-ray of calcaneus malunion showing plantar exostosis and pressure effect over heel fat pad.

♦ For bony protrusions, simple excision of protrusions will help in decompressing tendon, nerve, or ligament impingement (**Fig. 7.19**).
♦ Early malunions without subtalar arthritis are treated with only exostectomy and peroneal tendon tenolysis.

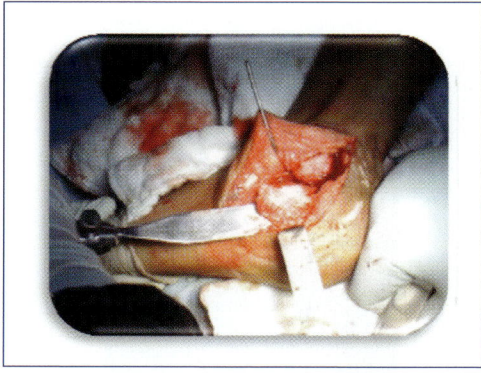

Fig. 7.19   Intraoperative picture of excision of lateral exostosis to decompress peroneal tendons and calcaneo-fibular ligament.

♦ Cases with subtalar arthritis are treated with subtalar fusion done in 0 to 5 degrees of valgus (**Figs. 7.20** and **7.21**).
♦ Those cases where over and above subtalar arthritis, heel is in varus or valgus, then corrective Dwyer osteotomy and medial calcaneal slide osteotomy are added, respectively, in addition to subtalar arthrodesis.

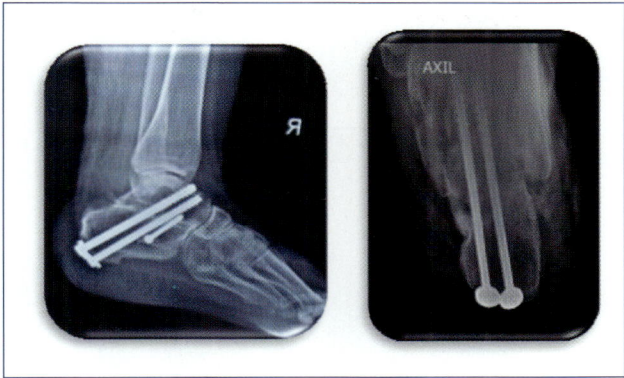

Fig. 7.20   Postoperative X-rays of subtalar fusion after malunited calcaneus fracture.

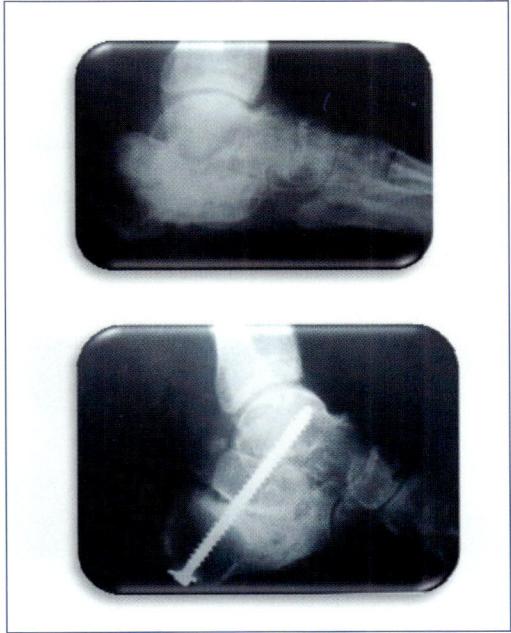

Fig. 7.21   Preoperative and postoperative X-rays of distraction subtalar fusion after malunited calcaneus fracture.

♦ Sural nerve decompression and correction of cavus, planus, and claw toe deformities may also be needed (**Fig. 7.22**).

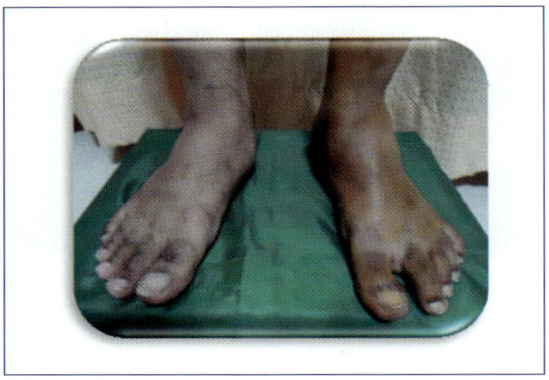

Fig. 7.22   Clinical picture of a patient with bilateral calcaneus malunion having claw toe deformities on the left side.

Talar Malunion

♦ Malunited dorsal fragment may block ankle dorsiflexion and just needs excision (**Fig. 7.23**).
♦ Talar head malunion with arthritis is best treated with fusion of talonavicular joint (**Fig. 7.24**).

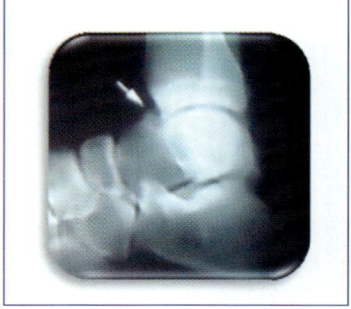

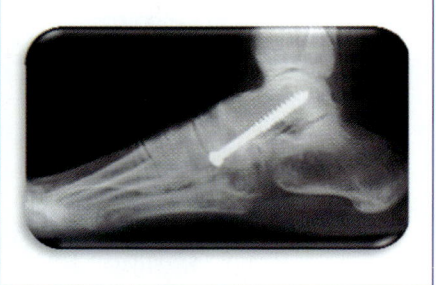

Fig. 7.23 Dorsal osteophyte after malunited talus fracture.

Fig. 7.24 X-ray showing malunion of talus head treated with talonavicular fusion.

♦ Peripheral process malunion need simple excision, except in cases where arthritis has set in, then arthrodesis is added (**Fig. 7.25**).
♦ Neck malunions are mostly in varus and cases without much arthritis can be corrected with corrective osteotomy, bone grafting, and fixation (**Figs. 7.26–7.28**).

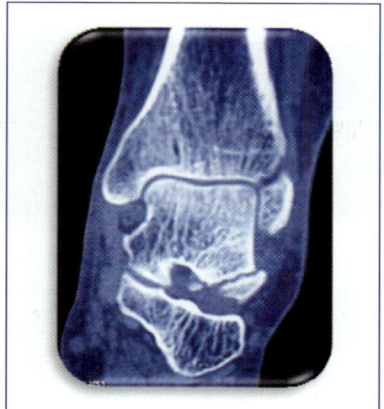

Fig. 7.25 CT scan showing malunited fracture of lateral talar process with arthritis of the subtalar joint where subtalar fusion was done.

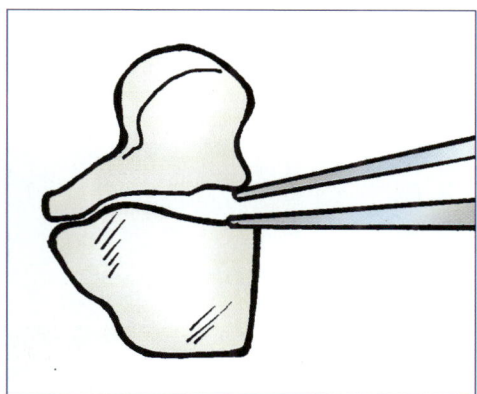

Fig. 7.26 Schematic representation of corrective osteotomy at the neck of talus.

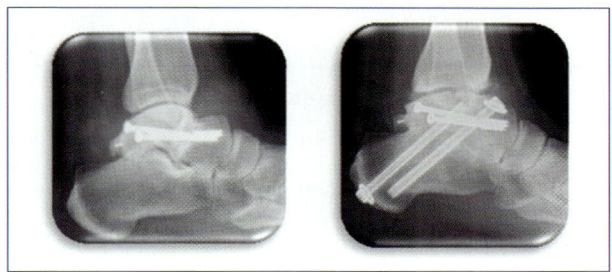

Fig. 7.27 Preoperative and postoperative X-rays of talus malunion treated with subtalar fusion.

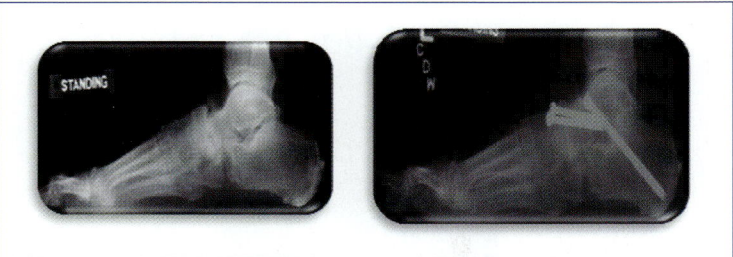

Fig. 7.28   Preoperative and postoperative X-rays showing corrective osteotomy and fusion for talar malunion.

◆ Late cases of varus neck malunion may need corrective arthrodesis.
◆ Avoid fusion of ankle joint as far as possible for talar malunion.
◆ Body malunion may need both ankle and subtalar fusion.
◆ Late presentations with arthritis in other joints may warrant triple arthrodesis (**Fig. 7.29**).

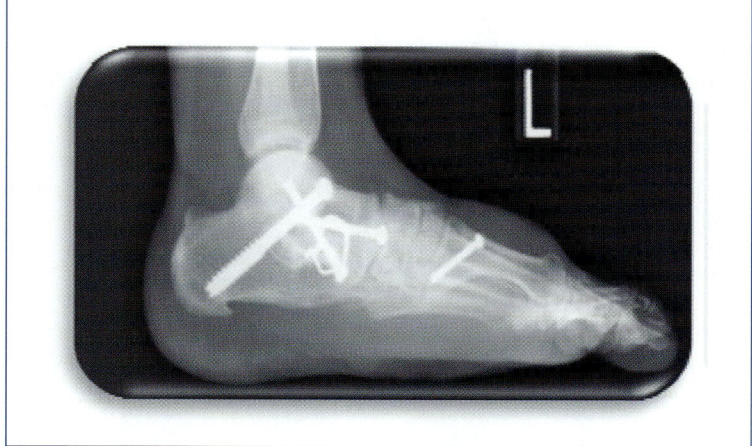

Fig. 7.29   X-ray showing triple fusion after talar malunion.

◆ Options such as ankle replacement and subtalar fusion can also be considered in young patients.
◆ For nonviable talar body, calcaneotibial arthrodesis is done (**Fig. 7.30**).

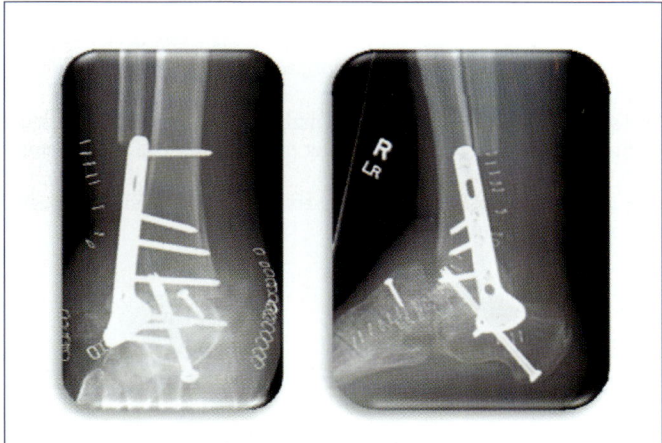

Fig. 7.30   Calcaneotibial arthrodesis.

Midfoot Malunion

♦ Conservative measures shall be tried as first line of care. Let patient earn surgery from surgeon.
♦ Corrective osteotomy or revision fixation has a lesser role to play in midfoot malunion because of small bones with multiple articulations with each other.
♦ Fusion is the gold standard but is always done with correction of deformities like adduction, abduction, plantar flexion, or dorsiflexion.
♦ The fourth and fifth tarsometatarsal joints are not good with fusion, and interposition arthroplasty is preferred.
♦ Appropriate wedges are removed for corrective fusion.
♦ Adjoining procedures such as plantar fascia and tendo-Achilles release may be required.

Forefoot Malunion

♦ First metatarsal malunion is least tolerated and acceptable. Early presentation needs correction and achieving the length with a distractor is advisable.
♦ Late presentations can be treated with lengthening osteotomy such as scarf osteotomy.
♦ Those cases where symptomatic arthritis has set in proximal or distal joints of first metatarsal, arthrodesis is inevitable.
♦ Malunion in lesser metatarsals is well tolerated as other metatarsals act as a splint.
♦ Shortening in lesser metatarsals can be corrected with Weil osteotomy.
♦ Head and neck malunion with plantar angulation may lead to pressure effects. Plantar angulation of metatarsal head can be corrected by distal oblique metatarsal osteotomy or with plantar condylectomy.

- Late cases shall be treated with excision arthroplasty maintaining parabolic arch of foot.
- Phalangeal malunion are usually nonsymptomatic and, if so, do not need any specific treatment.
- If they are symptomatic, then phalangeal malunion can be treated with orthotics.
- First proximal phalangeal malunion giving plantar pressure and keratosis needs correction with corrective osteotomy.
- Adjoining joint symptomatic arthritis is treated with excision arthroplasty or fusion in functional position.

Chapter

8

Deformity Correction: Foot and Ankle

*Planning, persistence and passion are three pillars
of foot and ankle deformity correction!*

This chapter describes the following commonly seen foot and ankle deformities in adult population.

- ◆ Sagittal plane deformities
  - Equinus
  - Dorsiflexion contracture
- ◆ Coronal plane deformities
  - Ankle varus
  - Ankle valgus
- ◆ Cavus

Evaluation of Foot and Ankle Deformity

The criteria for evaluation of foot and ankle deformities are listed below.

- ◆ Age and occupation
- ◆ Activity level
- ◆ Duration
- ◆ Causes: Posttraumatic, congenital, acquired and degenerative
- ◆ Comorbid conditions
- ◆ Joints above: Knee, hip, and spine
- ◆ Joints proximal
- ◆ Joints distal
- ◆ Neurological status of the limb
- ◆ Vascular status of the limb
- ◆ Pressure points

- Arches of the foot
- Skin and scars
- Presence of implants
- Presence of infection
- Soft tissue contractures: Tendo Achilles contracture is the most common
- Bone quality

Principles of Deformity Correction

- The aim is to achieve a plantigrade foot
- Correction proceeds from proximal to distal
- Soft tissue releases must precede bony correction
- Bony corrective procedures must precede tendon transfer
- Removal of bone for deformity correction must precede removal of articular cartilage at corrective arthrodesis
- In all indicated cases, supportive braces and orthotics must be planned and explained to a patient well in advance

Equinus Deformity

Management of equinus varies as regards the shape of talus, which is illustrated in **Flowchart 8.1**.

Tips and Tricks

The following points are needed to be considered for managing the equinus deformity:

- By flexing the knee, if the equinus is correctible either completely or partially, it signifies that the gastro-soleus is tight as it relaxes on knee flexion. If the deformity corrects completely on knee flexion, it is possible that a percutaneous tendo Achilles release may completely correct the deformity.
- White slide technique for percutaneous tendo Achilles release: Distal medial, middle lateral, and proximal medial incisions at the interval of few inches between them are made. The distal-most incision is taken a few inches above the tendo Achilles insertion. This is followed by forced ankle stretching in dorsiflexion and casting is put for 3 to 6 weeks.
- Take care not to damage the saphenous vein and sural nerve during this procedure.
- The incisions need to be modified as per the association of heel varus or valgus together with equinus, where, respectively, two medial, and one lateral incisions for heel varus and two lateral and one medial incisions for heel valgus are used.
- First choice is always to release posterior soft tissues.
- On lateral X-ray, presence of a round dome talus suggests that correction of equinus deformity is possible within ankle alone.
- If upon knee flexion the deformity is partially correctible, it may mean that not only is the tendo Achilles contracted, but also are some of the posterior soft tissues around the ankle. This needs *posterolateral soft tissue release.*
- *Important structures that need release are on the posterolateral aspect rather than on the posteromedial aspect.*

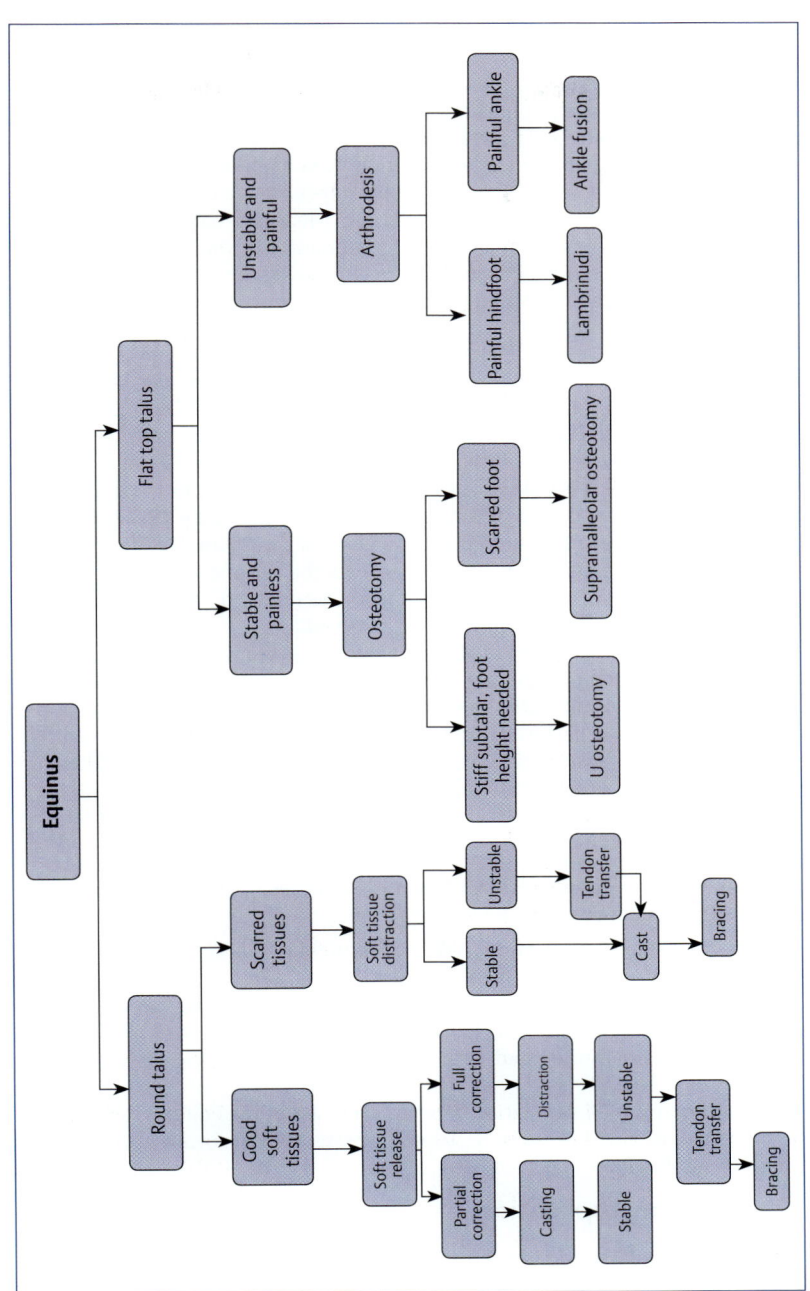

Flowchart 8.1 Management algorithm of equinus.

Posterolateral Release

A small curvilinear incision is made starting proximally and medially, crossing over the tendo Achilles, which ends with a gentle curve posterolaterally below the lateral malleolus. The paratenon of the tendo Achilles is neatly and carefully incised to prevent damage. A vertical split is made in the substance of the tendo Achilles. At its distal end the medial edge is cut, and at its proximal end the lateral edge is cut. Dorsiflexing the ankle will give some correction. Now the retractors are placed on the inner edges of the cut tendo Achilles and the edges are separated to gain deeper entry. The deep fascia is cut and the fat juts out. The flexor hallucis longus (FHL) tendon and muscle belly are retracted from the lateral side by the scalpel handle and retracted medially. The tendon of the FHL is key to saving the neurovascular structures at the posterior end of the ankle. It is visualized and retracted medially, taking the artery and nerve along with it.

This gives access to the entire posterior aspect of the ankle. The ankle capsule is released with a knife. In large deformities, the subtalar capsule may also be released. The lateral malleolus is palpated, and the knife is slid gently from distal to proximal in a gently curving arc to release the posterior syndesmotic ligament. As the anterior aspect of the talus is broader than the posterior one, sliding into the ankle mortise would not be possible unless the syndesmotic ligament is released, allowing the fibula to spring apart and allow the broader anterior part to extend into the tibio-talar joint.

The knife is now kept adjacent to the calcaneus and slid down laterally, releasing the calcaneofibular ligament. This ligament tethers the calcaneal tuberosity proximally and does not allow it to migrate distally unless released. This completes the soft tissue release and full correction may be achieved.

If correction is not fully achieved, it may indicate that tendons of the tibialis posterior and flexor digitorum longus are tight. After retracting the neurovascular bundle laterally, they are visible under the deep fascia through the proximal part of the wound. Z lengthening is performed of both the tendons and they are sutured. We preserve its paratenon by not going either medial or lateral to the tendo Achilles and ensure that there is no skin necrosis and wound dehiscence.

Soft Tissue Distraction

With a rounded talus but posterior soft tissues that may not be healthy or pliable, we can achieve correction with soft tissue distraction.

◆ The Ilizarov fixator is an ideal tool and has comprehensive capabilities under all clinical circumstances to achieve full correction
◆ A limited soft tissue release should be performed posterolaterally to achieve some correction before applying Ilizarov apparatus
◆ The Ilizarov fixator is mounted with two rings on the tibia, with two half pins and wires
◆ Configuration for the foot fixation depends on whether the equinus deformity is accompanied by cavus or varus or valgus or presence of deformity between the hindfoot and forefoot

Ilizarov Fixator Application

If there is no deformity within the foot, a horseshoe-shaped ring is used for foot fixation. A half pin is inserted in the calcaneum from the tuberosity from posterior to the anterior. One or two olive wires are inserted in the calcaneum from the postero-medial aspect from behind the neurovascular structures to exit laterally and distally. This may be sufficient fixation for the hindfoot. In more rigid deformities, additional wire is inserted from the anteromedial direction to engage in the sustentaculum, just underneath the tendons but dorsal to the neurovascular structures to exit posterolaterally. These two wires subtend a right angle to each other and hence offer very strong fixation.

At least two more wires are inserted in the mid- and forefoot. An olive wire from lateral aspect is inserted through the cuneiforms to exit medially. Just proximal to the MTP joints, an olive wire is inserted from medial side into the first metatarsal, passing underneath the second and the third and exiting laterally through the substance of the fourth and fifth metatarsals.

A wire is also inserted in the head–neck junction of the talus and an olive wire is inserted from the lateral side. This offers control over the talus. After tensioning, the foot frame becomes rigid.

Soft Tissue Distraction

Soft tissue distraction at the ankle may be performed using two principles:
1) Constrained correction
2) Unconstrained correction
Principle of correction of equinus by distraction is shown in **Fig. 8.1A** to **E.**

Constrained Correction

We may constrain the correction to occur around hinges placed in the apparatus. The center of rotation of the ankle is located around the lateral process of the talus. If we can locate the medial and lateral hinges to overlap accurately at this level, we can place the posterior distraction motor rods posteriorly anywhere conveniently. The rate of distraction is calculated depending on the distance between the posterior rods and hinge locations. The anterior rods do not perform compression. They are kept in "passive" mode; however, they are loosened just prior to posterior distraction and then locked in any new (slightly changed) position.

The distraction process is monitored with anteroposterior (AP) and lateral (LAT) X-rays to ensure that the tibio-talar joint remains congruent, that it is not overdistracted, and that cartilage is not crushed at the joint level.

Once correction is achieved, we aim to achieve overcorrection by a few degrees into dorsiflexion. The apparatus is maintained for a few more weeks in this mode. Extensions are made to the apparatus to enable the patient to walk with almost full weight bearing. After the apparatus is removed, a walking cast is applied for a few weeks and a brace is made to be worn at night to ensure there is no recurrence of deformity.

Equinus deformity in a patient who is treated with constrained correction is serially depicted in **Fig. 8.2A** to **G.**

Principles of correction of equinus by subluxation are shown in **Fig. 8.3A** to **D.**

Equinus deformity in a patient who is treated with equinocavus distraction is serially depicted in **Fig. 8.4A** to **K.**

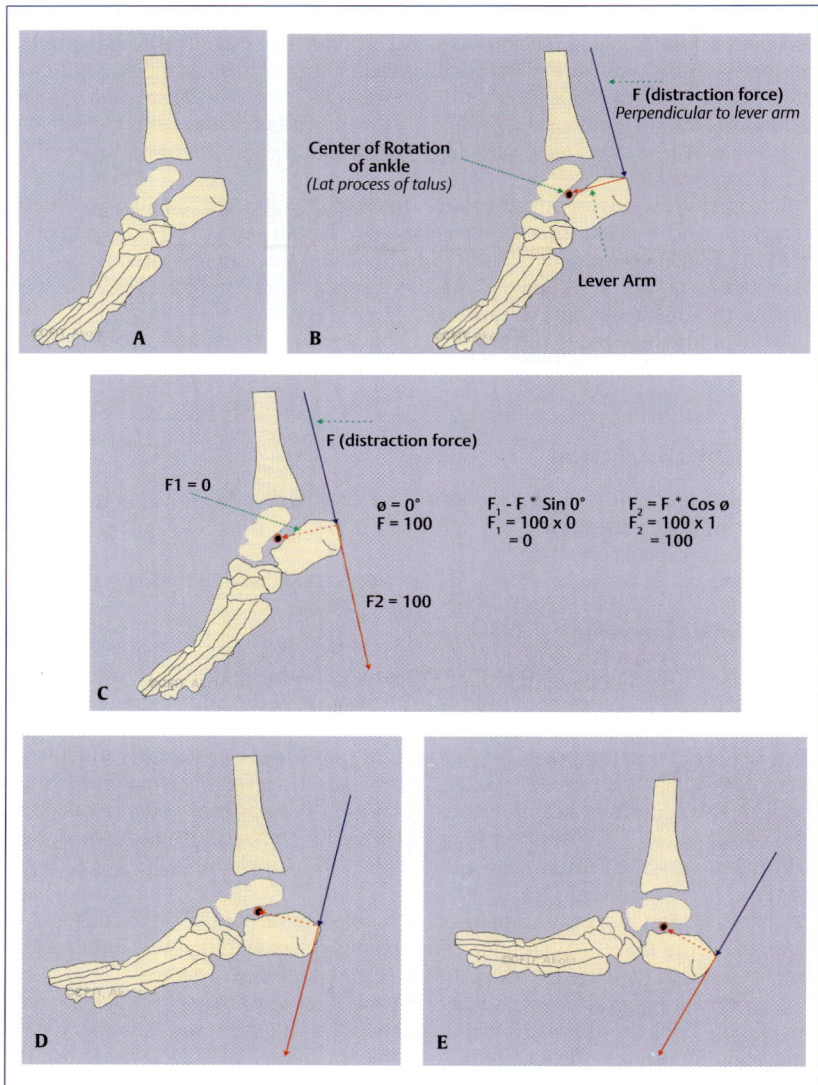

Fig. 8.1A to E Shows when the distraction motor is kept perpendicular to the lever arm at all times, there is no anterior force F1 component. Rotation occurs perfectly at the center of rotation of ankle and the ankle joint is preserved and accurately corrected.

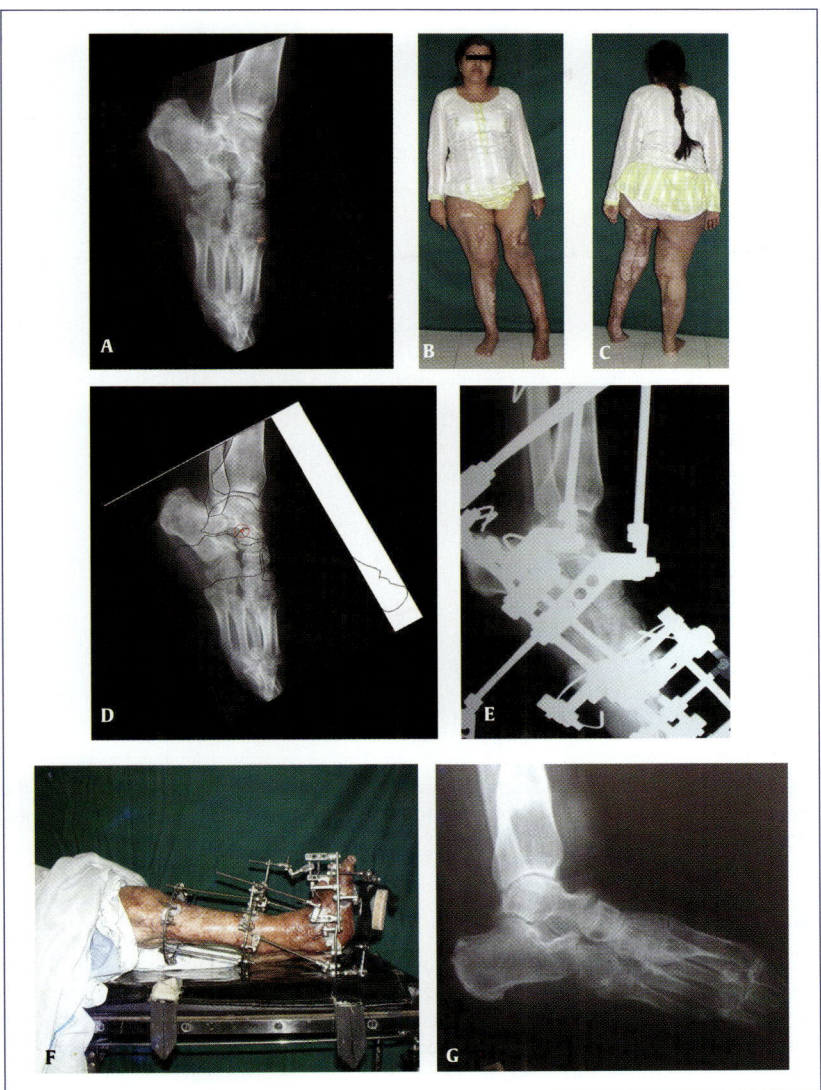

Figs. 8.2A to G   Postburns contracture with severe equinus and poor skin in a 45-year-old female. Simulation on a paper trace-out of the correction done with center of rotation located at the lateral process of talus, which results in correction without subluxing or damaging the ankle joint. Tibial block of fixation attached to the foot block with hinges accurately located at the center of rotation of ankle. Posterior motor for distraction angled such as to remain perpendicular to the lever arm of ankle. Correction seen in apparatus and postoperative X-ray showing full correction without subluxation of ankle, overdistraction or crushing of ankle articular cartilage.

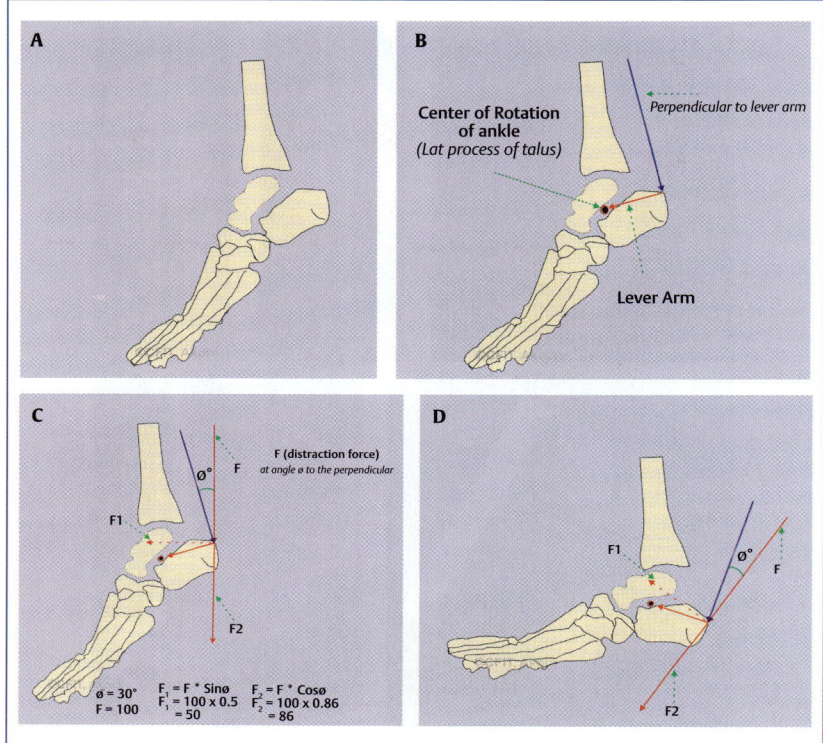

Fig. 8.3A to D When the distraction motor is at an angle ø° to the perpendicular to the lever (blue line) arm there is an anterior force F1 component, which pushes the talus anteriorly, subluxating the ankle.

Unconstrained Correction

In more complex corrections when equinus is accompanied by varus as in an uncorrected clubfoot, the better option is to perform unconstrained correction. Here there are no hinges that determine the exact center around which we are to rotate. The determinants of correction are the anatomical shape of the articular surfaces and the direction of the motor forces we apply.

In this method, the fixation of the tibia is the same as in above. The foot is fixed separately by two half rings, one for the hindfoot and the other for the forefoot. The hindfoot ring can have one half pin and two olive wires. The half ring can be extended by using a long connection plate, commonly placed laterally. This half ring remains horizontal and parallel to the floor. The forefoot half ring is perpendicular to the forefoot and is fixed with two wires. One is an olive wire inserted from medial side, which passes through the first and fifth metatarsals, while the second wire is inserted slightly proximal to the first and engages only the first and second metatarsals. The angle between the two is only 20°.

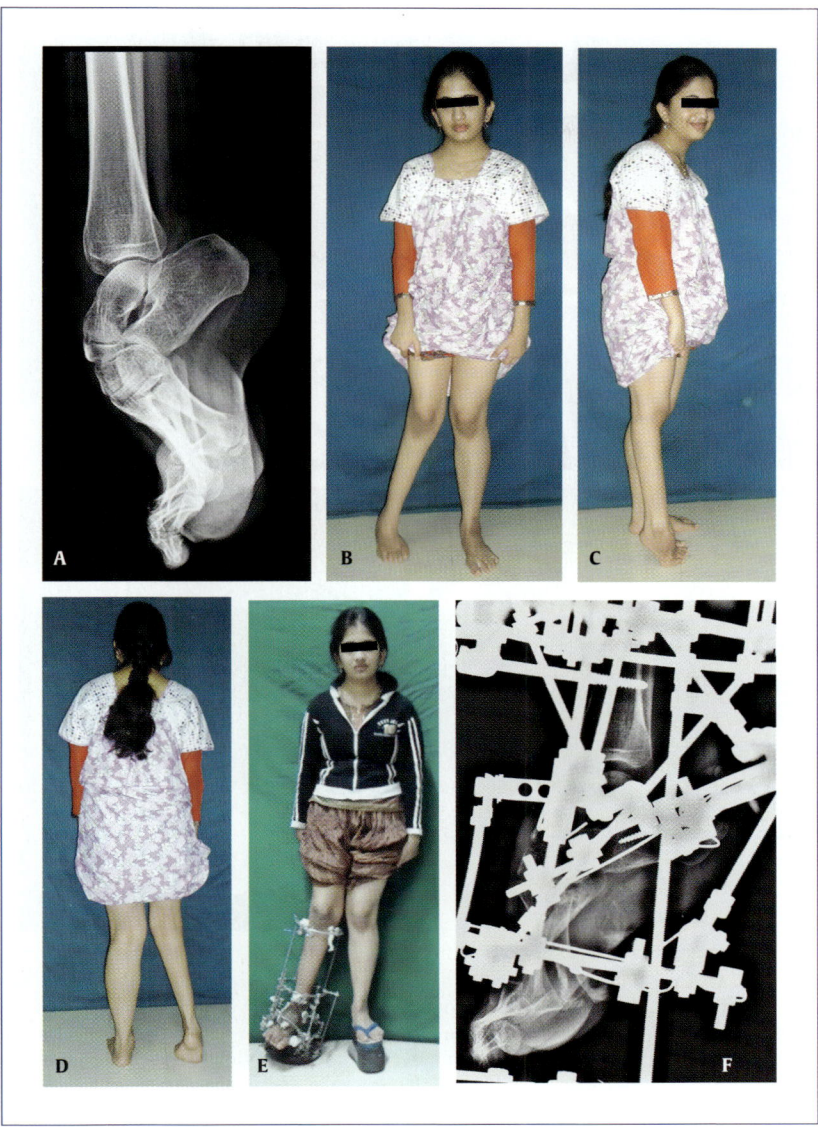

Fig. 8.4A to F   A 19-year-old patient with severe equinocavus deformity. Notice that the talus is round. Ilizarov fixator set up for distraction of the cavus as well as the equinus deformities. The hinges for cavus deformity correction are located at the apex of cavus. Distraction rods are inferior to this level at the sole. Patient gets a build-up below apparatus to enable walking. Ankle distraction set up in a nonconstrained manner. Notice the posterior motors are directed perpendicular to the lever arm. Excellent correction of both the deformities is seen.

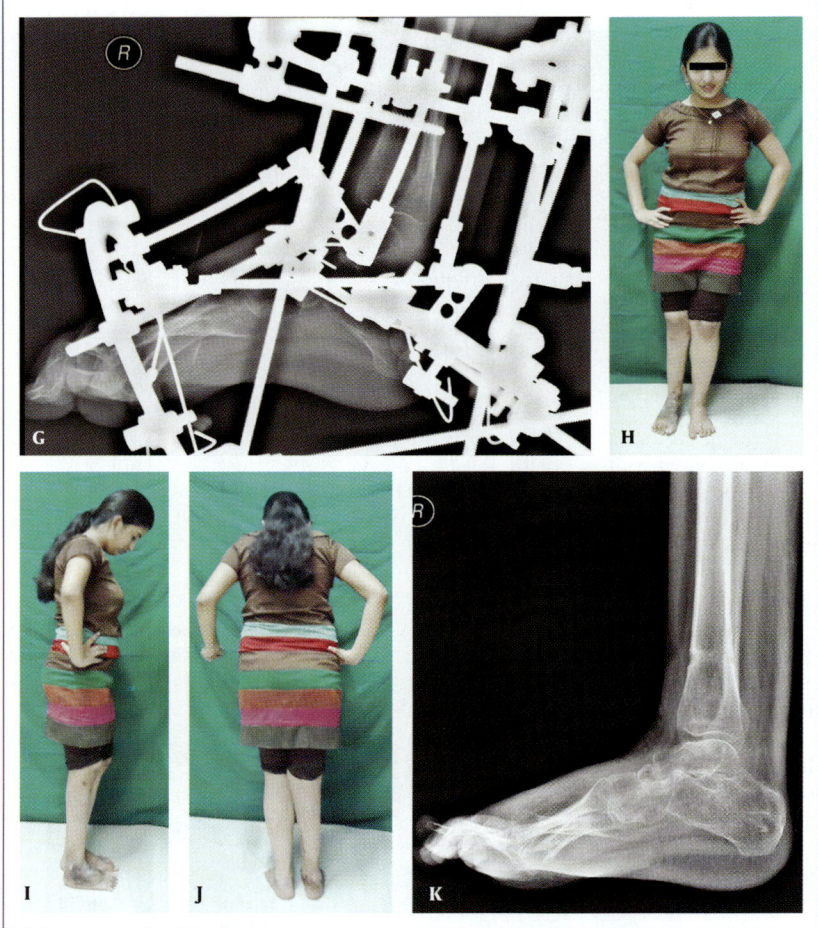

Fig. 8.4G to K *continued* A 19-year-old patient with severe equinocavus deformity. Notice that the talus is round. Ilizarov fixator set up for distraction of the cavus as well as the equinus deformities. The hinges for cavus deformity correction are located at the apex of cavus. Distraction rods are inferior to this level at the sole. Patient gets a build-up below apparatus to enable walking. Ankle distraction set up in a nonconstrained manner. Notice the posterior motors are directed perpendicular to the lever arm. Excellent correction of both the deformities is seen.

These two rings are tensioned using the manual method and can give very good stability. If the deformity is similar to an uncorrected clubfoot, the initial corrective maneuver is to match the supination of the hindfoot with that of the forefoot. The forefoot ring is supinated by using a force couple movement that raises the medial border of the foot cephalad and lowers the lateral border of the forefoot caudad. Once the forefoot and hindfoot supination match, the forefoot is abducted. The motors for this action are dropped off of the tibial assembly. The hindfoot ring during this correction is kept completely free. When the forefoot abducts, it transmits the forces to the anterior aspect of the calcaneus. The calcaneus now abducts, that is, the anterior aspect of the calcaneus rotates externally around an imaginary Z-axis running from cephalad to caudad. This, in turn, rotates the posterior aspect and tuberosity of the calcaneus so that it rotates away from the midline and toward the center.

After the rotation is complete, some inversion of the heel may remain before equinus can be corrected. Inversion of the heel can be corrected by distracting medially and keeping the lateral end passive.

Finally, the equinus can be corrected. The motors for equinus correction are posterior rods that are directed from anterior to posterior, connected over multiplane hinges attached to the tibial rings. The aim is to angle them in such a way as to remain perpendicular to the moment arm at the ankle.

The moment arm of the ankle is an imaginary line joining the center of rotation of the ankle with the posterior aspect of the tuberosity. Hence, the forces applied are accurately used to rotate the foot in the ankle without causing overdistraction, crushing at the ankle, or subluxation.

This motor rod is changed a few times as the correction progresses, always remaining perpendicular to the moment arm. As correction proceeds, the motor rod becomes more and more vertical. This correction is monitored by X-rays to ensure that ankle remains congruent and stable.

During the correction, outriggers can be attached to these foot rings to enable the patient to walk. This ensures that there is no osteoporosis and that the fixator remains stable. At the end of correction, casting is done and braces may be worn at night to prevent recurrence.

Principles of unconstrained correction of equinus deformity are shown in **Fig. 8.5A to J**.

Equino cavo varus distraction in a patient is serially depicted in **Fig. 8.6A to I**.

Focal dome correction of equinus by supramalleolar osteotomy (SMO) is depicted in **Fig. 8.7A to C**.

Dorsiflexion Contracture

Management of dorsiflexion contracture is illustrated in **Flowchart 8.2**.

Tips and Tricks

The following points hold importance for the effective management of dorsiflexion contracture:

♦ Dorsiflexion contractures are commonly seen after burns
♦ The simplest option would be to resect the contracted soft tissues and skin and to perform skin grafting
♦ Chronic contracture is better corrected gradually with soft tissue distraction

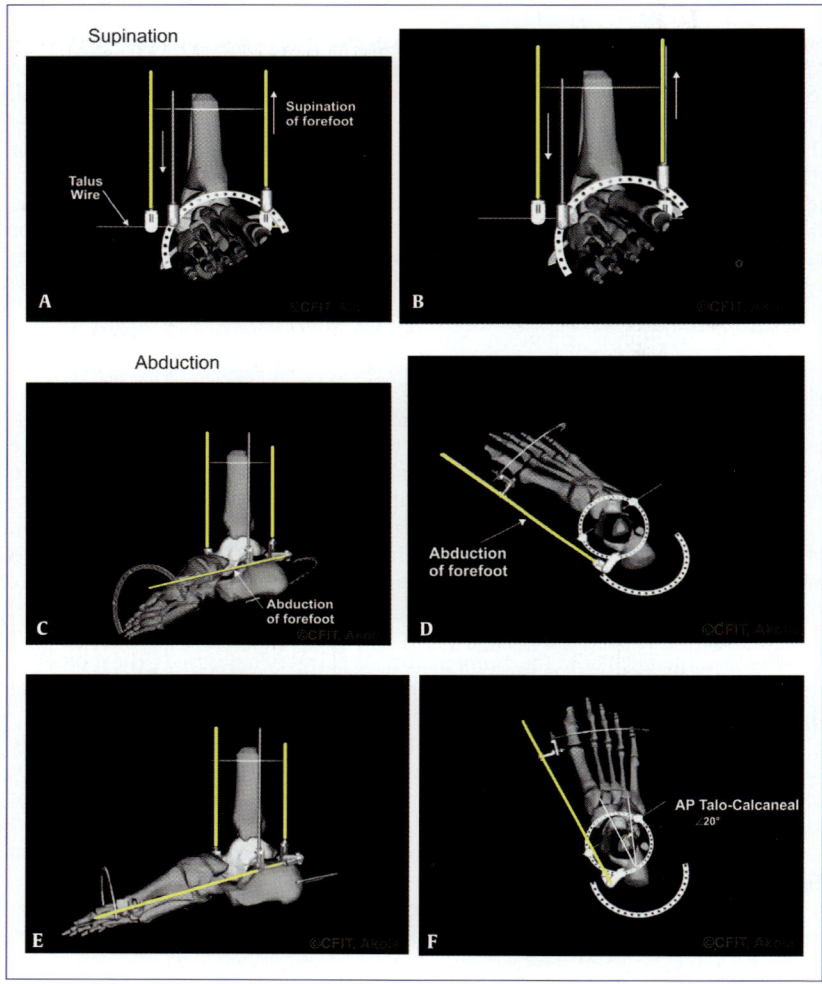

Fig. 8.5A to F   Unconstrained correction of clubfoot deformity. Tibial construct with two rings is not shown. Talus wire dropped off of tibial construct. Initial correction is of forefoot into supination. This is done by force couple action of the two parallel struts, inner bone pulling up and outer one pushing down. Once forefoot supination matches hindfoot supination, next step is to abduct the forefoot with a construct pushing from the tibial ring. View has shown alternating from inner and top views. Abduction is sufficient when anteroposterior (AP) talocalcaneal angle reaches 20°. During this step, the hindfoot ring is kept free and is not attached. Next is correction of inversion. Here, hindfoot force couple used with inner strut pushing down and outer strut pulling up. Finally, equinus correction begins. Here, the motor is angled so as to remain perpendicular to the lever arm (a line that joins the center of rotation of ankle with the tuberosity). This permits accurate correction of the equinus deformity without overdistraction, crushing of cartilage or subluxation of the joint.

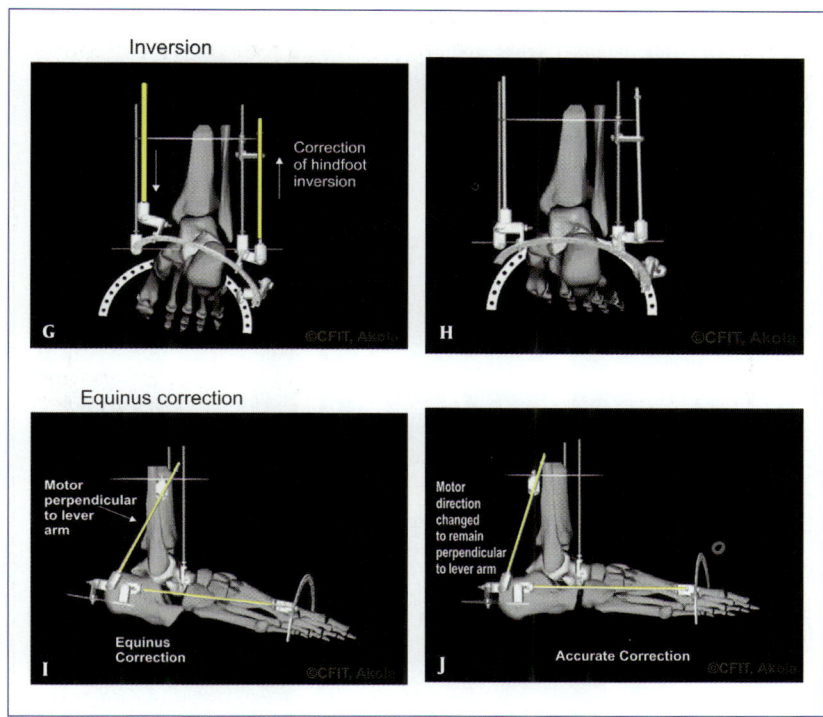

Fig. 8.5G to J *(continued)*   Unconstrained correction of clubfoot deformity. Tibial construct with two rings is not shown. Talus wire dropped off of tibial construct. Initial correction is of forefoot into supination. This is done by force couple action of the two parallel struts, inner bone pulling up and outer one pushing down. Once forefoot supination matches hindfoot supination, next step is to abduct the forefoot with a construct pushing from the tibial ring. View has shown alternating from inner and top views. Abduction is sufficient when anteroposterior (AP) talocalcaneal angle reaches 20°. During this step, the hindfoot ring is kept free and is not attached. Next is correction of inversion. Here, hindfoot force couple used with inner strut pushing down and outer strut pulling up. Finally, equinus correction begins. Here, the motor is angled so as to remain perpendicular to the lever arm (a line that joins the center of rotation of ankle with the tuberosity). This permits accurate correction of the equinus deformity without overdistraction, crushing of cartilage or subluxation of the joint.

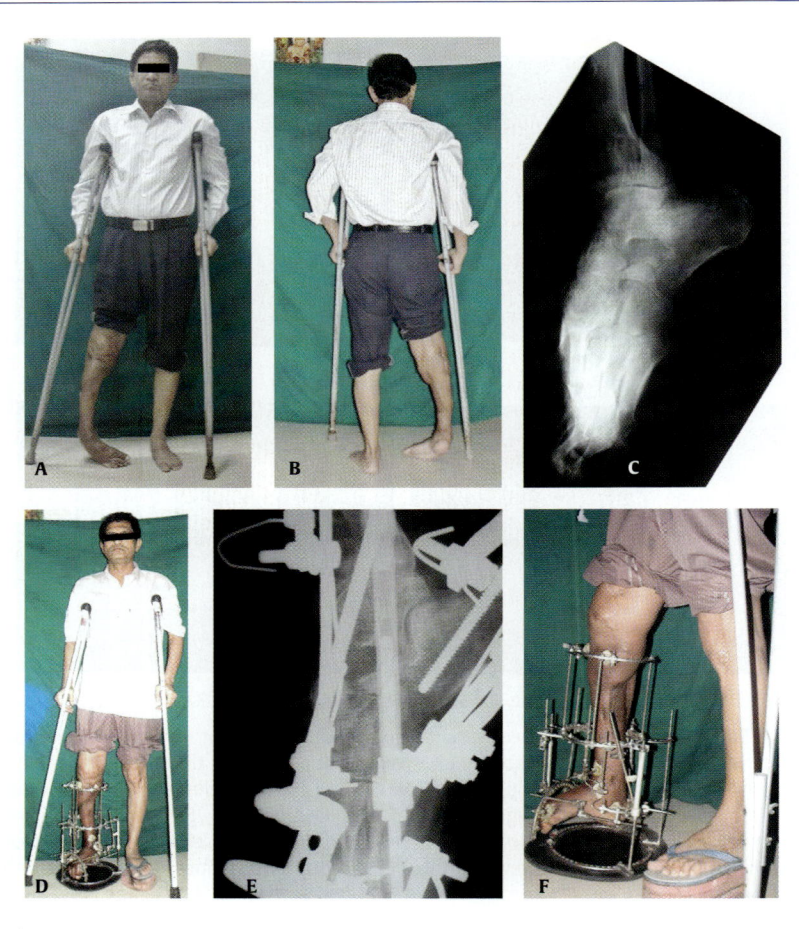

Fig. 8.6A to F A 50-year-old patient with posttraumatic severe equino-cavo-varus deformity. Talus is round in the ankle mortise. Soft tissue distraction of the ankle joint is done in a nonconstrained manner. Here the shape of the articular surfaces guides and constrains the correction, given that distraction forces are applied in appropriate direction. The deformities are corrected sequentially, with forefoot supination being dealt with initially, thereafter forefoot adduction and cavus being corrected. Hindfoot inversion and equinus are corrected last with motors that stay perpendicular to the lever arm (line joining center of rotation of ankle to the point where the distraction forces are being applied).

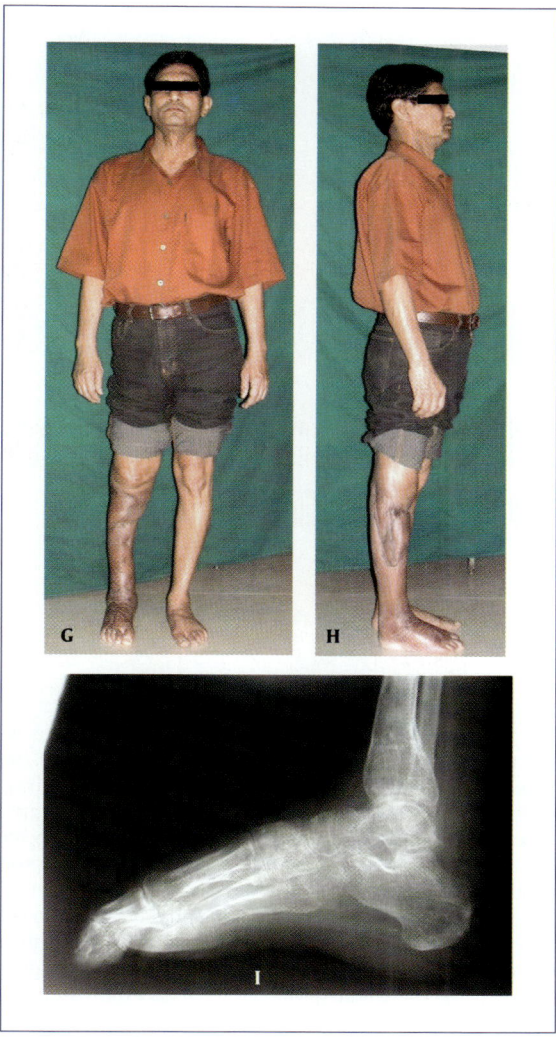

Fig. 8.6G to I *(continued)* A 50-year-old patient with posttraumatic severe equino-cavovarus deformity. Talus is round in the ankle mortise. Soft tissue distraction of the ankle joint is done in a nonconstrained manner. Here the shape of the articular surfaces guides and constrains the correction, given that distraction forces are applied in appropriate direction. The deformities are corrected sequentially, with forefoot supination being dealt with initially, thereafter forefoot adduction and cavus being corrected. Hindfoot inversion and equinus are corrected last with motors that stay perpendicular to the lever arm (line joining center of rotation of ankle to the point where the distraction forces are being applied).

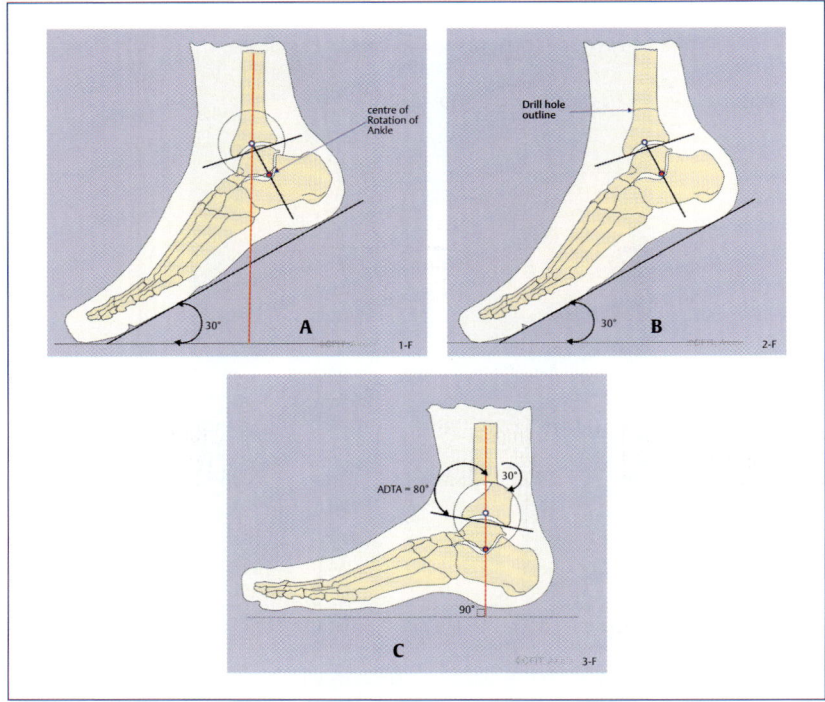

Fig. 8.7A to C This diagram represents the correction of an equinus deformity in the presence of a flat-top talus. A supramalleolar osteotomy is chosen for ease of approach and especially since there is no loss of hindfoot height or scarring at hindfoot level that precludes correction being performed at that level. A tarsal tunnel release has to be done initially with freeing of the posterior tibial nerve all the way distal to the origin of the abductor hallucis fascia. A fibular osteotomy is also performed as well as sometimes an os-tectomy of the fibula. An arcuate osteotomy outline is made with drill holes based on the center of rotation of ankle. Osteotomy is completed and then correction is achieved with the help of an external fixation device. It may be definitively treated with internal fixation using screws or a locking plate. Notice the translation of the distal fragment posteriorly. This is crucial to ensure that there is no unwanted secondary translation of the distal frag-ment anteriorly. A long stiff foot is a major handicap while walking. ADTA, anterior distal tibial angle.

♦ The assembly used is similar to that for clubfoot. Here the motor rods push the forefoot ring downward till they stretch out the anterior aspect of the ankle com-pletely.
♦ If the toes are contracted and dorsiflexed, it may be necessary to insert wires across the interphalangeal (IP) joints while the soft tissue distraction is progressing.
♦ The rate of distraction is monitored based on the response of the soft tissues.
♦ There is likely to be the need for fixing the talus and attaching the wire to fix the forefoot construct.

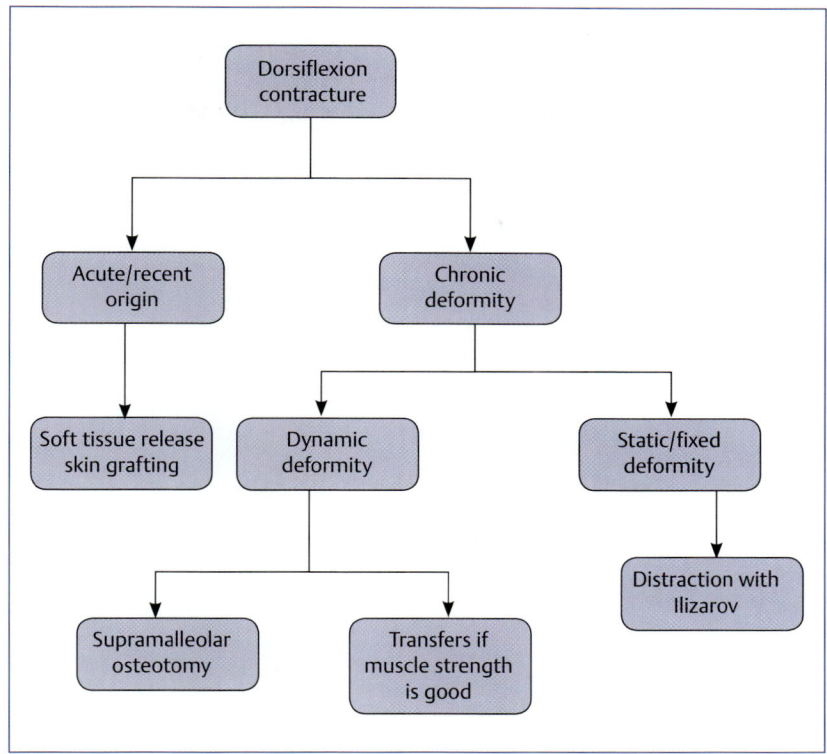

Flowchart 8.2   Management algorithm of dorsiflexion contracture.

♦ Dynamic ankle dorsiflexion deformities are seen in polio due to strong dorsiflexors and paralyzed tendo Achilles. This instability cannot be completely corrected by tendon transfers because of inadequate strength in the anterior muscles. Solution to this problem is to perform an SMO.

Supramalleolar Osteotomy

The point of contact of the dorsal talus with anterior lip of the lower tibia that happens in the recurvatum is changed so that full contact occurs in plantigrade position. Before performing the SMO, a tarsal tunnel release is performed prophylactically. The posterior tibial nerve is freed from under the tarsal tunnel as well as from under the sharp edge of the fascia deep to the abductor hallucis. The fibula is osteotomized just above the intended level of the SMO. The osteotomy is outlined with drill holes such that it describes an arc with its convexity proximally (**Fig. 8.8A and B**). The tibia is fixed with two half pins proximally and is fixed with two thin pediatric half pins distally along with two wires, one of which passes through the fibula as well. These are fixed to a carbon fiber half ring. After completion of the osteotomy, the ring is tilted so that the distal tibial fragment is brought out of recurvatum and is also translated anteriorly. The ankle is unable to go into dorsiflexion anymore and becomes stable in the plantigrade position.

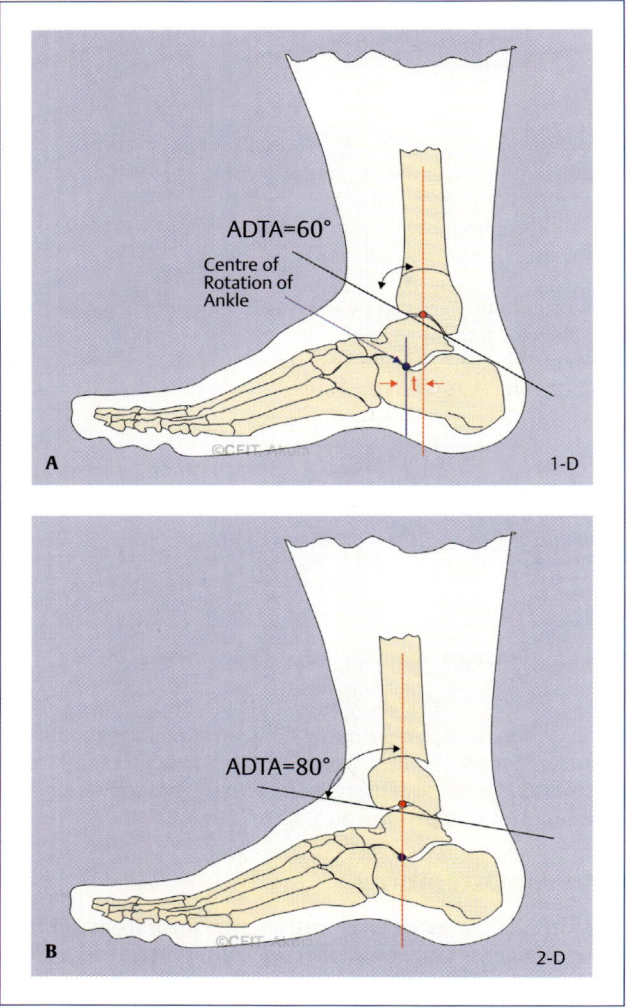

Fig. 8.8A and B   Recurvatum deformity in the ankle is also similar to a dorsiflexion contracture in polio where there is complete weakness of the tendo Achilles. Here we change the arc of rotation of the ankle using an arcuate supramalleolar osteotomy with its center of rotation at the level of lateral process of talus. A fibular osteotomy is also needed. A prophylactic tarsal tunnel release is also done at the start of surgery. In polio, the aim is to convert the arc of movement such that the ankle becomes stable in plantigrade position and is not allowed to collapse into dorsiflexion. ADTA, anterior distal tibial angle.

Ankle Valgus

Valgus deformity at the ankle may be caused by the following:

♦ Inclination of the tibial plafond
♦ Proximal migration of the fibula
♦ Extra-articular deformity at the supramalleolar level
♦ Valgus at the ankle joint itself due to a ball-and-socket ankle
♦ Hindfoot valgus deformity

Tips and Tricks

♦ An SMO with correction of the valgus can be performed as an open-wedge oste-otomy with its hinge point medially.
♦ The correction may be gradual and distracted apart with an external fixator or it may be opened acutely and fixed with a plate.
♦ A deformity that is located more proximally can be corrected as an angulation-translation osteotomy. This can be fixed with either an external fixation device or with a locking plate.
♦ The important thing is to ensure that the axis of the proximal and distal fragments line up (**Fig. 8.9**). This can happen when the proximal end of the distal fragment is translated laterally. Clubfoot correction in a patient is depicted serially in **Fig. 8.10A** to **I**.
♦ When the valgus is caused by a proximal migration of the fibula as can happen with a malunited ankle fracture, the ideal treatment is to bring down the fibula (**Fig. 8.11A** and **B**).
♦ For this to occur, the syndesmotic ligaments on the lateral side of the ankle must be released surgically. Thereafter, if fibular fracture has healed it must be

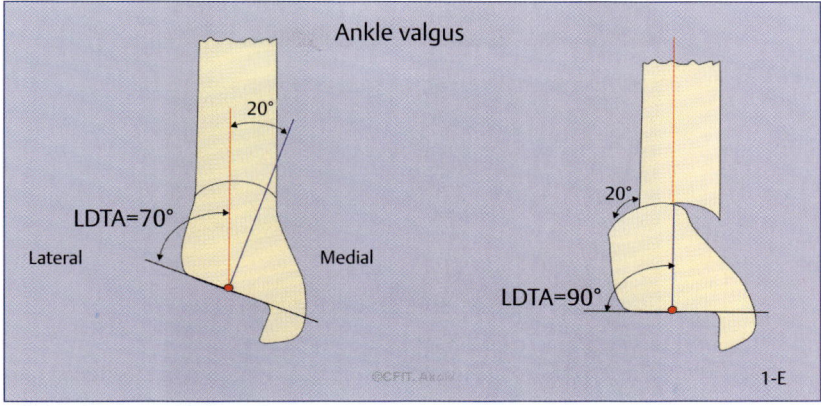

Fig. 8.9 Ankle valgus deformity shown here is with its center of rotation at the level of the joint. The osteotomy is outlined at the supramalleolar level with the hinge point at the level of joint. The arcuate cut is completed and there is a concomitant lateral translation of the distal fragment. This allows the center of proximal and distal fragments to line up.

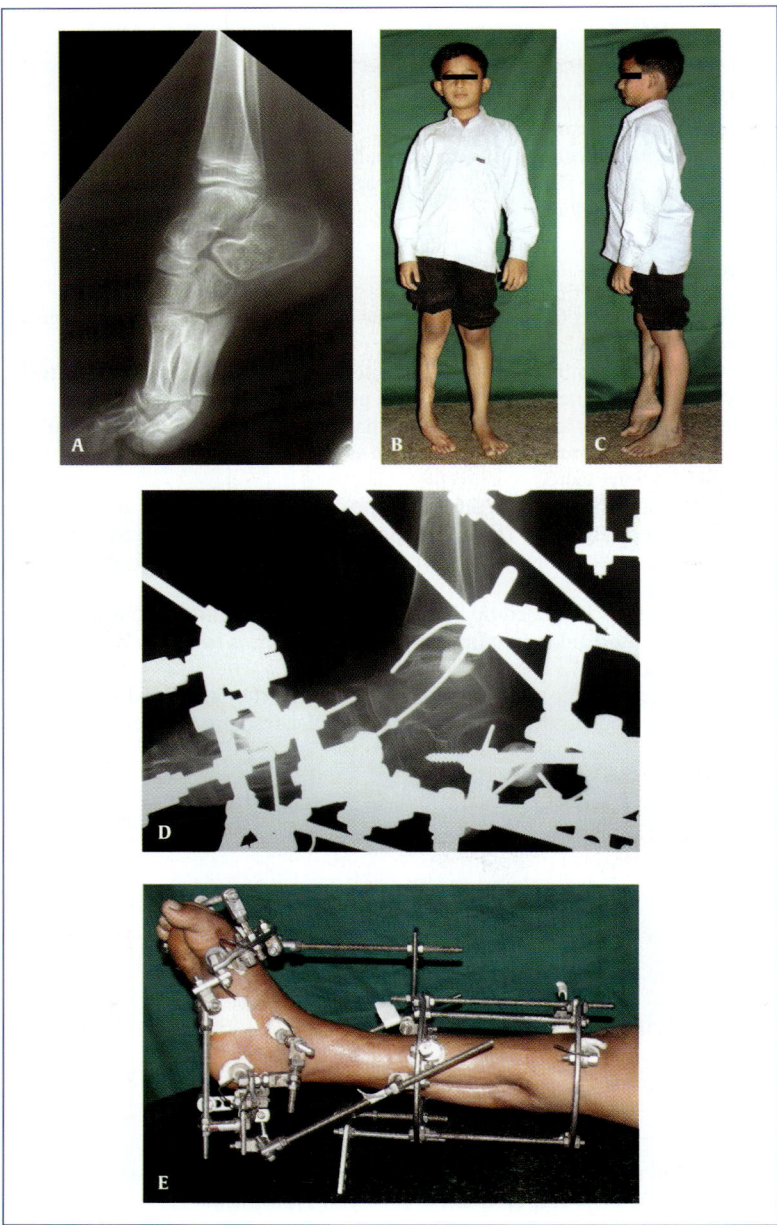

Figs. 8.10A to E   A 12-year-old with clubfoot secondary to sciatic nerve injury. The sequence of events has been explained in a diagram. The Ilizarov apparatus is applied in sequentially different montages to achieve full correction.

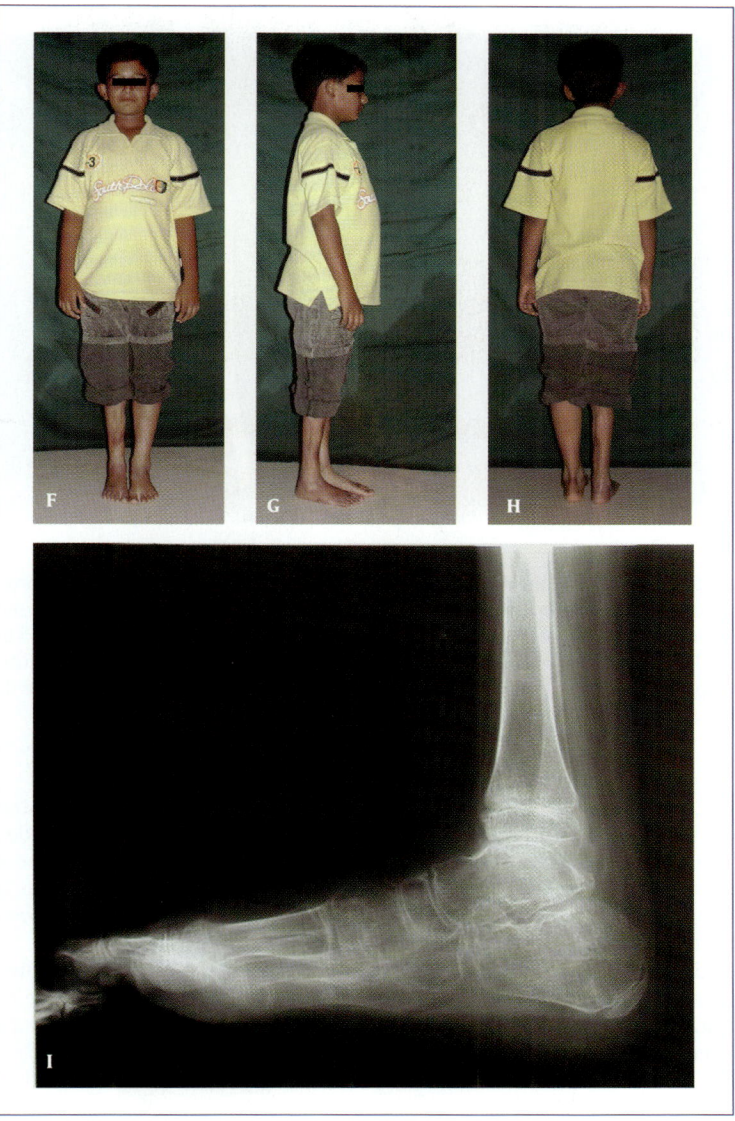

Figs. 8.10F to I *(continued)*   A 12-year-old with clubfoot secondary to sciatic nerve in-jury. The sequence of events has been explained in a diagram. The Ilizarov apparatus is applied in sequentially different montages to achieve full correction.

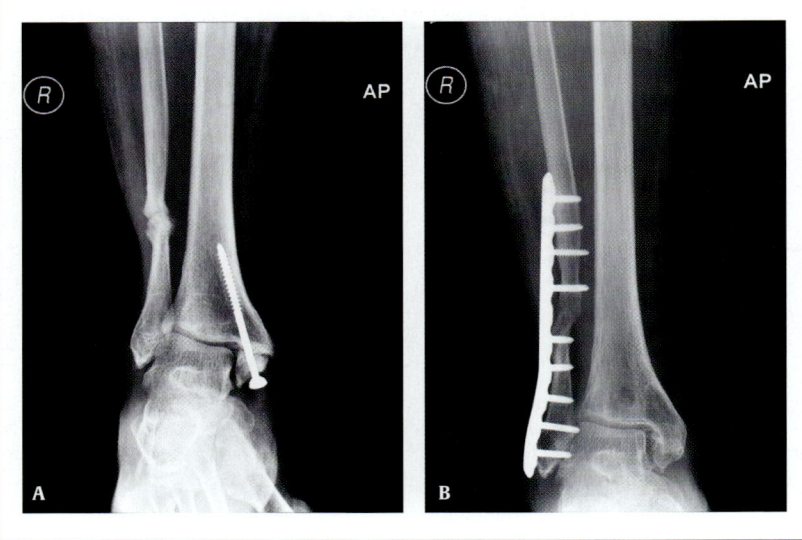

Fig. 8.11A and B Malunited ankle fracture with nonunion of medial malleolus, proximal overriding of the lateral malleolus, and valgus tilt of talus leading to valgus deformity at ankle. Surgery consists of releasing the syndesmotic ligaments, ankle release, and bringing the fibula down to a level similar to that of the opposite normal ankle. A distraction device helps bring it down and a strong plate is applied with a small bone graft in the fibular gap. Restoring fibular length in this case corrected the ankle valgus deformity.

re-osteotomized, and with a compression device, the fibula must be distracted and brought down till it comes to occupy the perfect position in the ankle. The fibula is now fixed with a locking plate and the gap reinforced with a bone graft.

♦ If the fibular valgus is caused by a chronic proximal migration, it needs to be brought down with a distractor, gradually and maintained with one or two syndesmotic screws.

♦ Hindfoot valgus may also be caused by subluxation of the calcaneum in the subtalar joint. This can be corrected with a posterolateral approach, release of the subtalar joint, tendo Achilles (TA) lengthening, and a subtalar fusion with a fibular graft or a screw inserted from the talar neck into the calcaneum.

♦ A medial displacement osteotomy of the calcaneum is also an ideal method for valgus deformity correction at hindfoot.

Varus Deformity

Varus deformity may be caused by the following:

♦ Malunited ankle or lower tibial fracture
♦ Residual effects of growth arrest due to physeal injury or osteomyelitis
♦ Neuromuscular imbalance

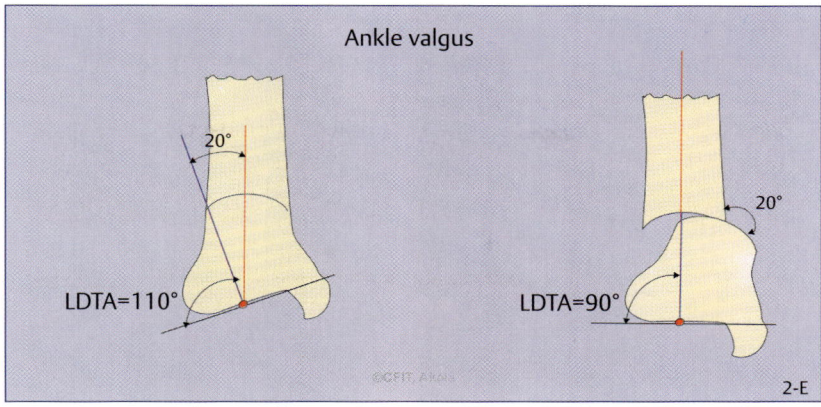

Ankle valgus

20°

LDTA=110°

20°

LDTA=90°

2-E

Fig. 8.12 Ankle varus deformity is with its center of rotation at the level of the joint. The osteotomy is outlined at the supramalleolar level with hinge point at the level of joint. The arcuate cut is completed and there is a concomitant medial translation of the distal fragment. This allows the center of proximal and distal fragments to line up.

Tips and Tricks

If the location of the varus deformity is at the ankle or supramalleolar level, it can be corrected with an osteotomy (**Fig. 8.12**).

◆ If accompanied by shortening, an open-wedge correction can be done and if there is no shortening, the deformity can be corrected as an angulation-translation osteotomy.

◆ Along with correction of the varus, the proximal end of the distal fragment must be translated laterally to enable the canals of the proximal and distal fragments to line up and hence prevent a secondary translational deformity.

◆ An open-wedge correction is done with the motor rods performing the correction, placed at right angles to the plane of the deformity. Hence, it may not be sufficient for the rods to be placed parallel to the tibia, but at dramatic angles perpendicular to the plane of the plafond. The motor rods can change their direction as the correction progresses. This will ensure the most mechanically sound correction.

◆ If there is a significant varus deformity with instability as seen in polio, the best solution may be to perform an ankle fusion.

◆ If there is concomitant shortening, a corticotomy lengthening should be added on along with fusion.

◆ This may be combined as a procedure done over an intramedullary nail inserted from the distal approach and an open fusion is combined with lengthening done just above the ankle-fusion level. This nail is locked distally and kept free proximally.

◆ External fixation devices can help motor the lengthening. As soon as the length is achieved, it can be locked proximally and the external device removed.

◆ Alternatively, ankle fusion as well as lengthening can be performed with an Ilizarov external fixator. This will enable giving sustained compression at the ankle fusion site.

Flowchart 8.3 differentiates between valgus and varus deformity in their occurrence and management.

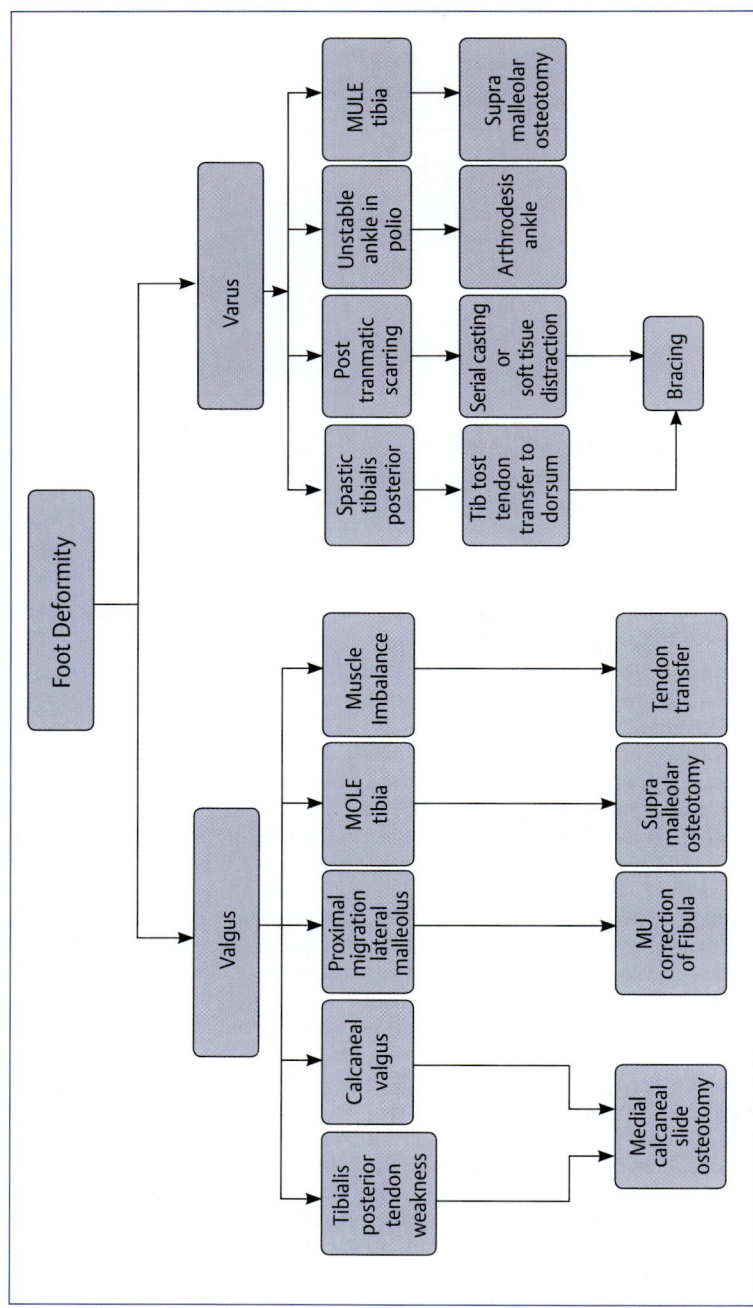

Flowchart 8.3   Valgus and varus deformity.

Cavus Deformity

The cavus deformity may be caused or exacerbated by tight plantar fascia. Management of cavus deformity is illustrated in **Flowchart 8.4**.

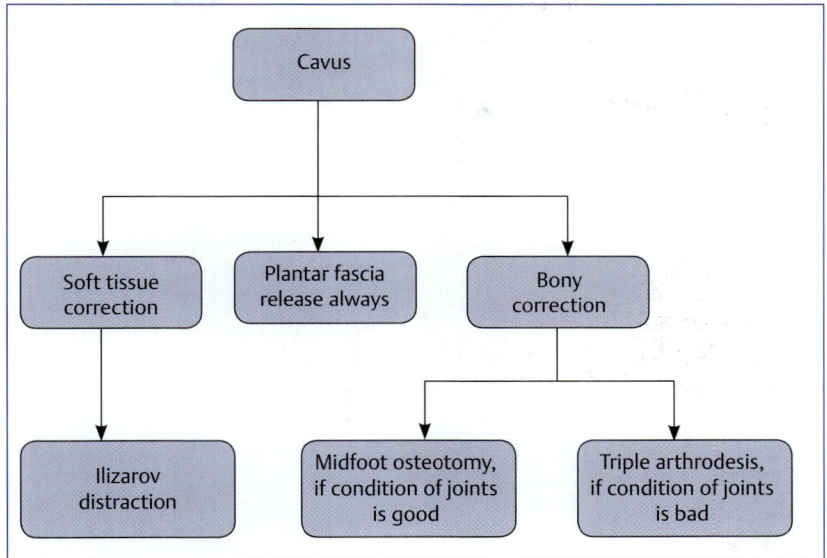

Flowchart 8.4 Management algorithm of equinus.

Tips and Tricks

The first step in correction of the cavus is to perform a Steindler's release of plantar fascia in the middle of the sole.

♦ Decision about correction is based on the possibility of correction using soft tissue distraction or by bony osteotomy.
♦ Soft tissue distraction is performed around a wire that is passed at the apex of the deformity as seen on a lateral X-ray.
♦ The hindfoot is fixed with a half ring and so is the forefoot. The two half rings are connected with strong plates, which meet at the intersection and rotate around the wire. This wire is passed at the apex, which can be placed at the level of cuneiforms or at the cuneiform–metatarsal junction. The distraction rods are inferior to these plates and help correct the cavus.
♦ It is better to overcorrect the deformity, and wait for a further 6 weeks in the apparatus to allow the soft tissues to mature in the frame. Later a walking cast is applied for 6 to 8 weeks and a brace is worn for a further 6 months at night.
♦ If the deformity cannot be corrected by soft tissue distraction, the best alternative is to perform an osteotomy correction (**Fig. 8.13A** to **D**).
♦ If the cavus is combined with a varus or valgus deformity, it is ideally corrected with a V osteotomy. The rear limb of the V osteotomy helps correct hindfoot

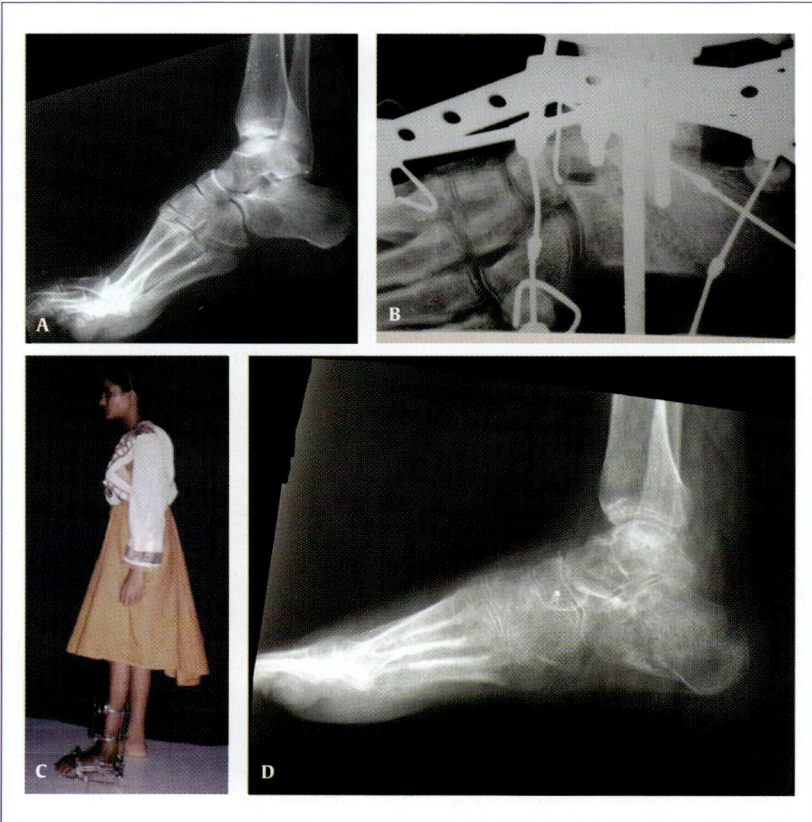

Fig. 8.13A to D A 17-year-old patient with rigid cavus deformity. This would not be correctible with soft tissue distraction. Hence, an osteotomy was performed at the level of the neck of talus and anterior part of calcaneus. This is the anterior part of the V osteotomy. The apex and hinges are located at the neck of the talus. A triangular regenerate bone is formed with its base inferiorly. This regenerate bone also fuses the subtalar joint and serves to prevent recurrence of deformity.

varus or valgus and the front arm of the V helps correct the sagittal plane deformity in the hindfoot–forefoot junction.

The Ilizarov Fixator-Assisted Cavus Correction

Montage in this condition is a block of two rings in the tibia. A half ring fixes the hindfoot and another fixes the forefoot. The essential part of the construct is a wire that passes in the neck of the talus and another wire that fixes the middle part of the calcaneus, avoiding the neurovascular structures. These two wires are attached to the tibial construct with a plate and stud assembly, mounted with its thin edge in the coronal plane. Hinges connect the hindfoot and forefoot half rings. The osteotomy itself is performed through two 2 cm incision over the lateral aspect of calcaneus, posterior to the peroneal tendons.

The anterior limb of the V is performed through a small incision parallel to the talo-navicular joint orientation, through the sinus tarsi. An image intensifier checks the position of the osteotome (**Fig. 8.14A** to **I**). A strong sense of feel prevents the osteotome from penetrating the medial cortex and endangering the medial neurovascular structures. Two osteotomes are stacked against each other to prise the osteotomy apart. The mobility at the bone ends must be checked under the image intensifier. Some distraction is built in into the osteotomy on the table itself as the osteotomy has a tendency to undergo premature consolidation.

Distracton is performed on both limbs of the V and monitored on X-rays. The aim is to correct the deformity by performing a gradual open-wedge correction. The regenerate is allowed to consolidate well enough before removing the apparatus.

♦ An alternative to all of the distraction osteotomies is of course the venerable and time-honored operation of triple arthrodesis.

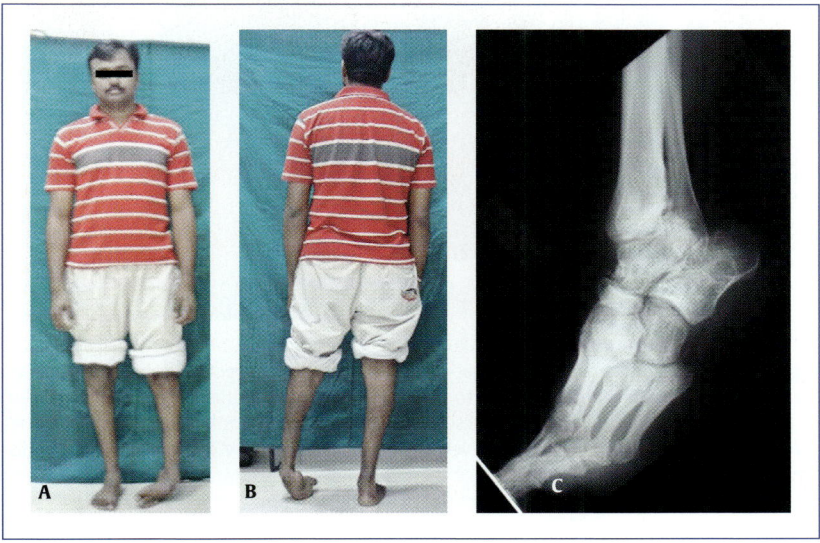

Fig. 8.14A to C   A 28-year-old patient with uncorrected clubfoot deformity. Notice that the talus is flattened due to multiple previous surgeries, and there is scarring of posterior soft tissues. Hence, soft tissue distraction is not an option. In this case, all deformities need to be corrected at the level of the hindfoot using a V osteotomy. The anterior limb of V passes down from the neck of the talus into the anterior part of the calcaneum. The posterior limb stays behind the subtalar joint. The anterior limb is distracted apart with apex superiorly and base of the regenerate bone is formed inferiorly. The posterior limb is distracted apart with its base inferiorly, with the base at superior level forming a triangular regenerate. The Ilizarov fixator is applied with two rings in tibia and one half ring each for the hindfoot and forefoot. There is a talus wire that helps to form the post against which the two osteotomies are distracted apart. Initial high rates of distraction are maintained to prevent premature consolidation. Complete correction of the deformity is seen in 3 months of fixator duration. The fusion at subtalar joint also prevents recurrence of the deformity.

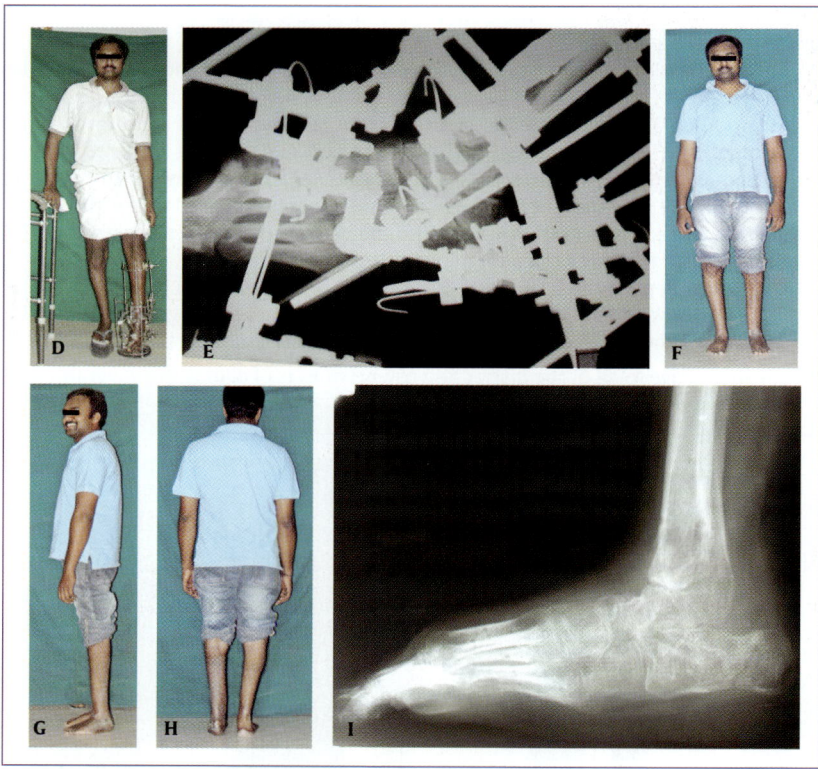

Fig. 8.14D to I (*Continued*)   A 28-year-old patient with uncorrected clubfoot deformity. Notice that the talus is flattened due to multiple previous surgeries, and there is scarring of posterior soft tissues. Hence, soft tissue distraction is not an option. In this case, all deformities need to be corrected at the level of the hindfoot using a V osteotomy. The anterior limb of V passes down from the neck of the talus into the anterior part of the calcaneum. The posterior limb stays behind the subtalar joint. The anterior limb is distracted apart with apex superiorly and base of the regenerate bone is formed inferiorly. The posterior limb is distracted apart with its base inferiorly, with the base at superior level forming a triangular regenerate. The Ilizarov fixator is applied with two rings in tibia and one half ring each for the hindfoot and forefoot. There is a talus wire that helps to form the post against which the two osteotomies are distracted apart. Initial high rates of distraction are maintained to prevent premature consolidation. Complete correction of the deformity is seen in 3 months of fixator duration. The fusion at subtalar joint also prevents recurrence of the deformity.

Short stiff foot is better than a long stiff foot.

◆ Hence, the V osteotomy and its analogue, like U osteotomy, performed for an equinus deformity can very well be avoided and substituted by a triple arthrodesis.

Chapter 9

Soft Tissues Are Equally Important!

Bone and joints are the trees, but its roots lie in soft tissues!

What Is Special about Soft Tissues in Foot and Ankle?

Important characteristics of skin and soft tissues in foot and ankle are represented in **Fig. 9.1**.

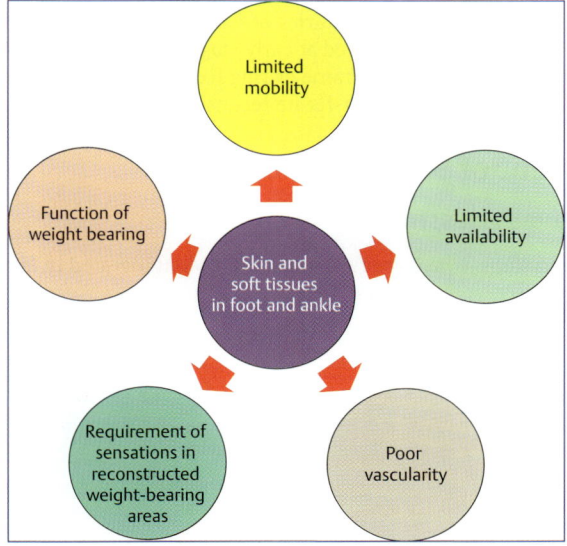

Fig. 9.1 Characteristics of skin and soft tissues in foot and ankle.

Prevention of Iatrogenic Foot and Ankle Soft-Tissue Damage

Some important tips and tricks for the prevention of iatrogenic soft-tissue damage at foot and ankle are enumerated below:

◆ Avoid putting small incisions
◆ Avoid vigorous retraction of skin
◆ Always take full-thickness flaps
◆ At tendo Achilles surgeries, incise skin and sheath together, and never create a plane between both of them
◆ A safe spacing of 4 to 6 cm between two incisions over midfoot and forefoot is mandatory to prevent skin ischemia and necrosis
◆ In an acute trauma setting, wait till wrinkles over the traumatized area are seen
◆ While waiting for wrinkles to appear and edema to settle down, always reduce subcutaneous bony prominences to prevent skin necrosis
◆ While waiting for skin condition to improve, a spanning fixator would be of help for ligamentotaxis and early settlement of edema
◆ Aspirate serous blister and wait for 3 to 5 days before operating through it
◆ Do not incise through blood-filled blisters; a healing time of 1 to 3 weeks before going in for surgery is mandatory
◆ Delicate skin flaps should be handled with blunt skin hooks and should be retracted with bent K-wires put in nearby normal bones
◆ Knots must be put outside the delicate skin flaps
◆ Anticipation of skin closure problems must be envisaged preoperatively and help and guidance of reconstructive plastic surgeon must be sought beforehand
◆ While dealing with compound injuries of foot and ankle, reconstructive plastic surgeon should always be involved at early stage for better outcome
◆ While putting external fixator frame or ring fixator, careful planning is required to not violate future areas of soft-tissue reconstruction

Management of Soft-Tissue Defects

Preoperative Assessment

It includes three steps, which are further separately enumerated in **Flowchart 9.1.**

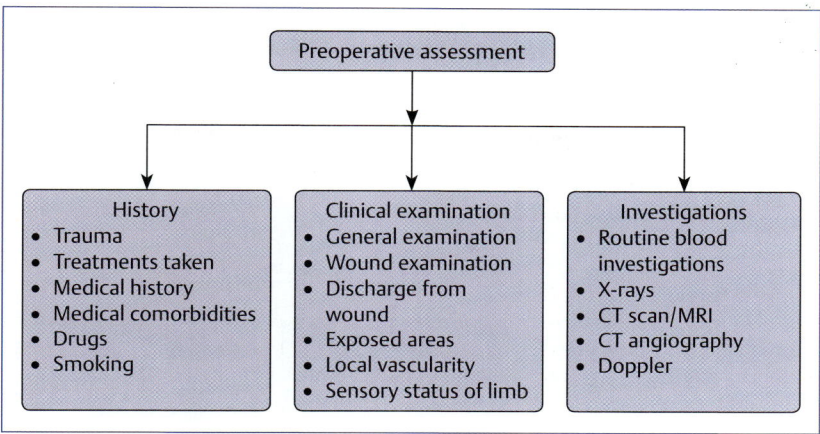

Flowchart 9.1 Preoperative assessment.

Prerequisites

Some of the prerequisites for the management of soft-tissue defects include:

♦ Sequential radical debridement
♦ Definitive or temporary skeletal stabilization
♦ Early soft-tissue coverage (**Flowchart 9.2**)

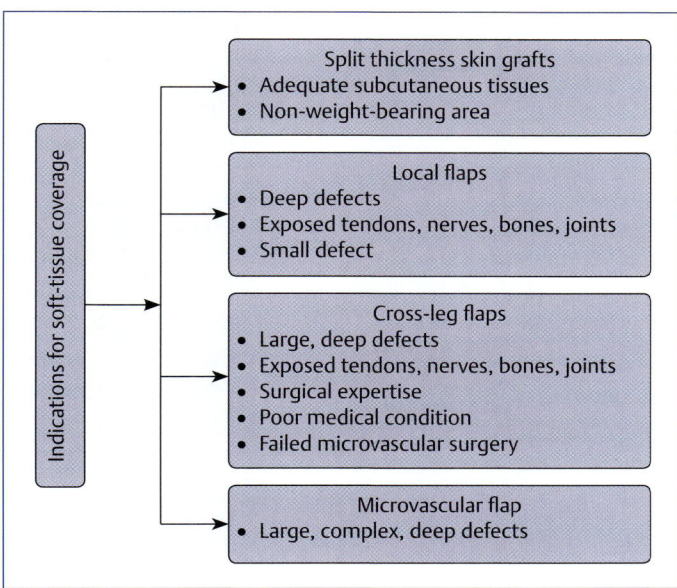

Flowchart 9.2 Soft-tissue coverage.

A brief overview of the soft-tissue defects is illustrated in **Flowcharts 9.3 to 9.5**.

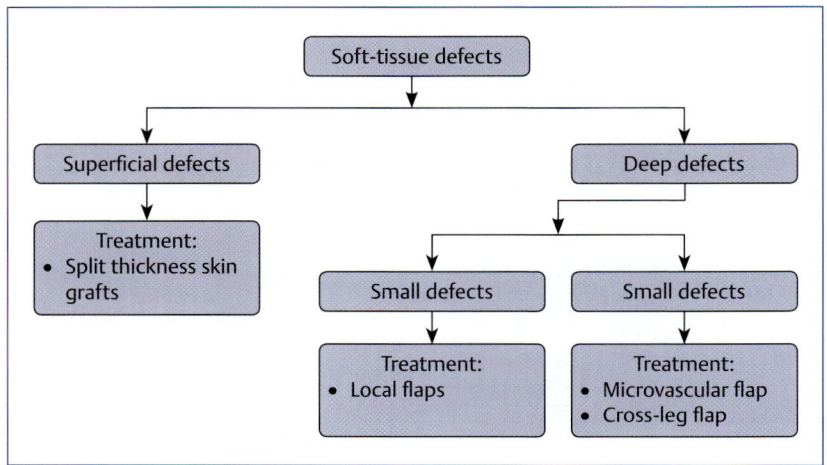

Flowchart 9.3 Overview of the soft-tissue defects.

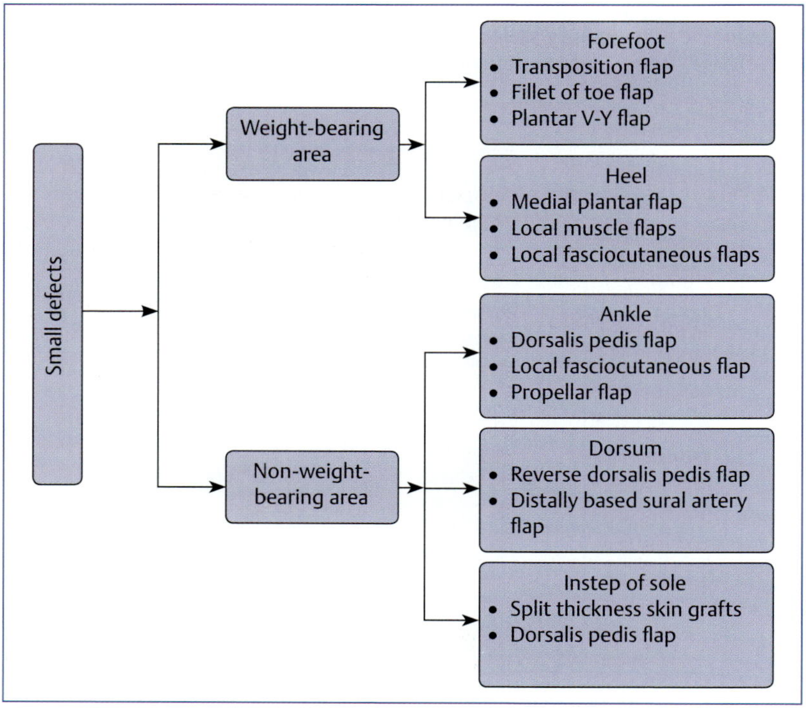

Flowchart 9.4 Overview of the soft-tissue coverage for small defects.

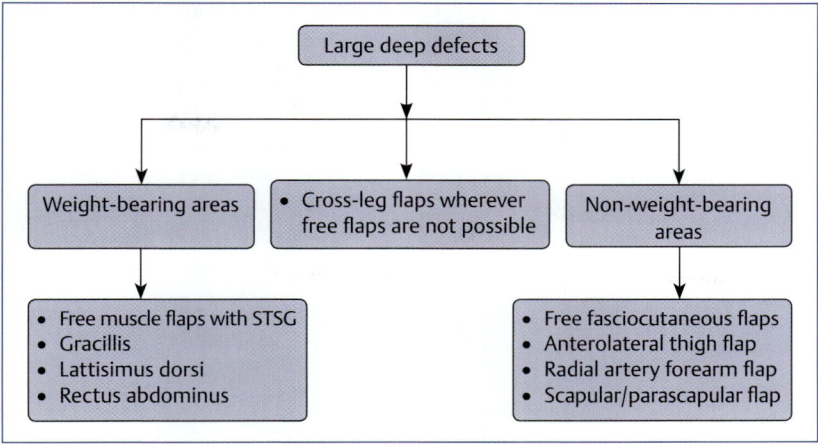

Flowchart 9.5   Overview of the soft-tissue coverage for large and deep defects.

Region-Wise Soft-Tissue Coverage Options

Ankle

♦ Local flaps: used for smaller defects
♦ Distant flaps: used for larger defects
Commonly used locoregional flaps for ankle are as follows:

1. *Distally based sural artery flap*: It is a fasciocutaneous flap that is elevated from the posterior aspect of the calf along with sural nerve and small saphenous vein. It is based on a perforator of the peroneal artery that emerges 5 cm proximal to the lateral malleolus and then runs cephalad. It can be raised as an island flap along with neurovascular bundle or as a pedicle flap. It is a very useful flap for lower one-third of leg and ankle defects. Disadvantages are visible donor defect at the calf and loss of sensations at the lateral border of the foot (**Fig. 9.2**).

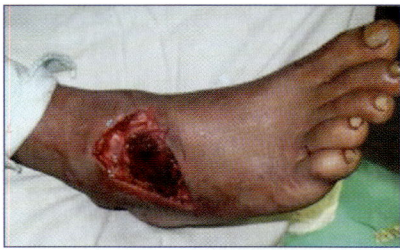
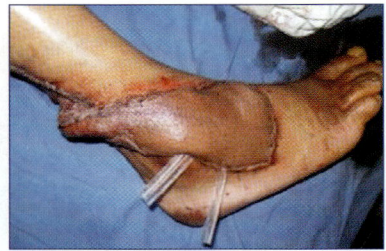
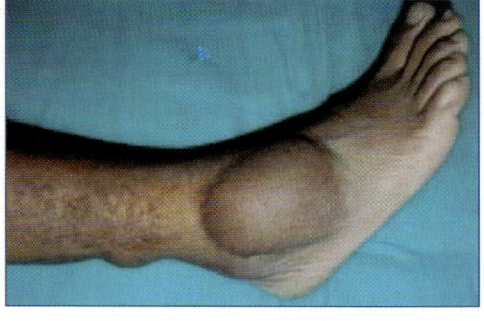

Fig. 9.2   Distally based sural artery flap for soft-tissue defect of anterolateral ankle region.

2. *Distally based fasciocutaneous saphenous flap*: A flap is raised from medial aspect of the lower leg. The pedicle contains saphenous vein, artery, and nerve. Distally based sural flap is preferred over it because of its perforator being at the more distal level, but one may need to use this flap in case of trauma in the region of sural flap perforator. As with other distally based flaps, it also has the disadvantages of the venous congestion and skin-grafted donor site (**Fig. 9.3**).

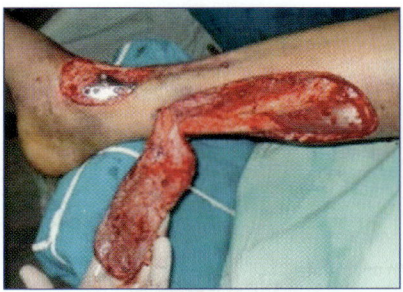
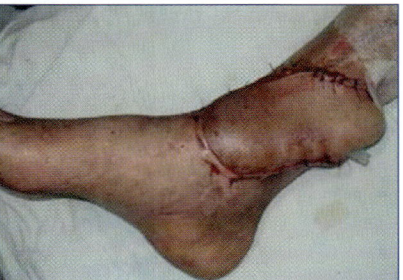
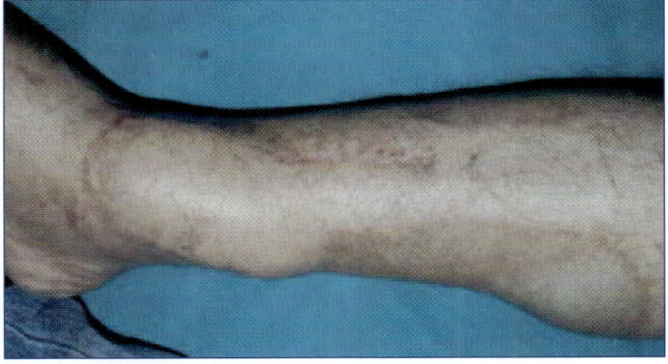

Fig. 9.3 Distally based fasciocutaneous saphenous flap for soft-tissue defect of antero-medial ankle region.

3. *Lateral supra malleolar flap*: This flap is based on anterior perforating branch of the peroneal artery that pierces the interosseous membrane approximately 5 cm above the lateral malleolus just proximal to tibiofibular ligaments. Problems associated with it are possible venous congestion and visible skin-grafted donor site.
4. *Lateral calcaneal artery flap*: This flap is based on pedicle containing the sural nerve, small saphenous vein, and lateral calcaneal branch of the peroneal artery. This can be used for smaller posterior ankle defects.
5. *Propeller flap*: Small defects can be covered with propeller flap based on one of the perforators of posterior tibial or peroneal vessels. The perforator is located

with handheld Doppler preoperatively. Dissection of the perforator is quite tedious and should be done under magnification (**Fig. 9.4**).

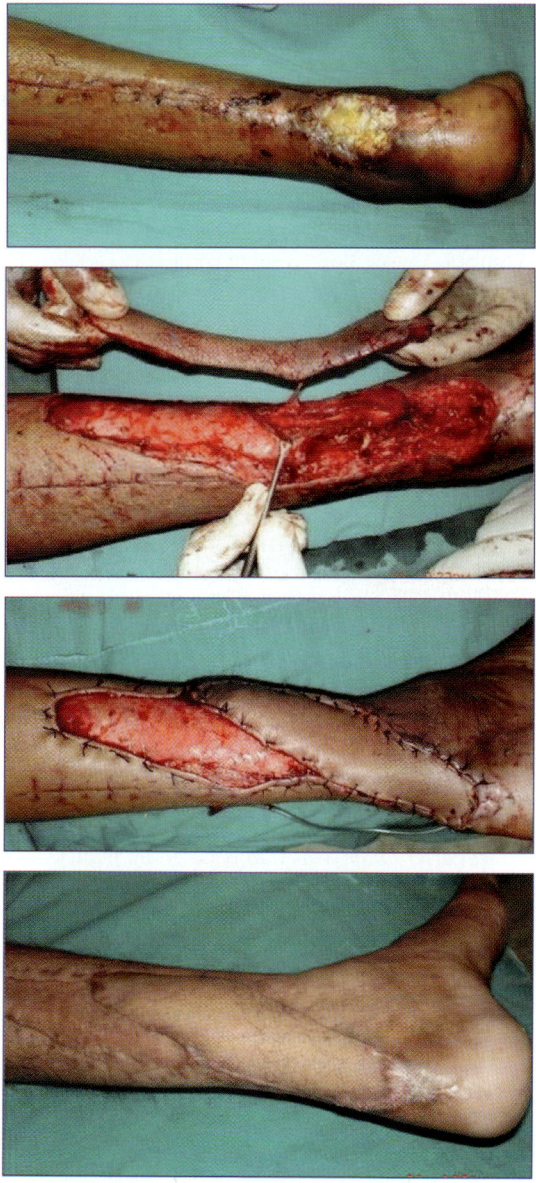

Fig. 9.4 Propeller flap for soft-tissue defect of tendo Achilles region.

6. *Dorsalis pedis flap*: This flap is raised from the dorsum of the foot, including dorsalis pedis artery. Large amount of tissue is available for coverage of lateral as well as medial malleolus region. Disadvantages include sacrifice of a major artery and superficial peroneal nerve with an undesirable donor defect. There is also loss of normal sensations on the dorsum of the foot. For these reasons, this flap should only be used if for some reason a free microvascular flap cannot be used.
7. *Local muscle flaps*: Local muscle flaps of the distal leg include extensor digitorum longus flap, soleus flap, flexor digitorum longus flap, peroneus brevis flap, and extensor hallucis longus flap. These are used for highly selective indications. These cannot be used in severely contused and traumatized limb.
8. *Extensor digitorum brevis muscle flap*: This flap may be transposed proximally to cover the anterior ankle and lateral malleolar wounds if there is no damage to the anterior tibial and dorsalis pedis arteries. This flap is useful only for small wounds measuring up to 4.5 or 6.0 cm in adults.

Dorsum of foot/midfoot

1. *Distally based sural artery flap*: This flap has limitation of inability to reach the forefoot area (**Fig. 9.5**).
2. *Saphenous flap*: This flap also has the limitation of inability to reach the forefoot area.

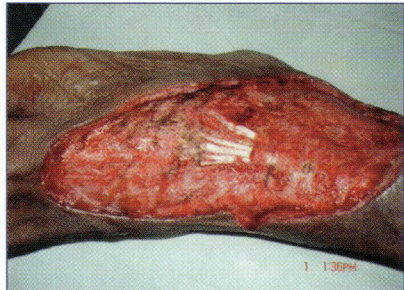
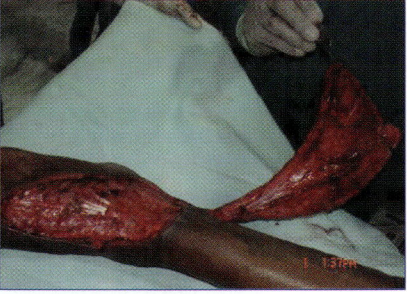
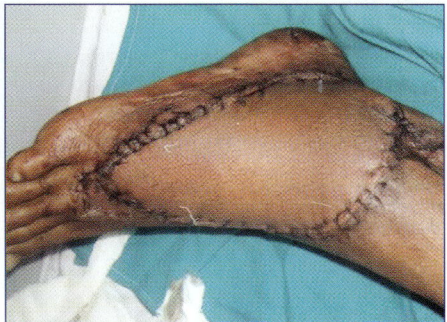

Fig. 9.5 Distally based sural artery flap for soft-tissue defect of dorsum of foot.

3. *Reverse-fashioned dorsalis pedis flap*: This flap should be done only after confirmation of patent communication between dorsalis pedis artery and first dorsal metatarsal artery.
4. *Cross-leg flap and free flaps*: These flaps are used for bigger defects.

Instep of sole

A localized defect of instep of sole should be skin grafted. In case a flap is required, one can use dorsalis pedis flap. For bigger defects involving weight-bearing area, a free flap is used.

For microvascular free flaps, fasciocutaneous flaps are preferred over muscle flaps as they provide gliding tissue for exposed tendons. Commonly used free fasciocutaneous flap is anterolateral thigh flap (**Fig. 9.6**), which is based on a perforator arising from a descending branch of the lateral circumflex artery. Smaller defects can be covered with gracilis muscle flap (**Figs. 9.7 and 9.8**).

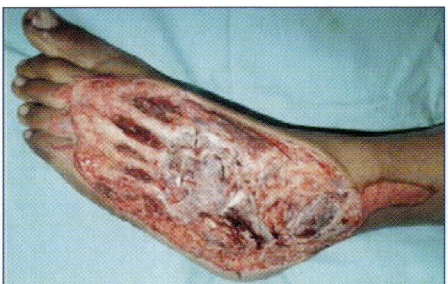
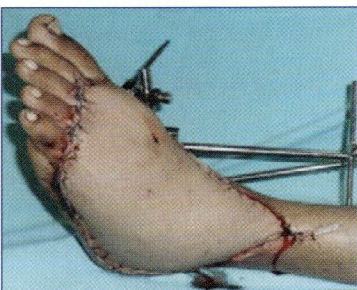
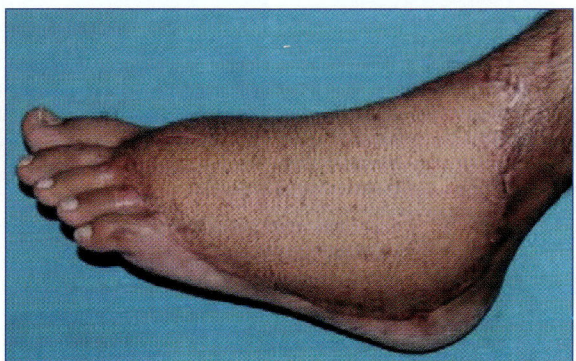

Fig. 9.6   Free microvascular anterolateral thigh flap for the soft-tissue defect of dorsum of foot.

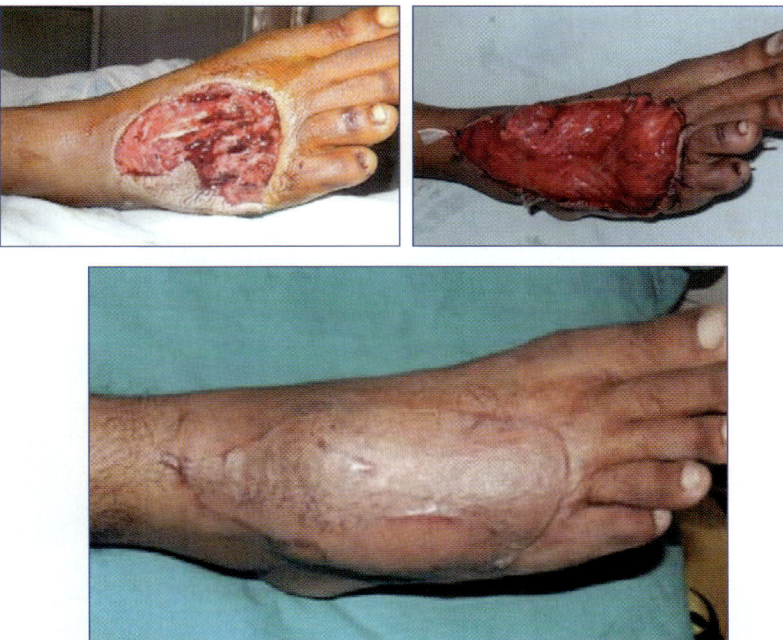

Fig. 9.7   Free microvascular gracilis flap for coverage of soft-tissue defect over dorsum of foot.

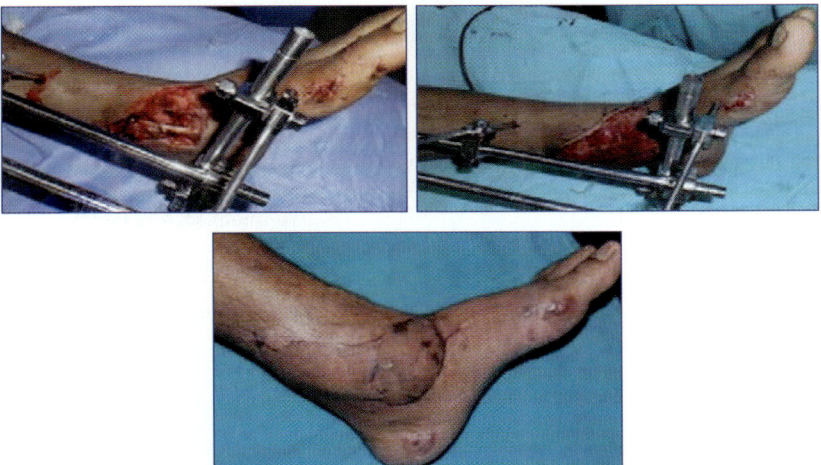

Fig. 9.8   Free microvascular gracilis flap for coverage of soft-tissue defect over medial aspect of ankle.

Forefoot plantar aspect

This is a weight-bearing area and needs special considerations. Transposition and rotation flaps are used for small defects. Fillet of toe flap is also used for coverage of small defects. Plantar V–Y flap is used for defects up to 2 cm in diameter. Larger defects require two such opposing flaps.

Heel

1. *Medial plantar artery flap or instep island flap*: This is an ideal flap for the heel as it provides similar sensate tissues. Defects as large as 4 to 5 cm in diameter can be closed. The flap is based on a medial plantar artery and can be raised as pedicled or an island flap. The donor area is skin grafted (**Fig. 9.9**).

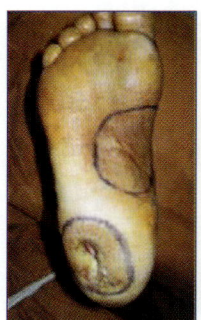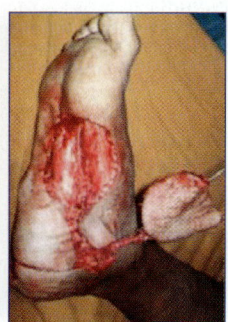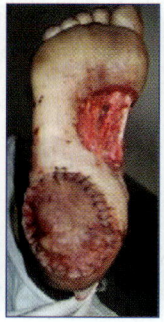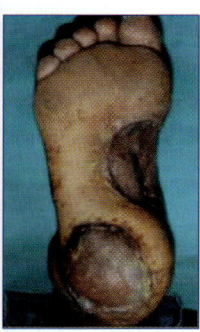

Fig. 9.9 Medial plantar artery flap for soft-tissue defect of the heel after excision of the trophic ulcer.

2. *Local muscle flaps*: Small defects of the heel can be covered with local muscle flaps such as abductor hallucis brevis, flexor digitorum brevis, and abductor digiti minimi flaps, which are further covered with skin graft.
3. *Lateral calcaneal flap, lateral supramalleolar flap, sural artery flap* (**Fig. 9.10**), *saphenous flap, or propeller flaps* based on perforators of posterior tibial or peroneal artery can also be used as second-line choices because of the problem of long-term stability of these flaps.

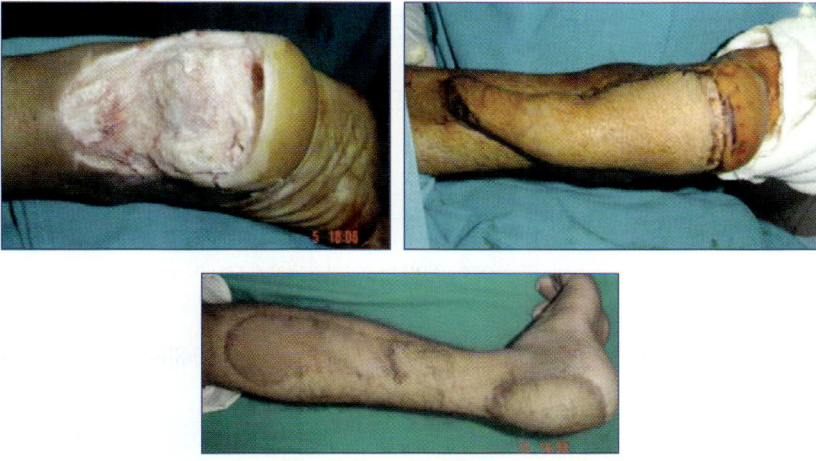

Fig. 9.10   Distally based sural artery based local flap for posterior aspect of heel and tendo Achilles.

4. *Microvascular flaps*: Large and complex soft-tissue defects of weight-bearing area of the foot can be covered with free microvascular flaps. Muscle flaps covered with skin graft are flaps of choice for weight-bearing areas as walking on the muscle flap is easier than on a fasciocutaneous flap. Latissimus dorsi (**Fig. 9.11**)

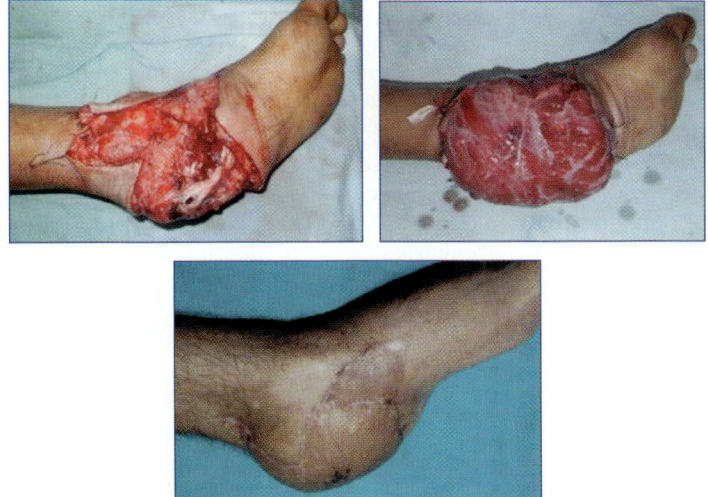

Fig. 9.11   Free microvascular latissimuss dorsi muscle flap for posttraumatic heel defect.

is the most commonly used muscle flap. Gracilis muscle can also be used for relatively smaller defects. For narrow and longitudinal defects, rectus abdominis muscle flap (**Fig. 9.12**) can be used. Muscle flaps bring more vascularity to the area, which helps in control of infection.

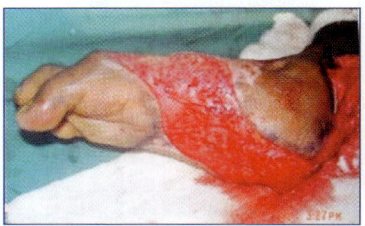
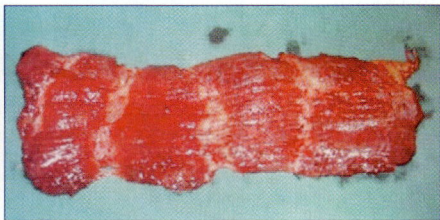
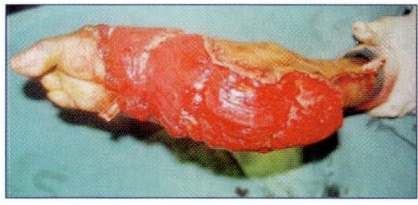
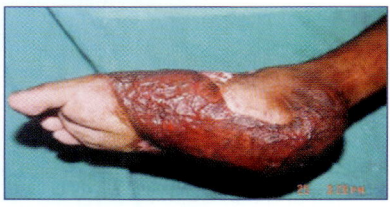

Fig. 9.12   Free microvascular rectus abdominis muscle flap for soft-tissue of the sole.

5. *Use of cross-leg flap in foot and ankle reconstruction:* Cross-leg flaps are still a very relevant option in situations where microvascular flaps cannot be done. The most common indication in developing countries is nonavailability of a microvascular surgeon. A cross-leg flap comes as a rescue flap in case of nonavailability of a suitable vessel for anastomosis, in a patient medically unfit for long surgery, economic reasons in an uninsured patient, or after failure of a microvascular flap.

A cross-leg flap can be raised as medially based conventional cross-leg flap (**Fig. 9.13**), proximally based (**Fig. 9.14**), or distally based (**Fig. 9.15**) cross-leg fasciocutaneous flaps. Inconvenience caused by cross-leg flaps has been considerably reduced with the use of external fixators.

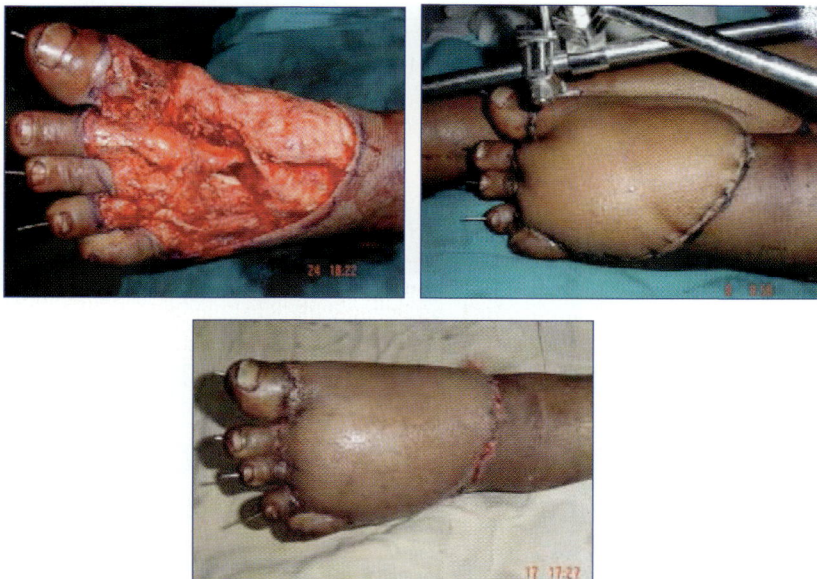

Fig. 9.13 Medially based conventional cross leg flap for soft-tissue defect of dorsum of the foot.

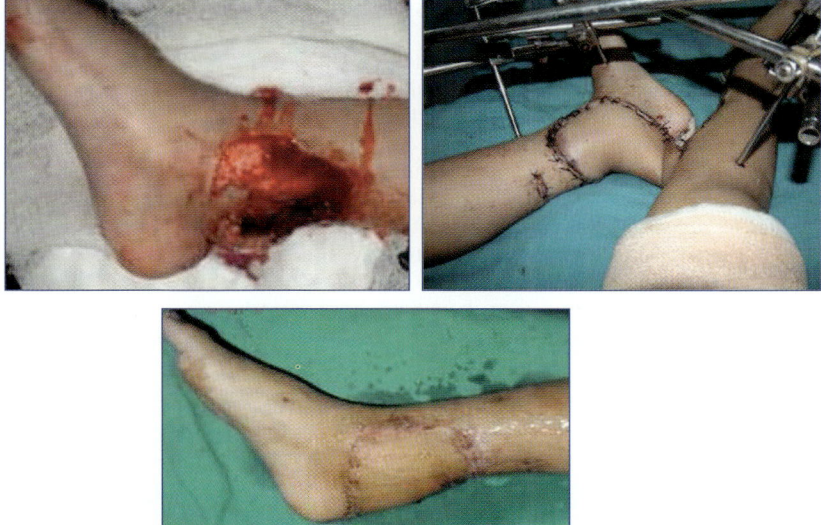

Fig. 9.14 Proximally based cross-leg flap for soft-tissue defect of posteromedial region of ankle.

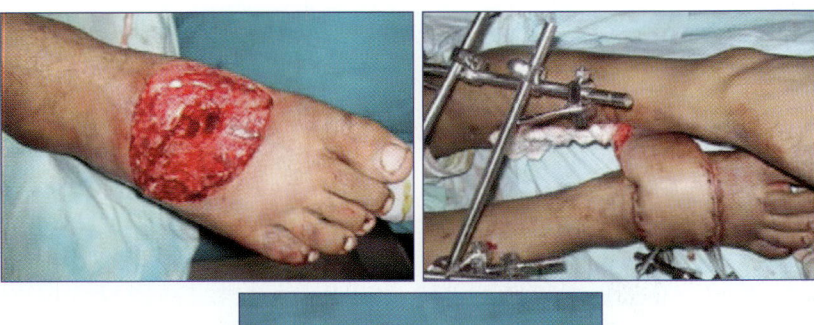

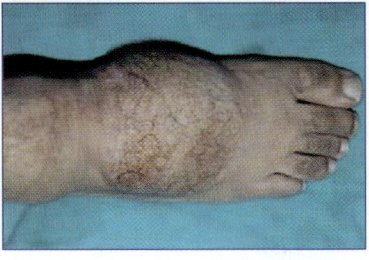

Fig. 9.15 Distally based cross-leg flap for soft-tissue defect of dorsum of foot.

Tips and Tricks

♦ Before embarking upon soft-tissue coverage, radical wound debridement should be done under loupe magnification.
♦ Proper planning of local and regional flaps is the key to success.
♦ Suturing of the flap under tension, kinking, or compression of the pedicle are the important causes of failure and should be avoided.
♦ Inadequate hemostasis can also be a cause of compression.
♦ In case of a free flap, anastomosis should be done outside the zone of trauma.
♦ Maintenance of postoperative immobilization with an external fixator or splintage for at least 3 weeks is very important.
♦ Compression stockings or crepe bandages are used after the wounds have completely healed in about 2 to 3 weeks and are continued for about 6 months.
♦ Weight bearing is started after about 6 weeks of surgery.
♦ Proper foot care and use of adequate footwear is crucial to prevent repeated ulcerations.

Plantar Heel Pain

Plantar heel pain is not the diagnosis! Clinician must aim to arrive at etiological diagnosis!

Diagnosis of Plantar Heel Pain

To arrive at a correct diagnosis, answers should be sought for the following three questions:

Question 1: Is heel pain referred from same joint or not?
Answer: Refer to **Box 10.1.**

Box 10.1   Causes of heel pain.

♦ Local cause
♦ Distant cause/Referred pain from:
  • Spine and sacroiliac (SI) joint
  • Knee
  • Hip

Points of Differential Diagnosis

♦ Signs and symptoms of original condition such as back, knee, or hip pain is predominant than foot and ankle pain
♦ Foot and ankle examination is normal
♦ Pain is in the specific dermatome
♦ Investigations help in the diagnosis

Question 2: What is the underlying pathology of heel pain?
Answer: Refer to **Box 10.2**.

Box 10.2	Underlying pathology heel pain.

♦ Local pathology (foot and ankle)
♦ Systemic pathology

Point of Differential Diagnosis

♦ Heel pain due to systemic etiology would be mostly bilateral

Question 3: What is the etiology for locally originating heel pain?
Answer: Refer to **Box 10.3**.

Box 10.3	Etiology of heel pain

♦ Mechanical
♦ Neuritic
♦ Bony
♦ Infective
♦ Combined

Points of Differential Diagnosis

♦ Mechanical—abnormal foot and ankle mechanics in the form of pes planus, pes cavus or deformed foot
♦ Neurological—neuritic pain that also radiates
♦ Bony—bony abnormality such as plantar exostosis following malunited fracture calcaneus
♦ Infective—foot and ankle infection such as osteomyelitis, Madura mycosis or tuberculous sinuses
♦ Combined—more than two problems may be associated as cause for plantar heel pain

Points of Significance in History

♦ Bilateral heel pain suggests systemic etiology
♦ Pain in other joints in the body suggests systemic etiology
♦ Night pain suggests infective or neoplastic etiology
♦ Burning pain or tingling numbness suggests neuritic etiology
♦ Pain at heel strike can be due to fat pad atrophy or stress fracture of calcaneus
♦ Pain at toe off can be due to plantar fasciitis
♦ Pain at the back of heel can be due to tendo Achilles disorders
♦ Painful first step in the morning suggests plantar fasciitis

♦ Radiation of pain suggests neuritic etiology
♦ History of amount of weight-bearing time spent is equally important as the amount of weight gained
♦ History of recent change in the activities and weight gain is important

Points of Significance in Clinical Examination

♦ *Location of pain*: This is the key feature. Ask the patient to point out at the location of pain (**Fig. 10.1**). The precise location of pain will help the examiner in deducing a probable cause for the pain (**Table 10.1**).

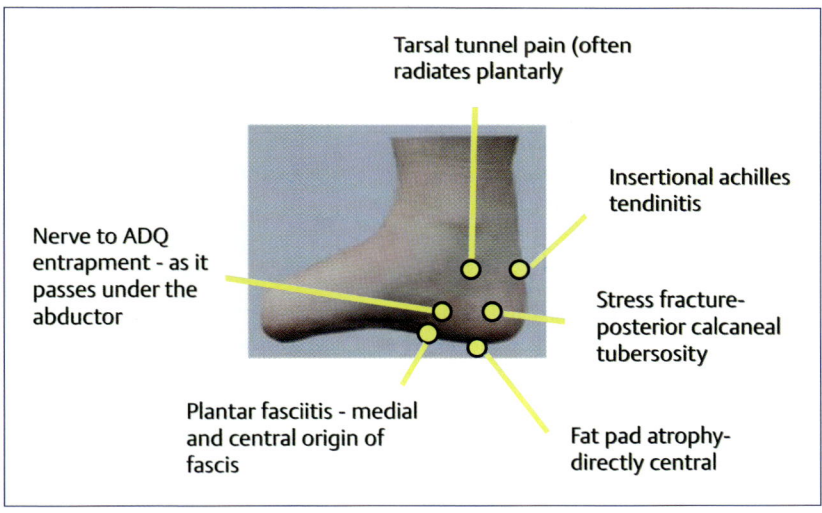

Fig. 10.1   Various locations of pain can direct examiner toward possible cause. ADQ, abductor digiti quinti.

Table 10.1   Location of heel pain and probable cause

Location of pain	Probable cause
Medial calcaneal tubercle	Proximal plantar fasciitis
Distal aspect of plantar fascia	Distal plantar fasciitis
Body of calcaneus	Stress fracture
Lateral border of heel	Entrapment of nerve to abductor digiti quinti
Central plantar aspect of heel	Fat pad atrophy
Posterior aspect of heel	Tendo Achilles tendinopathies
Master knot of Henry	Flexor hallucis longus (FHL) tendinitis
Medial side of ankle	Tarsal tunnel syndrome
Central part of plantar fascia	Plantar fibromatosis

♦ Tenderness at body of calcaneus suggests stress fracture.
♦ Shifting tenderness suggests neuritic etiology.
♦ Standing examination is done to rule out arch problems as well as to diagnose dynamic deformities.
♦ General examination is aimed at looking for pathologies in spine, hips, knees, and other joints.
♦ No examination is complete without looking at orthotics and footwear.

Investigations

♦ Hemogram, ESR, and serum investigations such as RA test, uric acid, ANA, and HLAB-27
♦ Nerve conduction studies and electromyogram
♦ Plain X-rays: look for Haglund's deformity, heel spur, osteoporosis, old fractures, tumors, etc
♦ USG: posterior heel pathologies
♦ MRI: posterior heel pathologies, stress fracture, plantar fasciitis
♦ Bone scan: stress fracture

Spot Differential Diagnosis

♦ Distal heel pain suggests distal plantar fasciitis
♦ Atrophied heel in elderly patient suggests fat pad syndrome
♦ Pain and tenderness on lateral side of heel suggest entrapment of nerve to abductor digiti quinti
♦ Doughy swelling in front of and above insertion of tendo Achilles suggests retrocalcaneal bursitis
♦ Doughy swelling at back of heel at insertion of tendo Achilles suggests Achilles bursitis
♦ Sudden acute knife-like pain with history of trauma or sprain with ecchymosis suggests plantar fascia rupture
♦ Trivial trauma or strain with acute heel pain with history of previous local injections suggests plantar fascia rupture
♦ Diffuse symptoms of dull or burning pain increasing on activities suggest tarsal tunnel syndrome
♦ Pain with weight-bearing worsening on prolonged standing suggests stress fracture of calcaneus
♦ Deep bone pain more during night without any relationship with activities with or without constitutional symptoms suggests the presence of a tumor

Sample Etiological Diagnosis

♦ Diagnosis 1—Plantar heel pain due to proximal plantar fasciitis plus compression of nerve to abductor digiti minimi in a case of adult acquired flat foot deformity plus obesity.

♦ Diagnosis 2—Plantar heel pain due to distal plantar fasciitis with gout and associated posttrauma midfoot deformity.

Management

Treatment is directed at etiological diagnosis!
The three-step protocol of heel pain management are as follows:

Step 1: Primary conservative treatment modalities

♦ Treatment of systemic disease
♦ Physical treatment by ultrasound, laser, massage, hot fomentation, or contrast bath
♦ Reduction of weight-bearing activities
♦ Modification of training for athletes
♦ Total non–weight bearing in few cases or a weight-bearing walking below knee plaster cast
♦ Lifestyle modification and weight reduction
♦ Plantar fascia, tendo-Achilles, and hamstrings stretching exercises (**Fig. 10.2**)

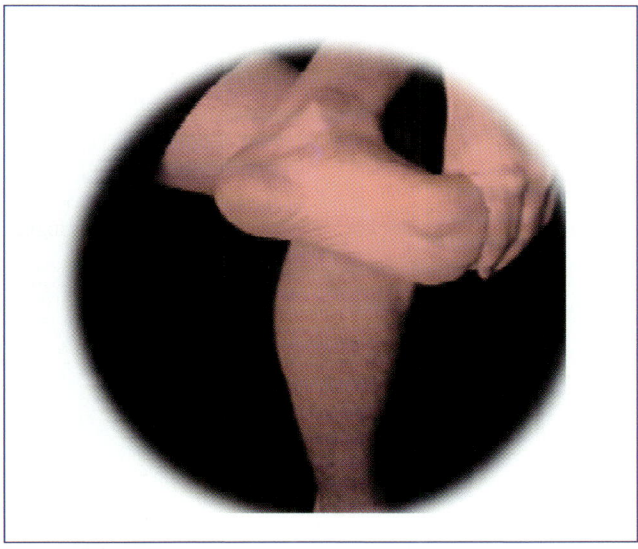

Fig. 10.2   Typical plantar fascia stretching exercise.

♦ Drugs: nonsteroidal anti-inflammatory drugs (NSAIDs) and neurotropic drugs
♦ Orthosis—heel lift or soft heel pad, medial longitudinal arch support, deep heel cup
♦ Night splints—Ankle foot orthosis (AFO) in 5° of dorsiflexion (**Fig. 10.3**)

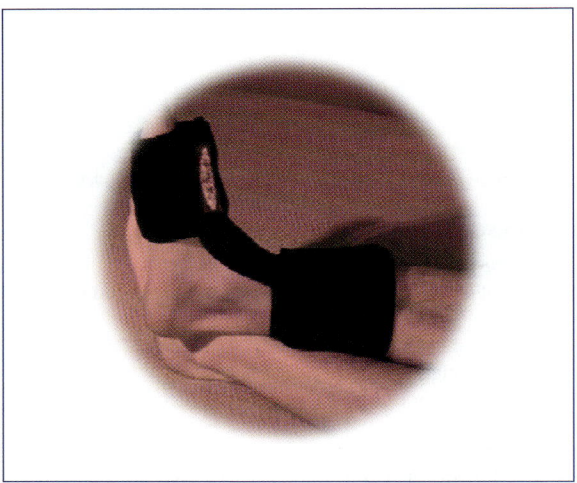

Fig. 10.3   AFO in 5° of dorsiflexion.

♦ Cane rolling exercises at home to increase flexibility of plantar fascia (**Fig. 10.4**).

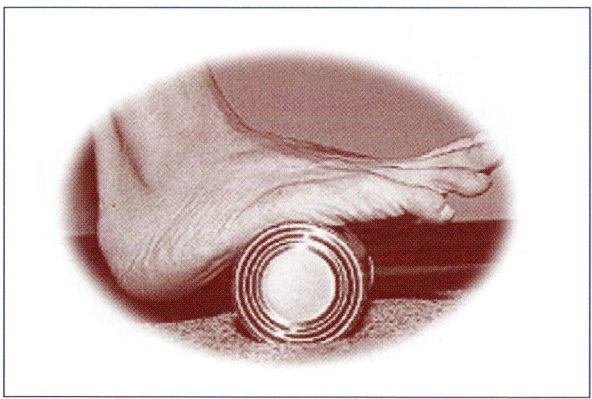

Fig. 10.4   Cane rolling exercise.

♦ Rarely local steroids—Thumb rule is to inject dorsal to spur and never inject in plantar fascia or in heel fat pad. Place the needle superior to fascia from the medial side so that the solution spreads across fascial layer and avoids nerves and fat pad. (**Fig. 10.5**)

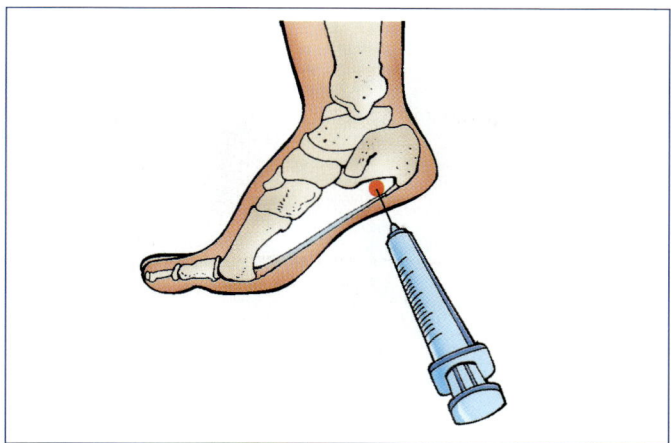

Fig.10.5   Method of giving local steroid injection for heel pain.

Primary conservative treatment modalities are continued for 3 to 6 months.

Reassurance that heel pain is self-limiting plays important role in mental outlook of patient!

Step 2: Secondary conservative treatment modalities

◆ Posterior tibial nerve block
◆ Extracorporeal shock wave therapy (ESWNL) (**Fig. 10.6**)
◆ Radiofrequency (RF) coblation (**Fig. 10.7**)
◆ Cast, cam walker for 4 to 6 weeks
◆ Platelet-rich plasma (PRP) injections
◆ Gastrocnemius recession

Secondary conservative treatment modalities are tried for 6 to 12 months.

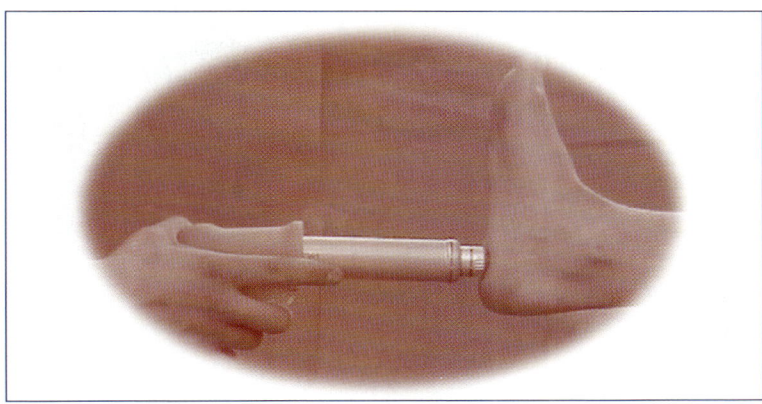

Fig. 10.6   Extracorporeal shockwave being applied to heel.

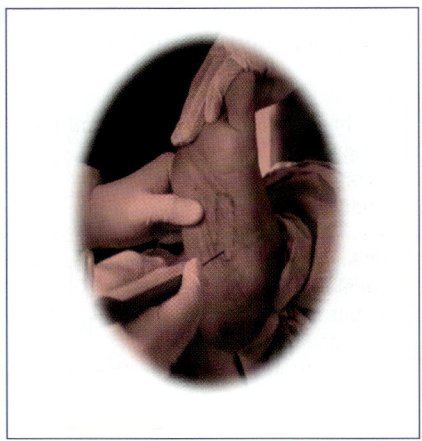

Fig. 10.7 Radiofrequency probe being inserted for the treatment of distal plantar fasciitis.

Step 3: Surgical treatment modality

♦ Surgery is advised after failure of all conservative treatment modalities tried for 12 months

♦ Plantar fascia release from the bone is aimed as a soft tissue procedure

♦ Decompression of first branch of lateral plantar nerve as a neurological procedure (**Fig. 10.8**)

♦ Excision of heel spur as a bony procedure (which is controversial)

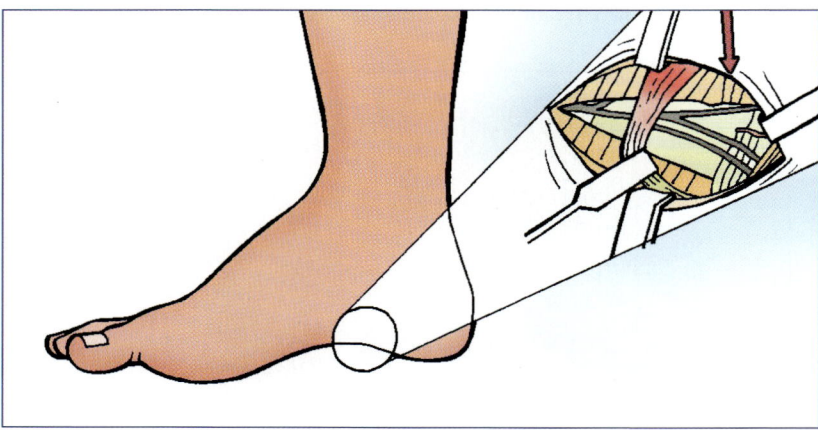

Fig. 10.8 Line diagram demonstrating release of nerve and plantar fascia excision.

◆ Supine position with lowering of head at the end of a table will help a lot
◆ Use of tourniquet, 2.5 magnification, and strong illumination at foot end is mandatory
◆ Ligation of all varicosities encountered is very important
◆ Retraction of abductor hallucis muscle dorsally and plantarward is a must for complete neural decompression
◆ Use freer dissector to confirm precise decompression
◆ Rectangular piece of medial plantar fascia is excised
◆ Spur may not be the cause of pain, but at surgery it may be worthwhile to excise heel spur. In the context of developing countries, most patients have a set notion of spur being the cause of heel pain
◆ Always release tourniquet to check for capillary feeling of decompressed nerves and for meticulous hemostasis
◆ Early postoperative mobilization is the key to success
◆ In some noncompliant patients, a post-suture-removal below knee walking plaster cast may help to gain confidence
◆ Postoperative neuritic pain is expected to last up to 3 to 4 months
◆ Surgery can be done through endoscopic method but this procedure has a steep learning curve

Growing with Flat Feet: Childhood to Adulthood

Replace ignorance with aggression for treatment of adult flat foot! Replace aggression with reassurance for treatment of paediatric flat foot!

Adult Flat Foot

Every adult flat foot is not due to tibialis posterior insufficiency!
Insufficiency of tibialis posterior (TP) is the most common cause of flat feet in adults!

Diagnostic Algorithm

To reach at a correct diagnosis, the examiner needs to have answers for the following questions:

Question 1: Is there a flat foot?

Answer: History, clinical examination, and radiology would help in answering this question.

Question 2: What is the cause of flat feet?

Answer: Six basic sets of causes are found for adult flat feet.

1. Adult flexible flat foot
2. Adult acquired flat foot deformity (AAFD) or posterior tibial tendon dysfunction (PTTD) (**Fig. 11.1**)
3. Tarsal coalition (**Fig. 11.2**)
4. Posttraumatic, arthritic, or iatrogenic flat foot (**Fig. 11.3**)
5. Charcot flat foot (**Fig. 11.4**)
6. Neuromuscular flat foot
   Cause-specific diagnostic features of flat foot are displayed in **Table 11.1**.

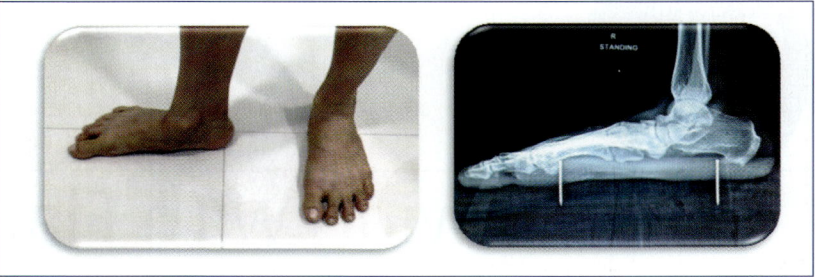

Fig. 11.1 Clinical and standing X-ray picture of a patient with adult acquired flat foot.

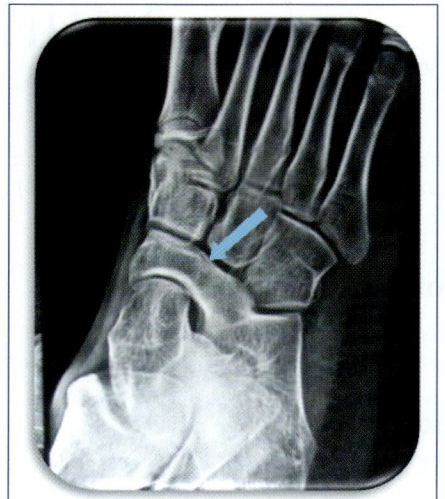

Fig. 11.2 X-ray picture of calcaneonavicular coalition.

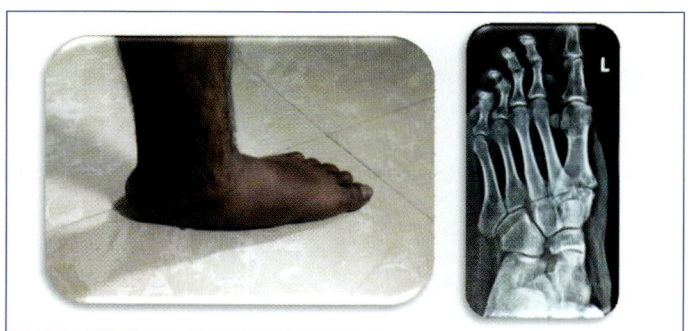

Fig. 11.3 Clinical and X-ray picture of flat foot due to arthritis of midfoot.

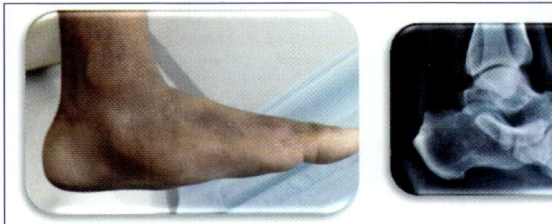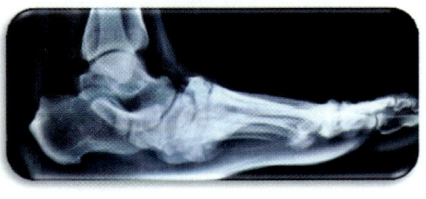

Fig. 11.4: Clinical picture and X-ray of flat foot due to midfoot Charcot.

Table 11.1	Cause-specific diagnostic features of flat foot	
S. No.	**Specific-cause of flat foot**	**Cause-specific diagnostic features**
1	TP tendon dysfunction	• Tender TP • Flat arch • Forefoot deformity • Hindfoot deformity • Too many toes sign +ve • Single heel raise test +ve • Radiological signs
2	Non-PTTD flat feet	• Postural complaints • Arch pain • Heel pain • Symptomatic weight bearing • TP intact • Foot flexible • Angle changes in radiology
3	Arthritic, post-traumatic, and iatrogenic flat foot	• History of trauma or • prior surgery • RA or seronegative arthritides • Joint pain along with effusion • Radiology shows implant, arthrosis, malalignment
4	Tarsal coalition	• Adolescent age • Symptoms ± • Reduced motion of hindfoot • Peroneal spasm • Rigid flat foot • Radiology • CT Scan
5	Charcot foot	• History of swelling and deformity • Neuropathy • Radiology shows joint destruction, osteolysis, fractures, and vascular calcifications
6	Adult neuromuscular flat foot	• History of trauma, or prior surgery • Pain on ambulation • Gait abnormalities • Neuromuscular dysfunction • Radiology shows anomalies and malalignment

Question 3: Which is the stage of adult acquired flat feet (AAFD)?
Answer: Stage-specific diagnostic algorithm is displayed in **Flowchart 11.1**. Stage-specific flat foot is well depicted in **Figs. 11.5** to **11.13**.

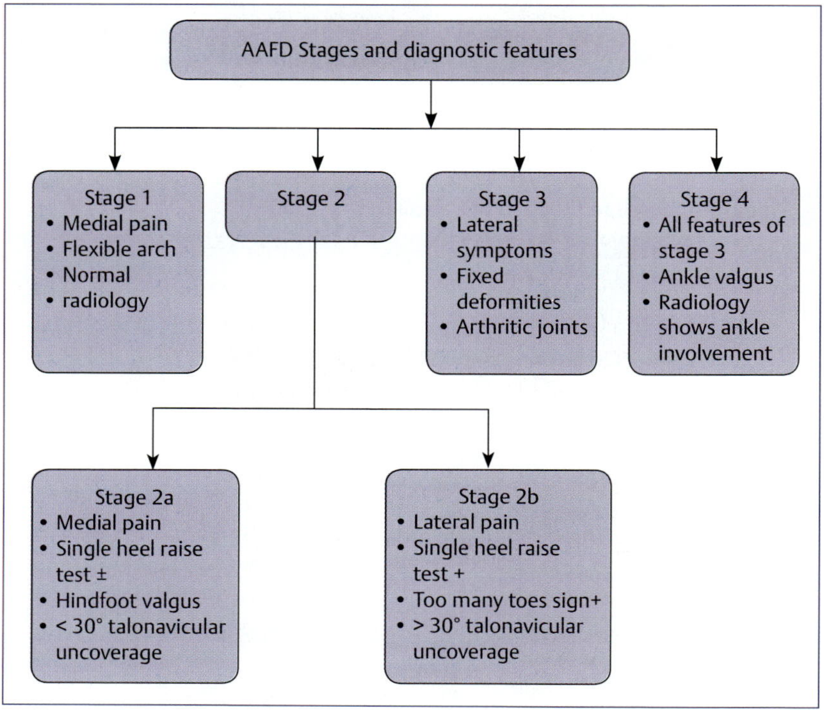

```
                    AAFD Stages and diagnostic features

    ┌──────────────┬──────────────┬──────────────┬──────────────┐

    Stage 1          Stage 2          Stage 3          Stage 4
  • Medial pain                     • Lateral         • All features of
  • Flexible arch                     symptoms          stage 3
  • Normal                          • Fixed           • Ankle valgus
  • radiology                         deformities     • Radiology
                                    • Arthritic joints  shows ankle
                                                        involvement

            ┌──────────────┴──────────────┐

        Stage 2a                      Stage 2b
      • Medial pain                 • Lateral pain
      • Single heel raise           • Single heel raise
        test ±                        test +
      • Hindfoot valgus             • Too many toes sign+
      • < 30° talonavicular         • > 30° talonavicular
        uncoverage                    uncoverage
```

Flowchart 11.1   Adult acquired flat feet Stages and diagnostic features.

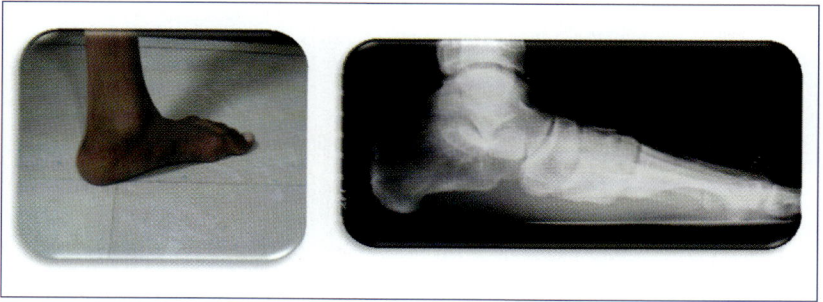

Fig. 11.5   Clinical and X-ray picture of Stage 1 adult acquired flat feet.

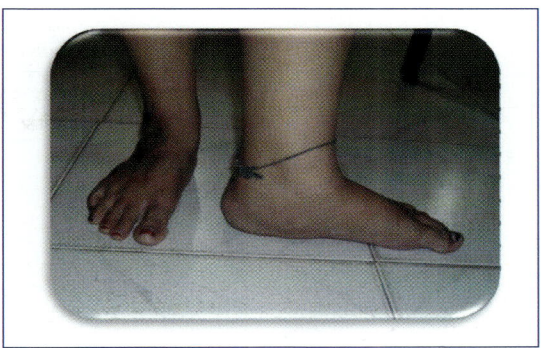

Fig. 11.6   Clinical picture of Stage 2 adult acquired flat feet.

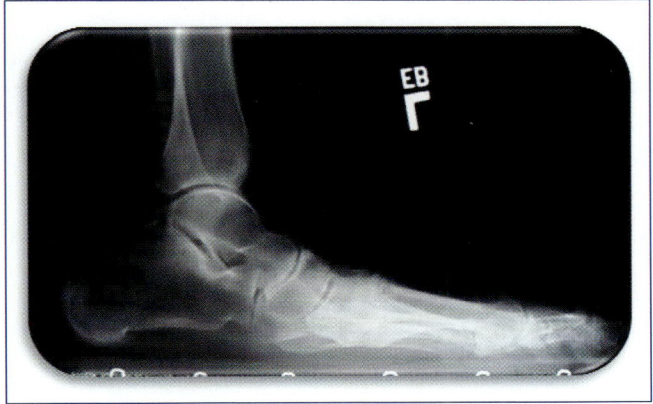

Fig. 11.7   X-ray picture of Stage 2 adult acquired flat feet.

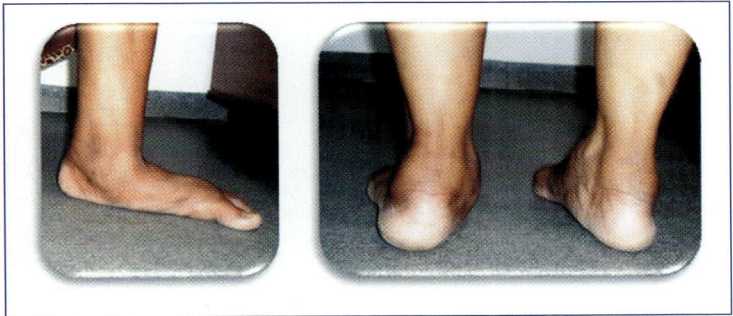

Fig. 11.8   Clinical picture of Stage 2b adult acquired flat feet with heel valgus.

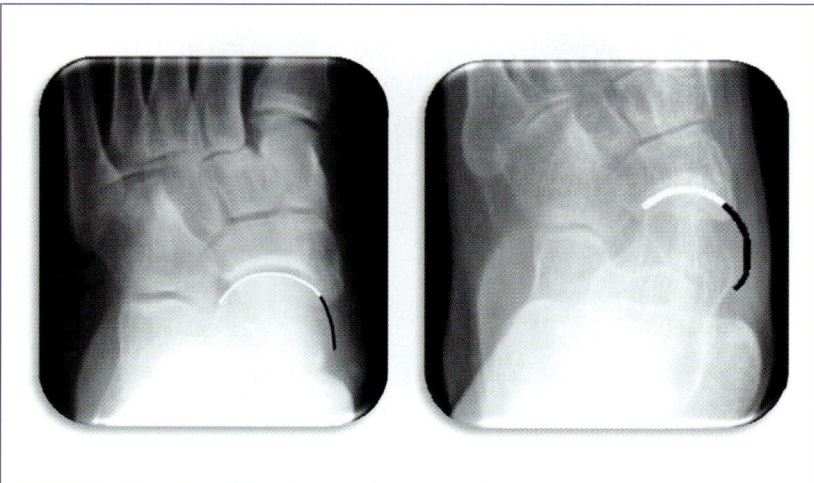

Fig. 11.9 X-ray pictures showing differentiation between a Stage 2a and Stage 2b adult acquired flat feet.

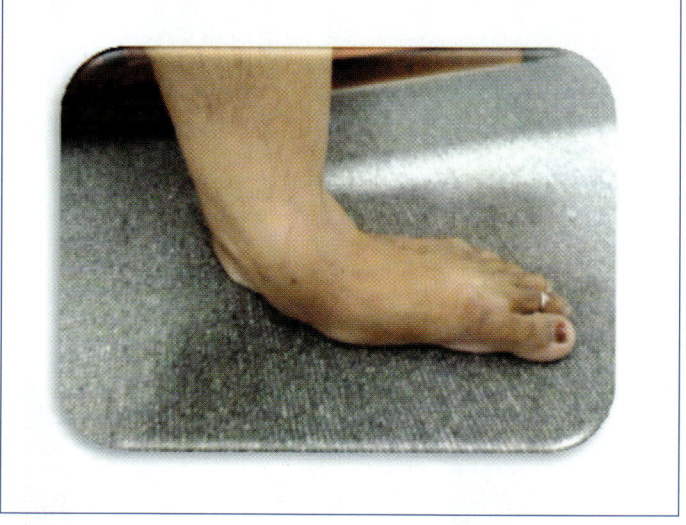

Fig. 11.10 Clinical picture of Stage 3 adult acquired flat feet.

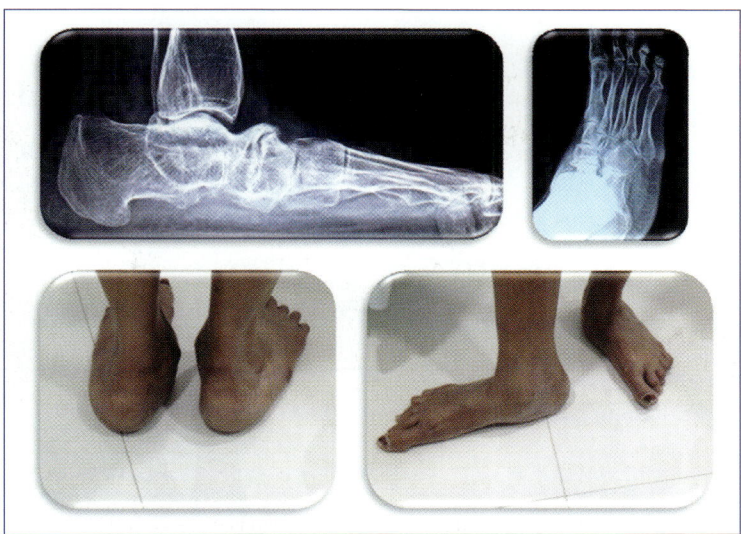

Fig. 11.11   Clinical and X-ray pictures of Stage 3 adult acquired flat feet.

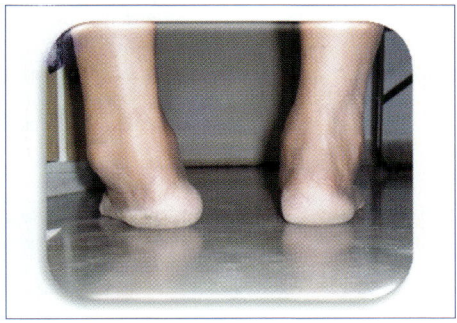

Fig. 11.12   Clinical picture of Stage 4 adult acquired flat feet.

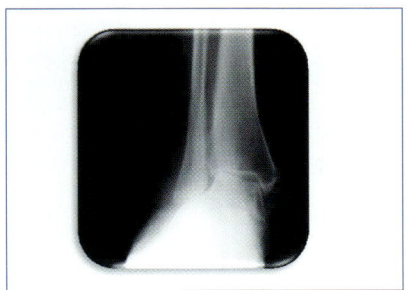

Fig. 11.13   X-ray picture of Stage 4 adult acquired flat feet.

Treatment

Treatment is directed toward specific cause of adult flat foot.

Cause-specific treatment of adult flat foot is explained in **Flowcharts 11.2** to **11.6**.

Stage-specific treatment of flat foot is explained in **Flowcharts 11.7** to **11.9**.

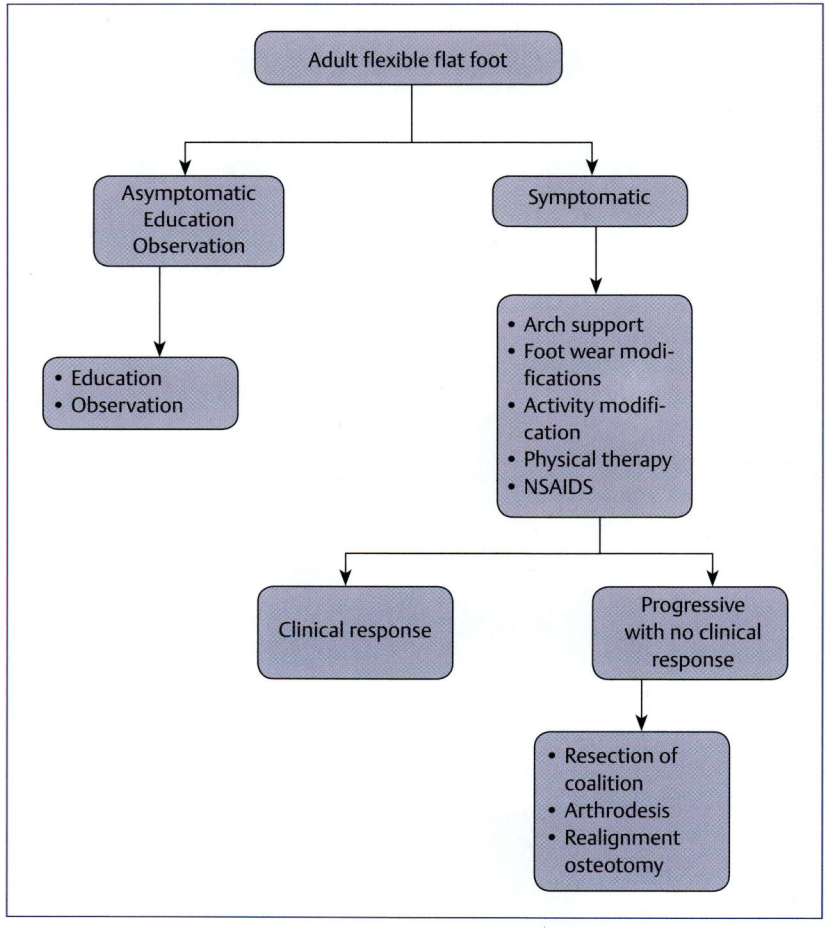

Flowchart 11.2   Treatment of adult flexible flat foot.

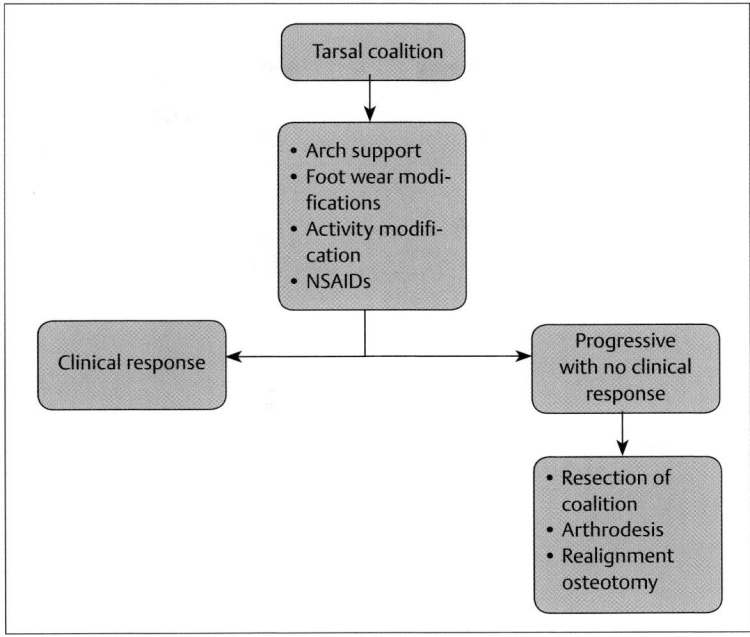

Flowchart 11.3   Treatment of tarsal coalition.

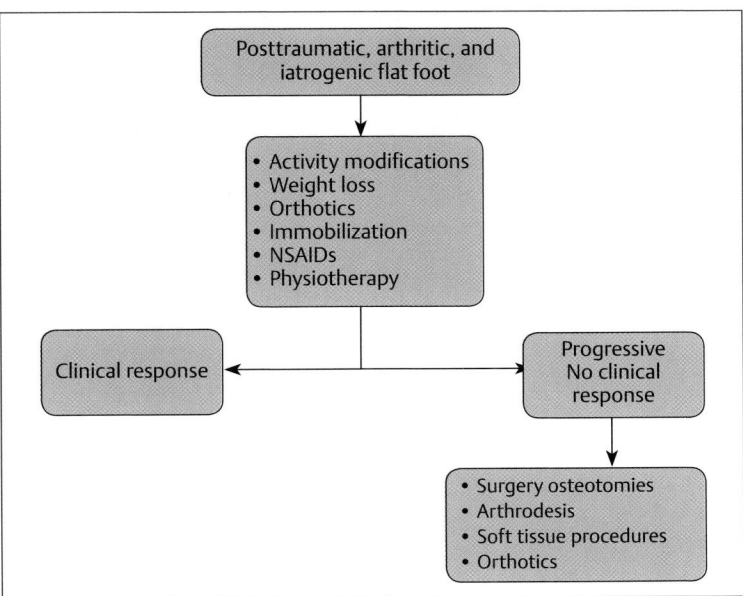

Flowchart 11.4   Treatment of posttraumatic, arthritic, and iatrogenic flat foot.

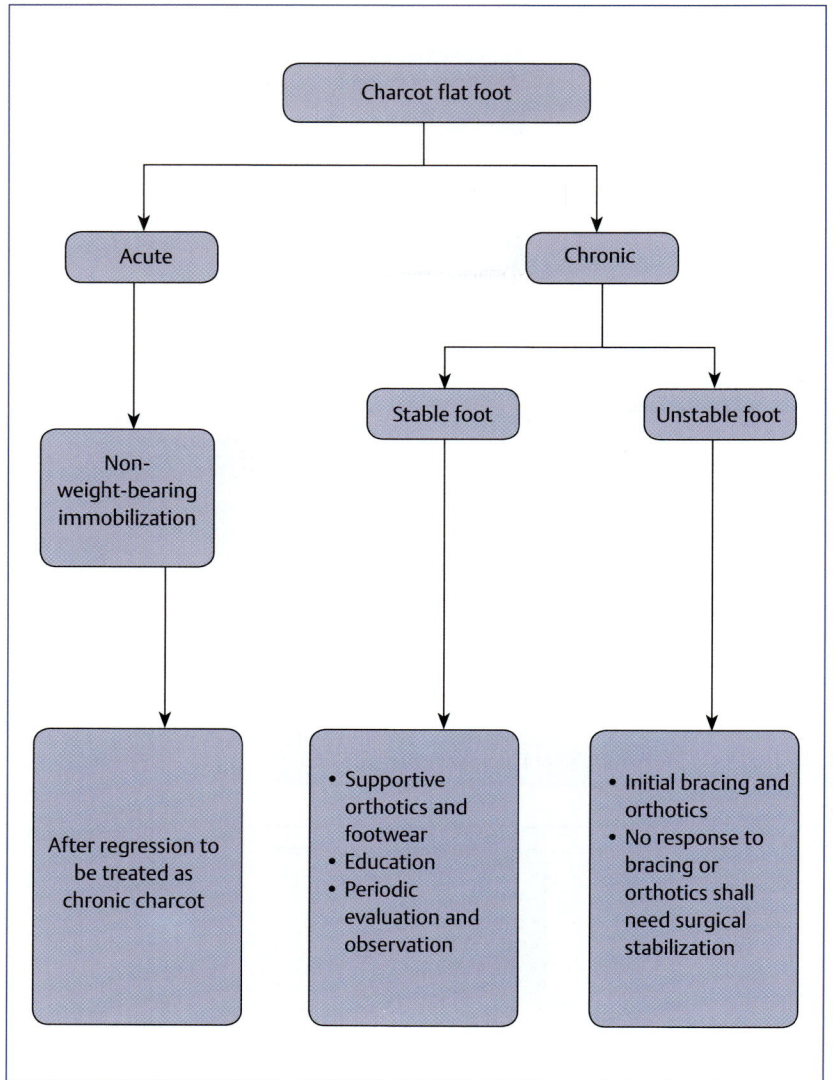

Flowchart 11.5 Treatment of charcot flat foot.

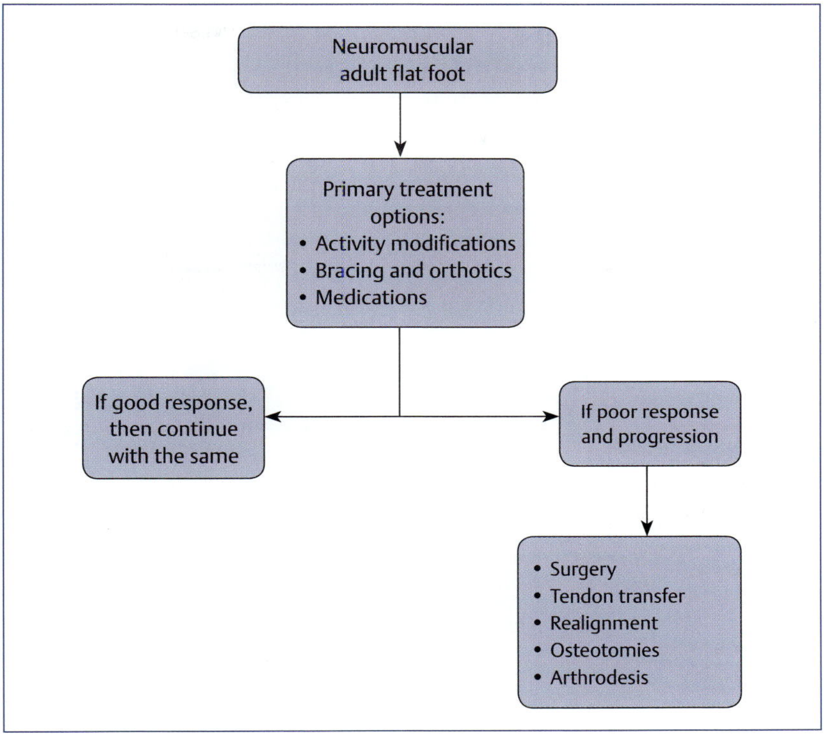

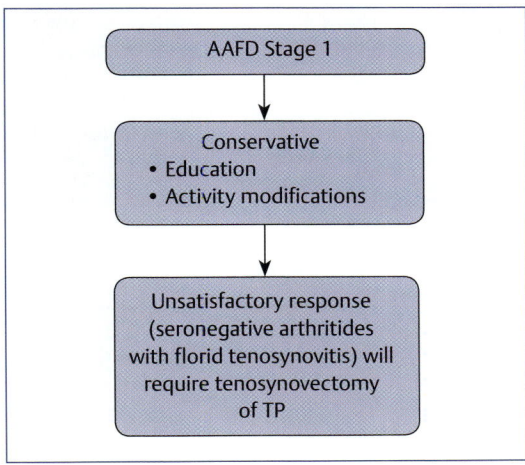

Flowchart 11.6   Treatment of neuromuscular flat foot.

Flowchart 11.7   Treatment options for Stage 1 adult acquired flat feet. TP, tibialis posterior.

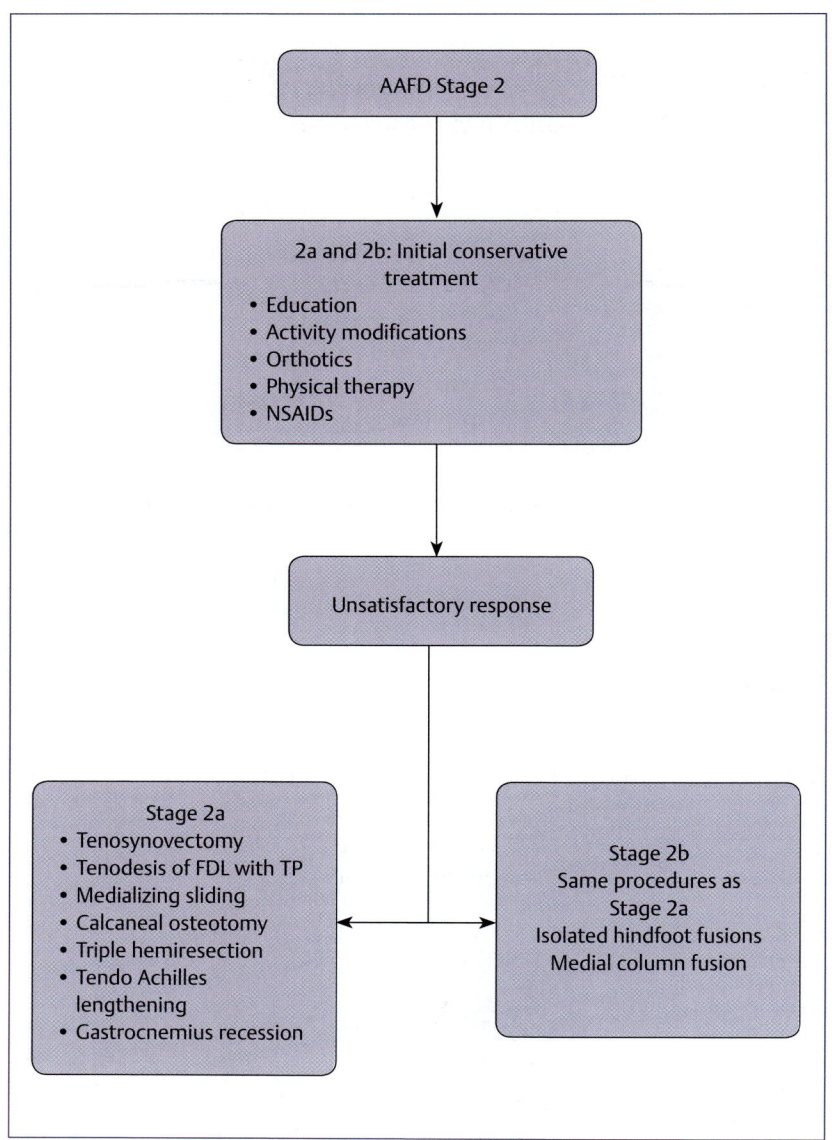

Flowchart 11.8 Treatment options for Stage 2 adult acquired flat feet.

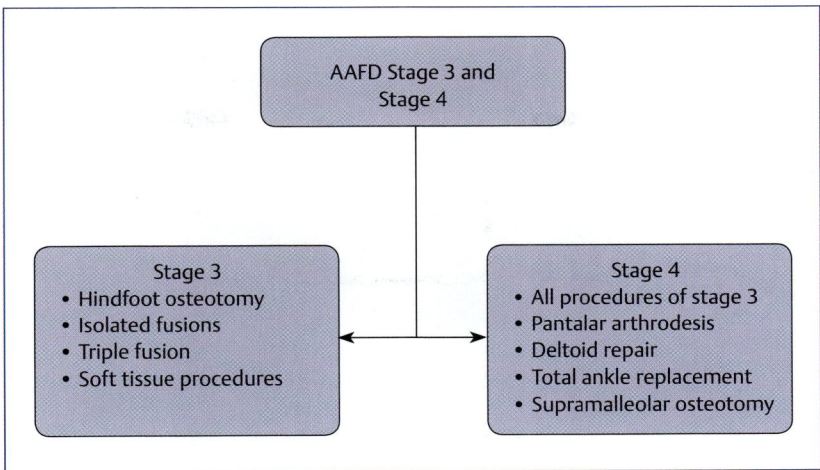

Flowchart 11.9 Treatment options for Stages 3 and 4 adult acquired flat feet.

Tips and Tricks

The following tips should be considered while opting for common adult acquired flat feet treatment procedures:

Tenosynovectomy of TP

1. Look at the undersurface of the tendon for a commonly missed tear.
2. Look at the turning of tendon at the medial malleolus for tear.
3. Always check the excursion of tendon before and after surgery.
4. Always close the retinaculum for prevention of snapping of tendon.
5. *Be prepared to change the procedure on looking at tendon's morphology, intraoperatively!*

Tenodesis and Transfer for TP

1. Use of bipolar coagulation is a must for many venous tributaries near the crossing of tendons of flexor digitorum longus (FDL) and flexor hallucis longus (FHL).
2. Doubly check tendon of FDL by passively flexing the four lateral toes.
3. Tension the transfer in maximum possible foot inversion.
4. Tenodesis of proximal cut end of TP tendon is done with tendon of FDL (**Figs. 11.14** and **11.16**).

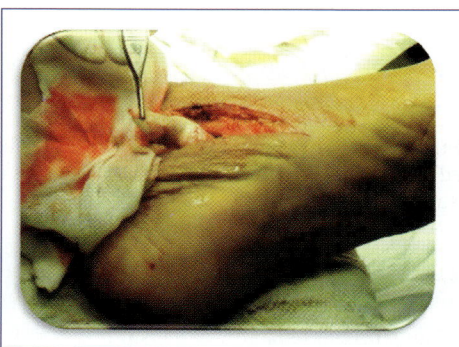

Fig. 11.14 Picture showing complete rupture of TP tendon at surgery.

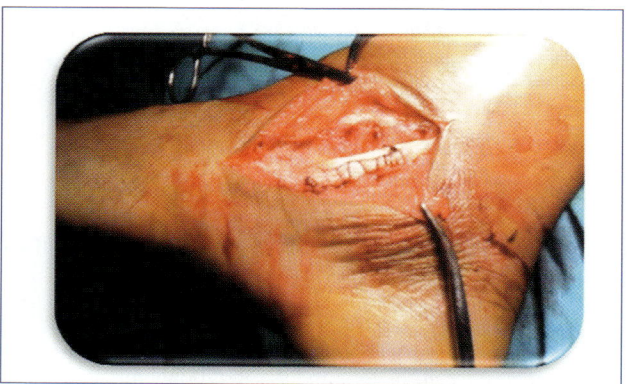

Fig.11.15 Operative picture showing tenodesis of TP with FDL tendon.

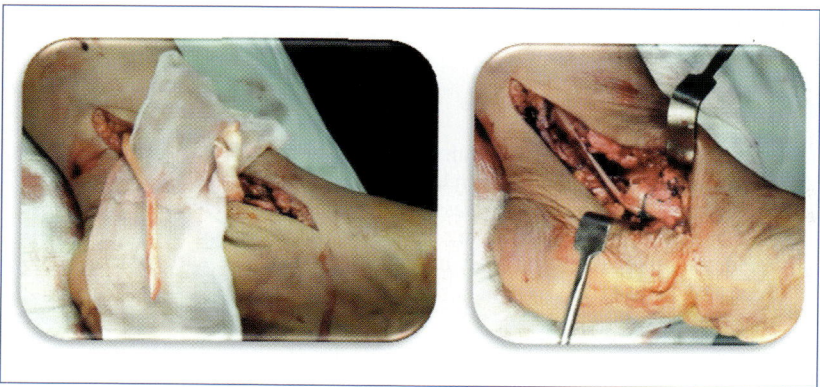

Fig.11.16 Operative pictures showing transfer of FDL to TP.

Medializing Calcaneal Slide Osteotomy

1. Identify and isolate the branch of sural nerve after the incision.
2. Two Holman retractors are used to protect, respectively, the tendo Achilles tendon and plantar structures during osteotomy.
3. Smooth lamina spreader is used to open up osteotomy. This allows surgeons to complete medial side of osteotomy under vision, thereby damage to important medial structures is prevented.
4. A 5-mm osteotome is used to pierce the medial side taking care to avoid injuring the medial neurovascular structures.
5. Fixation of screws must be from the non-weight-bearing area of the heel (**Fig. 11.17**).
6. After completion of osteotomy, the sharp lateral border of proximal fragment is tamped to make the bony edges smooth.

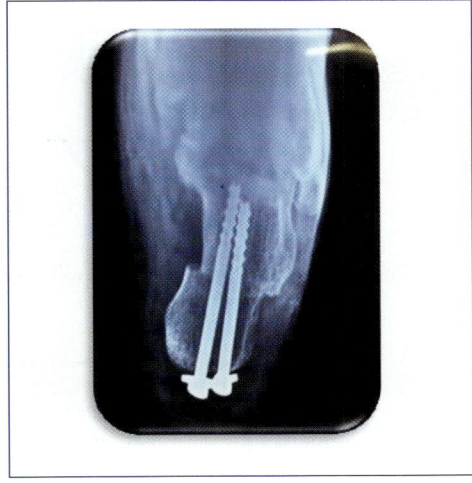

Fig. 11.17   Postoperative X-rays showing medializing calcaneal sliding osteotomy.

Tendo Achilles Procedures

♦ *Almost every flat foot surgery would need a tendo Achilles procedure!*
♦ During gastrocnemius recession procedure, utmost care in exploring and identifying the sural nerve is taken to prevent injury to the nerve (**Fig. 11.18**).
♦ Care is also taken to identify tendo Achilles and to complete the procedure of percutaneous lengthening of tendo Achilles while continuous dorsiflexion at the ankle is maintained (**Fig. 11.19**).

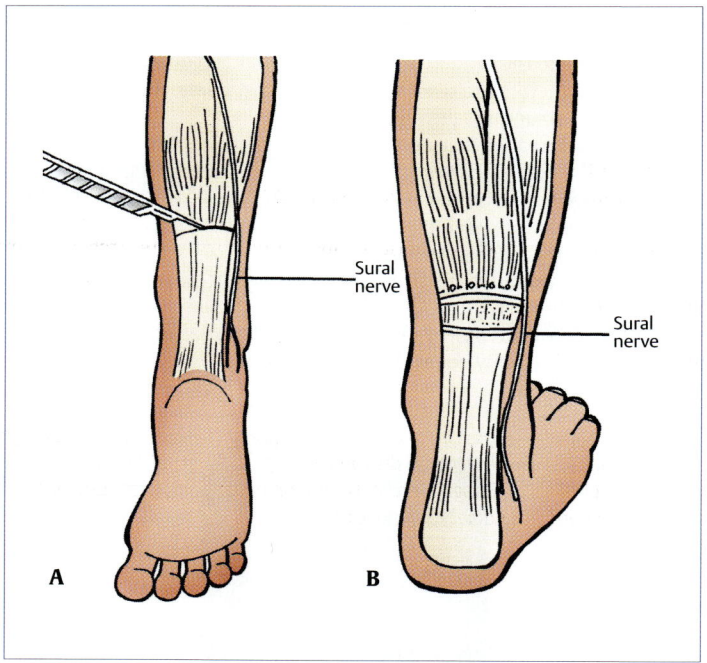

Fig. 11.18   Diagrammatic representation showing gastrorecession.

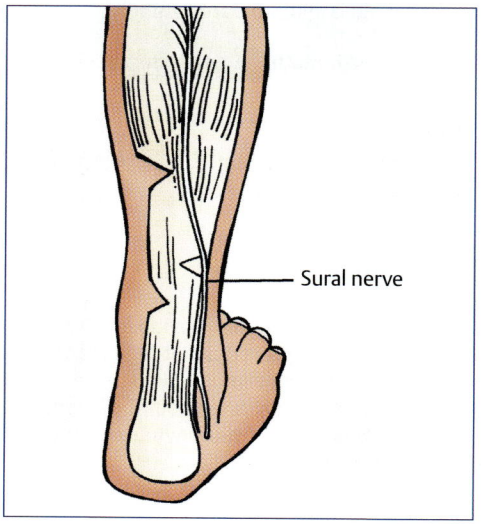

Fig. 11.19   Diagrammatic representation showing percutaneous tendo Achilles release.

Pediatric Flat Foot: Managing It Is an Art or Science?

We all are born with flat foot!

Facts

♦ We all are born with a flat foot!
♦ Full development of the arch occurs usually by 5 years, but may take up to 10 years!
♦ There is no evidence that orthotic support will formulate arch of a growing child's feet!
♦ Asymptomatic child does not need treatment for flat feet.
♦ For a symptomatic child, use of orthotics is justified!
♦ Same surgical principles apply to children as those for adults.
♦ *What can be done with an asymptomatic child with severe flat foot deformity is a gray zone!*
♦ *Orthopedician must possess the art to differentiate between a normal, benign variant versus one that would lead to disability if left untreated! Surgeon should have scientific insight of avoiding overtreatment of benign variant and not avoiding treatment of potentially disabling variant!*
♦ *Treatment of pediatric flexible flat foot is both art as well as science!*

Four Questions at Help

Question 1: Whether foot is flexible or rigid?

Question 2: Whether flexible foot is a normal anatomical benign variant or one that would lead to disability?

Question 3: Whether the child is symptomatic or not?

Question 4: Does the child need treatment or reassurance?

Treatment

Management of pediatric flat foot is explained in **Flowchart 11.10**.

Accessory navicular excision is depicted in **Fig. 11.20** and is explained in **Flowchart 11.11**.

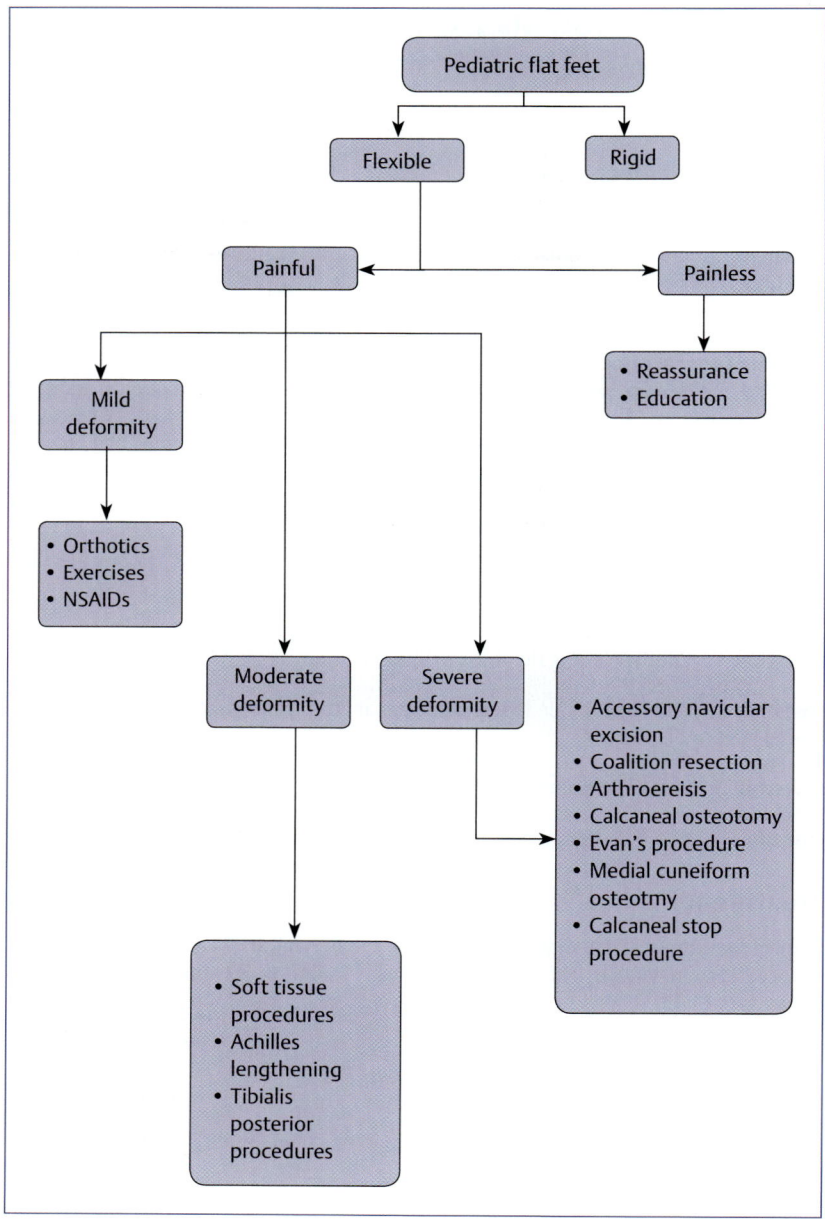

Flowchart 11.10 Management of pediatric flat foot.

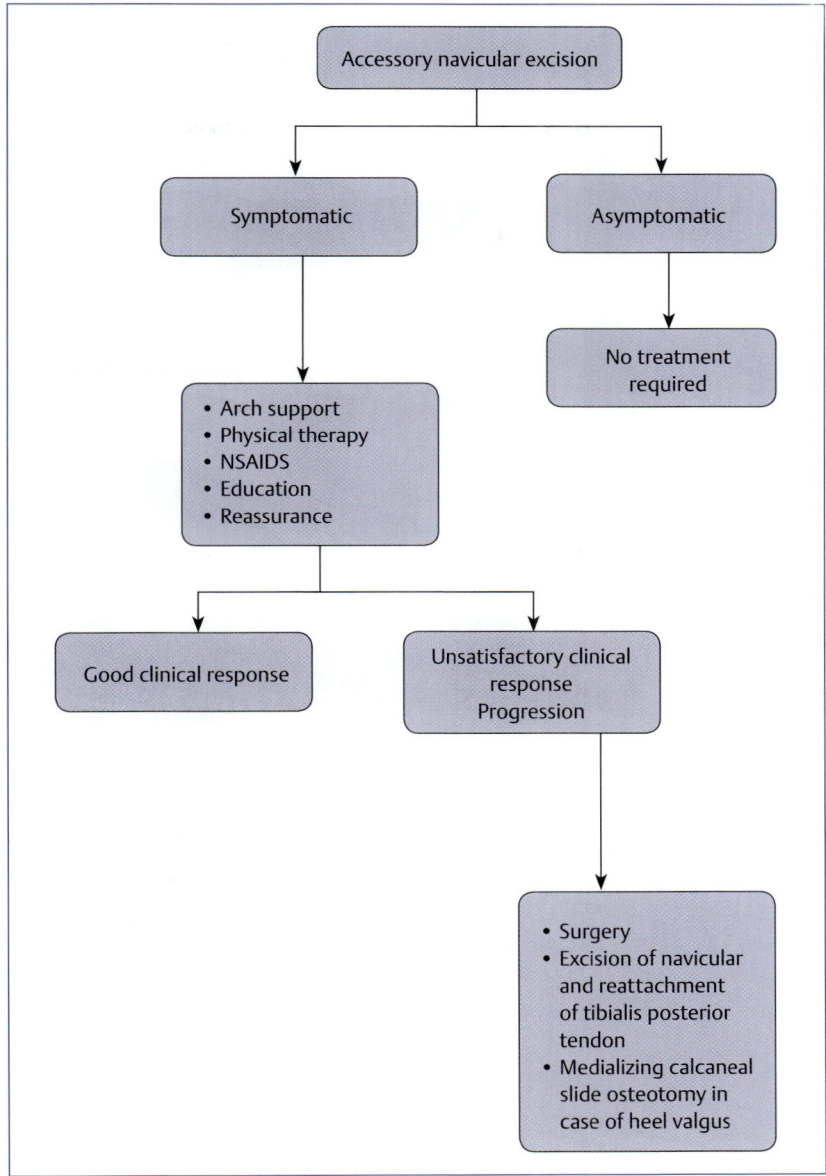

Flowchart 11.11   Accessory navicular excision.

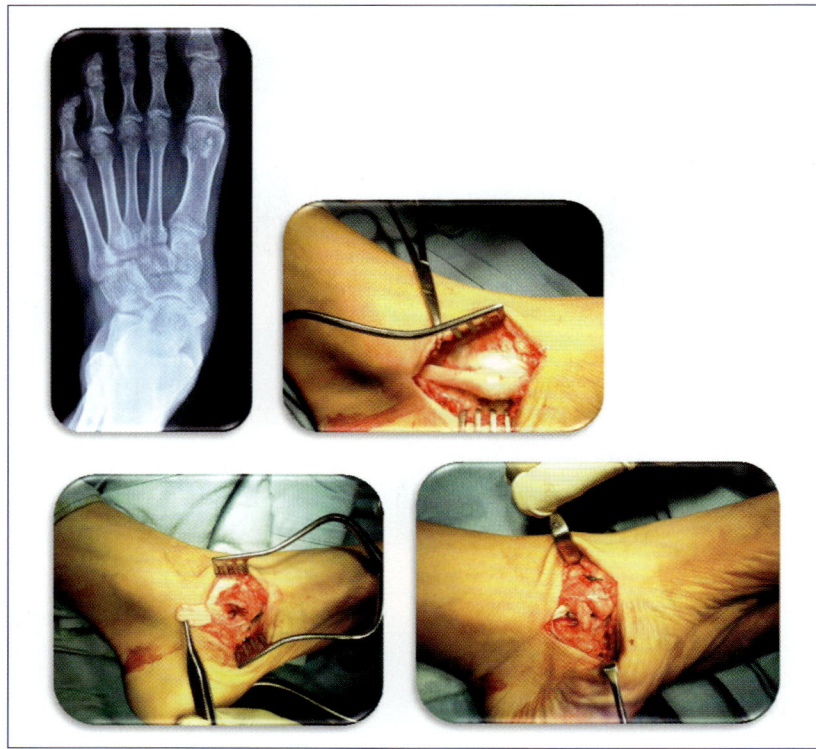

Fig. 11.20 Intraoperative photographs of a case with excision of accessory navicular and reattachment of tendon of TP.

Lucid Approach and Simplistic Management of Diabetic Foot

India is the diabetic capital of the world!

Alarming Facts about Diabetic Foot

♦ More than 135 million diabetics worldwide
♦ Number would reach up to 300 million by 2025
♦ India has second largest (70 million) diabetic population after China
♦ India would overtake China by 2025
♦ India has 35 million prediabetes patients
♦ 15% of confirmed diabetic patients will get ulcers once in their lifetime
♦ 1% will undergo higher-level amputation
♦ 200,000 higher-level amputations per year are done in India for infected diabetic foot ulcers/wounds and gangrene
♦ 50% of people who have amputation of one limb would need amputation of the other limb within 5 years
♦ Mortality rate following amputation is
  • 13% to 40% at 1 year
  • 35% to 65% at 3 years
  • 39% to 80% at 5 years
♦ 85% of these amputations can be completely prevented by simple cost-effective measures

Strategy to prevent an ulcer is to preserve and protect epidermal barrier in the presence of advancing neuropathy, vasculopathy, and loss of pain sensations!

Fig. 12.1 shows the reasons for ulcers in diabetic foot.

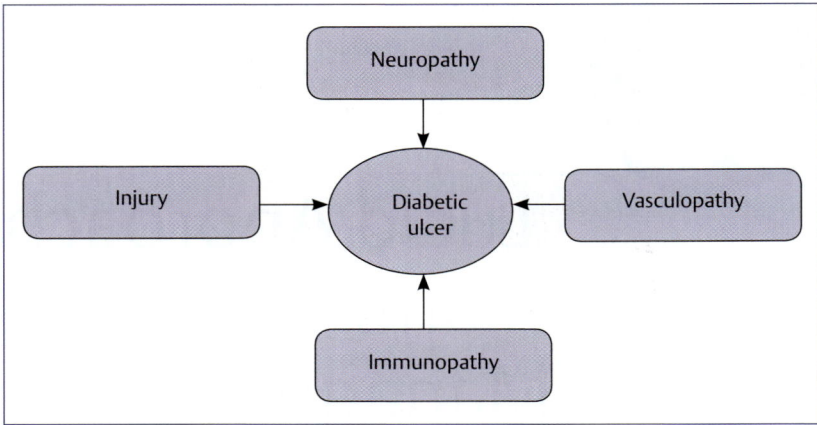

Fig. 12.1 Causes of ulcers in diabetic foot.

Clinical Examination of Foot to Assess the Risk of Ulcer

Three types of clinical examination can be done as shown in **Box 12.1**.

Box 12.1	Types of clinical examination of diabetic foot.

♦ **2-minute examination**
  - Vascular examination
  - Web space examination
  - Status of foot skin
  - Examination of ulcer
  - Foot wear examination
♦ **5-minute examination**
  - All examinations as in 2 minutes
  - Monofilament test (**Fig. 12.2**)
  - Test to check status of intrinsic muscles
  - Measurement of 1st toe extension with go niometer (**Fig. 12.5**)
♦ **10-minute examination**
  - All examinations as in 2 + 5 minutes
  - Ankle–brachial index
  - Test for heat andcold sensations
  - Test for vibration perception

The following are the tests done in case of diabetic foot ulcer.
♦ *Monofilament test*: Monofilament pressure testing of the sole of the foot is the simplistic means of diagnosis of neuropathy. Lack of feeling of pressure is the neuropathy (**Fig. 12.2**).

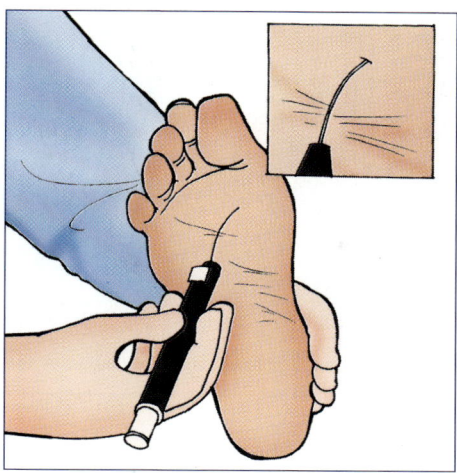

Fig. 12.2 Monofilament test.

◆ *Test for vibratory sense*: Biothesiometer measures vibratory sense. The probe is put at various areas of the sole of the foot to evaluate the perception of vibrations. Vibratory sensations are lost very early in the setting of neuropathy (**Fig. 12.3**).

◆ *Test for the evaluation of blood flow:* Vascular Doppler will evaluate the blood flow patterns in dorsalis pedis and posterior tibial arteries of foot and ankle. The kind of flow waves and the pattern of flow give an idea about the vascular status of the limb (**Fig. 12.4**).

◆ *Test to measure movements*: Goniometer is used to measure the movements of forefoot joints. In diabetics, loss of these movements would be an early predictor

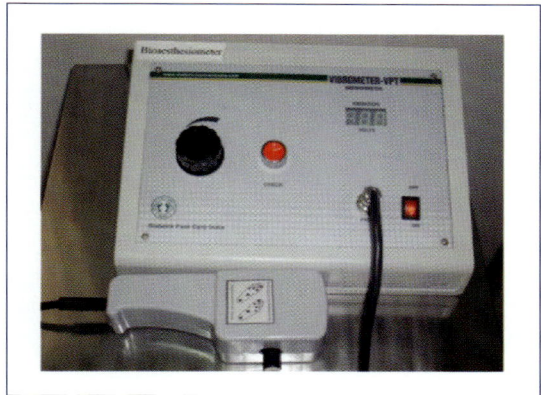

Fig. 12.3 Biothesiometer.

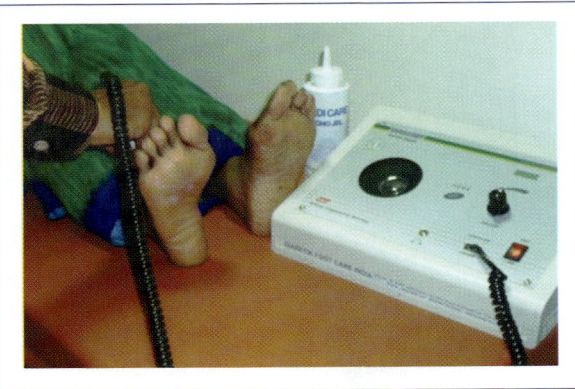

Fig. 12.4 Vascular Doppler.

of development of stiffness and deformities, which in turn may lead to ulcers. **Fig.12.5** shows the method of measurement of first metatarsophalangeal (MTP) joint extension with a goniometer.

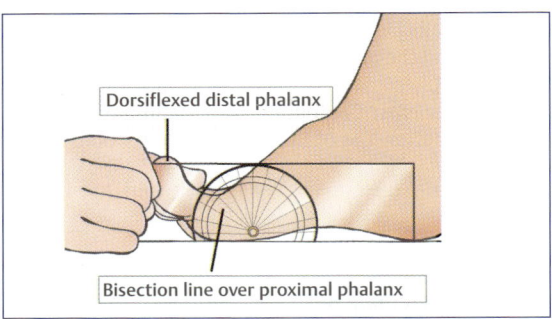

Dorsiflexed distal phalanx

Bisection line over proximal phalanx

Fig. 12.5 Test to measure movements.

Radiology

♦ Plain X-rays:
  • *Active infection in soft tissues*: Depicted in the form of swelling, fat plane obliteration, gas in cases with abscess or cellulitis due to gas-forming organisms (**Fig. 12.6**)
  • *Ulcer*: A soft tissue defect
  • *Bony lesions*: Bony erosions, osteomyelitis, Charcot neuroarthropathy, and arthritis of joint (**Fig. 12.7–12.9**).

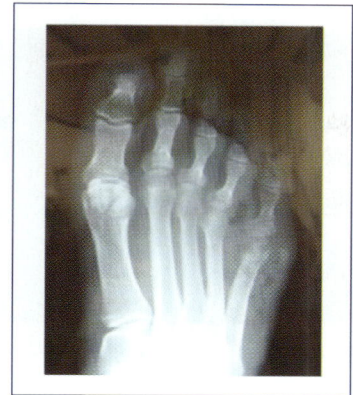

Fig.12.6   Diabetic foot infection with cellulitis showing gas in the soft tissues around the lateral aspect of foot in radiograph.

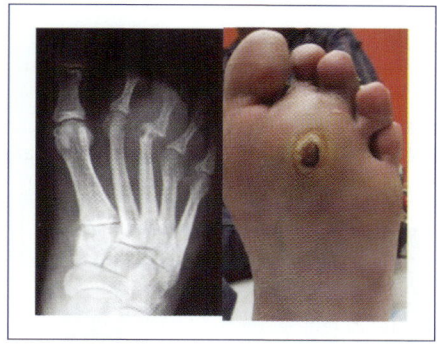

Fig. 12.7   Radiograph showing erosions in the head of third metatarsal in a patient with diabetic foot ulcer.

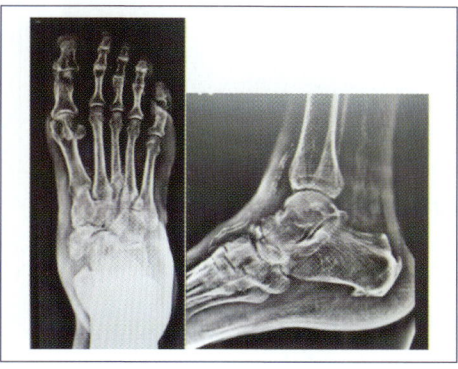

Fig. 12.8   X-ray showing Charcot midfoot.

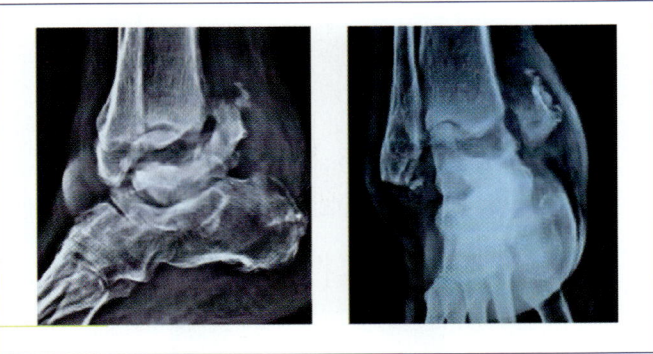

Fig. 12.9 X-ray showing hindfoot Charcot.

- Ultrasound:
  - Examination of masses: Either solid or fluid filled
  - Aspiration of abscess.
- Bone scan: Diagnosis of soft tissue versus bony infections.
- CT scan: Bone architecture.
- MRI (**Fig. 12.10**):
  - Abscess: Increased signal in T2, dark in T1.
  - Bone infection: Marrow edema bright in STIR, reduced marrow brightness in T1.

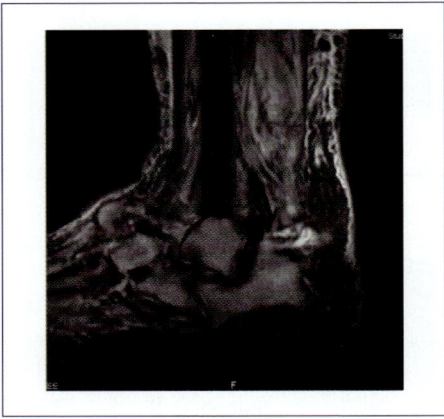

Fig. 12.10 MRI of diabetic Charcot arthropathy.

Treatment

Diabetic Ulcer and Wounds

Conservative treatment plan for diabetic foot ulcers is enumerated in **Flowchart 12.1**. Contact cast for diabetic ulcer is shown in **Fig. 12.11**.

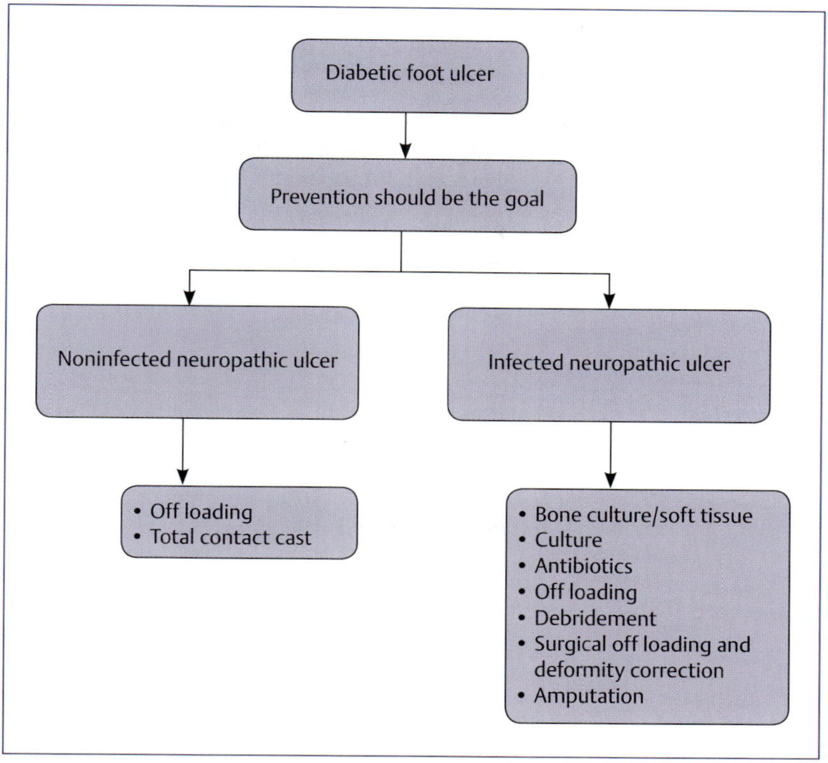

```
                    ┌─────────────────────────┐
                    │    Diabetic foot ulcer   │
                    └─────────────────────────┘
                                 │
                                 ▼
                    ┌─────────────────────────┐
                    │ Prevention should be the goal │
                    └─────────────────────────┘
                         │               │
          ┌──────────────┘               └──────────────┐
          ▼                                              ▼
┌───────────────────────────┐          ┌───────────────────────────┐
│ Noninfected neuropathic ulcer │      │  Infected neuropathic ulcer   │
└───────────────────────────┘          └───────────────────────────┘
          │                                              │
          ▼                                              ▼
┌───────────────────────┐              ┌───────────────────────────┐
│ • Off loading          │             │ • Bone culture/soft tissue   │
│ • Total contact cast   │             │ • Culture                    │
└───────────────────────┘             │ • Antibiotics                │
                                       │ • Off loading                │
                                       │ • Debridement                │
                                       │ • Surgical off loading and   │
                                       │   deformity correction       │
                                       │ • Amputation                 │
                                       └───────────────────────────┘
```

Flowchart 12.1   Conservative treatment plan for diabetic foot ulcer.

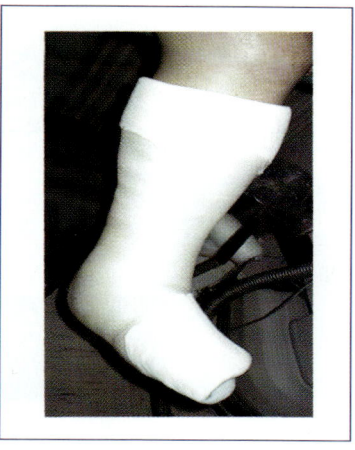

Fig. 12.11   Picture showing total contact cast for diabetic ulcer.

Newer modalities of diabetic wound care are listed below:

♦ Platelet-derived growth factor and epidermal growth factor
♦ Foam dressings
♦ Negative pressure wound therapy (VAC)
♦ Skin substitutes
♦ Jetflo debrider
♦ Ultrasonic debrider
♦ Versa jet debrider
♦ Maggot therapy
♦ CO_2 laser therapy
♦ Hyperbaric oxygen
♦ Biodegradable antibiotic granules
♦ Stem cell therapy
♦ Platelet-rich plasma therapy

The corrective surgeries used in the case of diabetic foot with deformities are listed below:

♦ Tendoachilles lengthening–percutaneous
♦ Flexor tenotomy for toe deformities
♦ IP excision arthroplasty for rigid deformity
♦ Excision of metatarsal head
♦ Dorsal wedge correction osteotomy for 1st MTP ulcers
♦ Transfer of tibialis anterior for inversion deformity

Dorsiflexion wedge correction osteotomy, midfoot exostectomy, and corrective hind foot arthrodesis as a means of surgical offloading are serially depicted in **Figs. 12.12** to **12.14**.

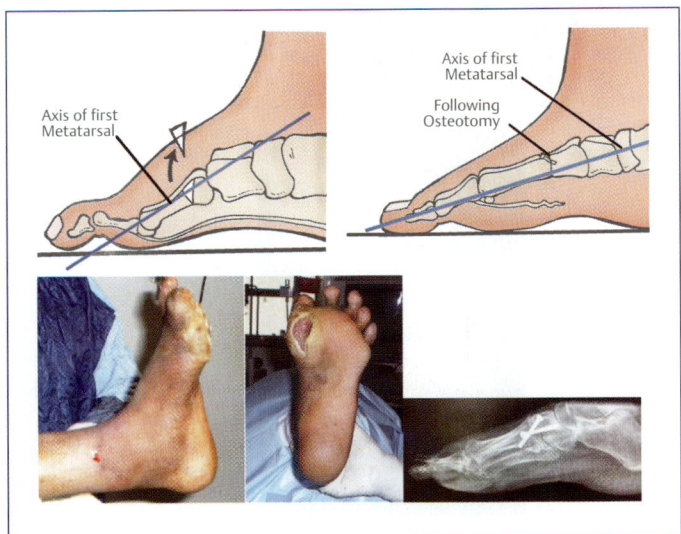

Fig. 12.12   Dorsiflexion wedge correction osteotomy of first metatarsal for diabetic ulcer.

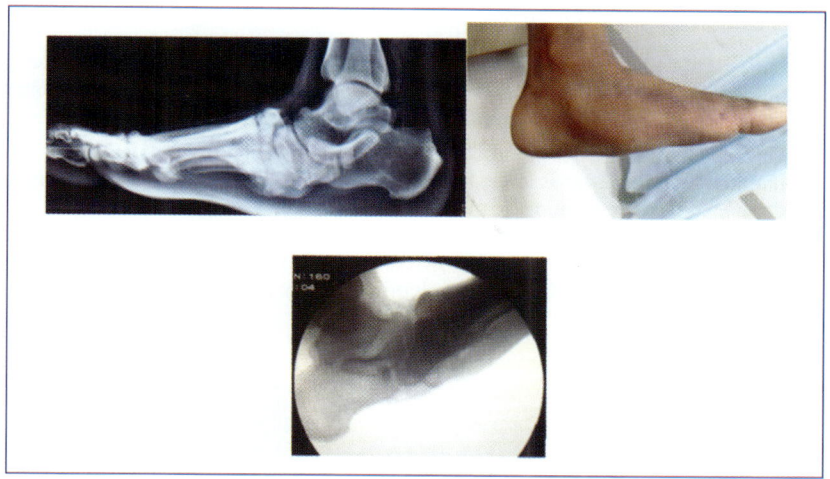

Fig. 12.13   Midfoot exosectomy

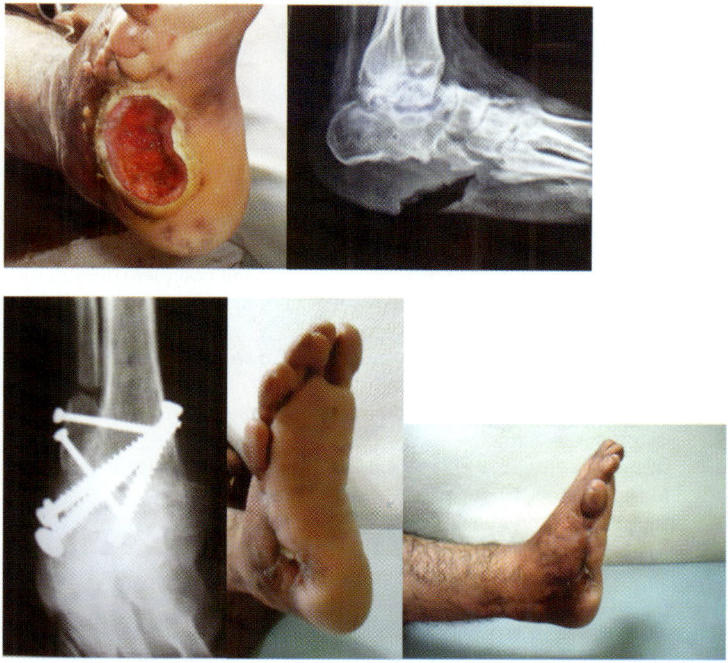

Fig. 12.14   Hindfoot corrective arthrodesis for nonhealing ulcer.

Tips and Tricks

For surgery of diabetic foot wounds and ulcers, following points hold importance:

Diabetic ulcer is a mechanical problem and no amount of antibiotics or dressings are going to heal it unless the pressure is reduced!

♦ Complete vascular assessment before surgery even in acute cases is a must
♦ If ankle–brachial index is lower than 0.7, then reconstructive vascular surgery is done before major orthopedic procedure
♦ Local debridement must be done before vascular reconstruction and total debridement should be done after vascular reconstruction
♦ Always probe the ulcer to know the depth and bony involvement (**Fig. 12.15**)

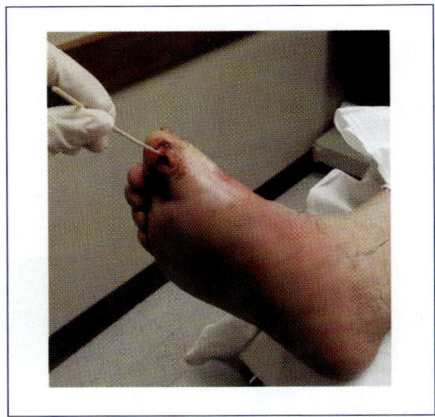

Fig. 12.15   Picture showing probing of ulcer.

♦ Concept of foot spaces should be used for proper and complete debridement
♦ To drain a particular web space widely by way of deroofing, many a times a normal-looking toe needs to be removed
♦ Tendon sheath must be followed and explored for complete clearance of infection as infection spreads via the tendon sheaths
♦ Maintenance of optimum serum albumin level more than 3.5 mg is a must for good postoperative outcome
♦ Moist wound healing concepts and wound bed healing concepts should be followed for healing of diabetic ulcers and wounds
♦ Concept of TIME should be followed
  • T = Tissue debridement (**Fig. 12. 16**)
  • I = Infection and inflammation control
  • M = Moisture control
  • E = Edge of the ulcer, education of the patient
♦ Sutures should not be removed early because of possibility of wound dehiscence and infection
♦ Offloading must be continued till complete wound healing

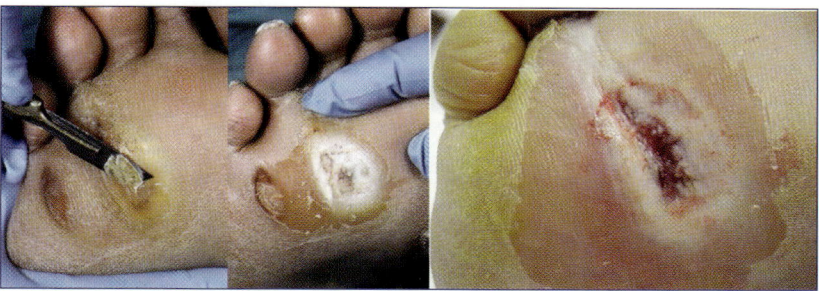

Fig. 12.16   Series of pictures showing how to debride callus.

♦ VAC: Vacuum-assisted treatment of diabetic ulcer gives most gratifying results (**Fig. 12.17**).
Flowchart 12.2 displays ideal method of dressing diabetic wounds and ulcers.

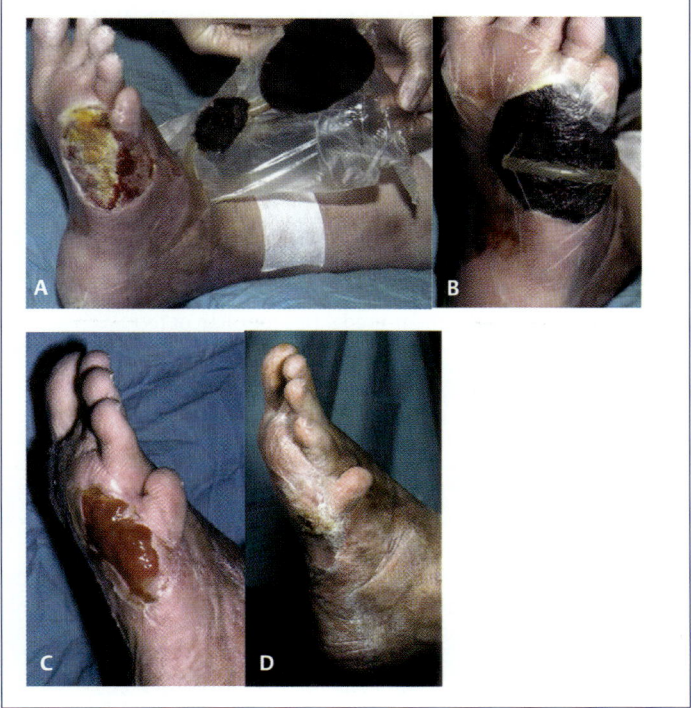

Fig. 12.17 (A-D)   Pictures showing **(A)** diabetic ulcer **(B)** coverage of ulcer with vacuum application **(C)** picture after three vacuum applications **(D)** final healing.

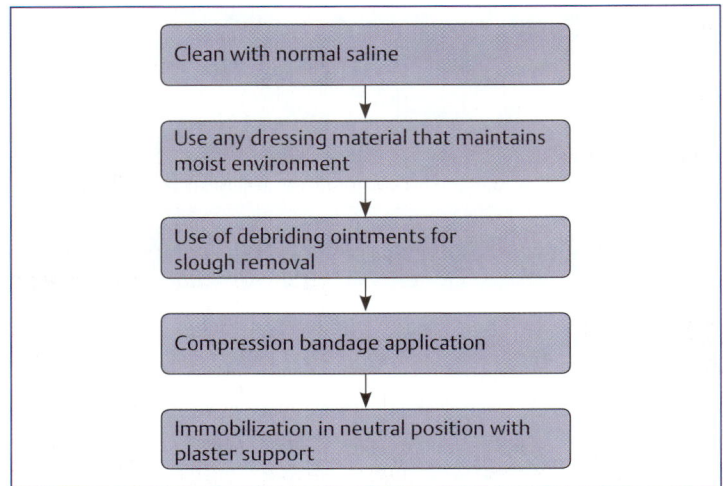

Flowchart 12.2 Method of dressing diabetic wounds and ulcers

Agents causing delay in wound healing in diabetes are listed below:

◆ Chlorhexidine—2%
◆ Povidone iodine
◆ EUSOL solution
◆ Hydrogen peroxide
◆ Neomycin sulphate
◆ Liquid detergents
◆ Corticosteroids and Nitrofurantoin

Charcot Foot

Flowchart 12.3 shows management modalities for Charcot foot.

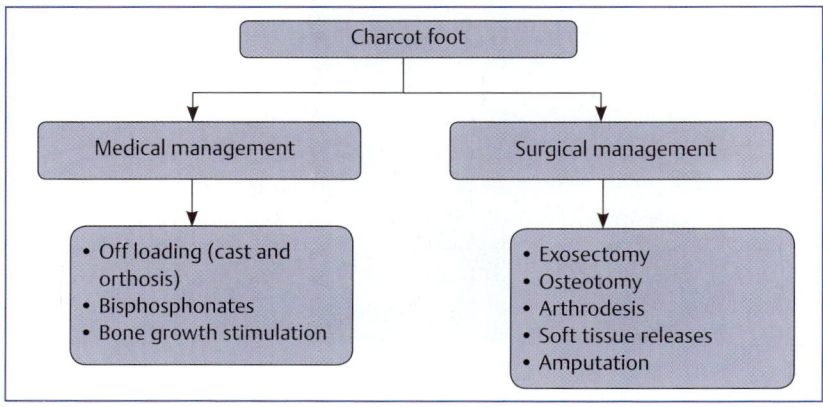

Flowchart 12.3 Treatment modalities for Charcot foot.

Tips and Tricks

For diabetic Charcot management, the following points hold importance:

◆ Goal is to always give plantigrade foot
◆ Correction of deformity is a must
◆ Never fuse *in situ*
◆ Fusion needs longer, stronger, and combination fixations (**Fig.12.18**)

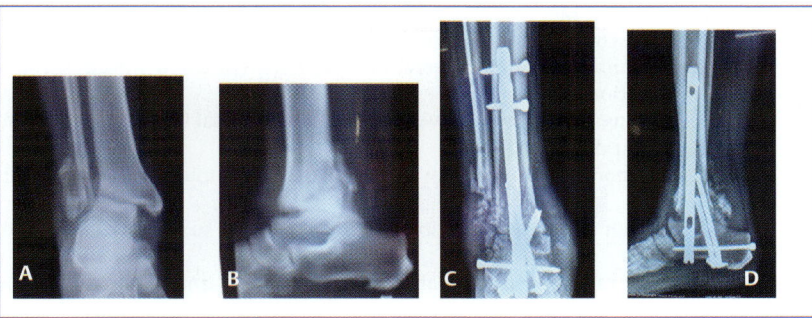

Fig. 12.18 (A-D)   (A) AP **(B)** lateral image of Charcot ankle. Treated with arthrodesis of ankle and subtalar joints tibiotalocalcaneal nail **(C)** AP postoperative view and **(D)** lateral postoperative view.

◆ Fixations need to span and cross the joints for better stability (**Fig.12.19**)
◆ Adjuvant soft tissue releases are a must
◆ Immobilization is doubled
◆ Weight bearing is delayed
◆ Postprocedure brace or orthotic support is continued for 12 to 18 months

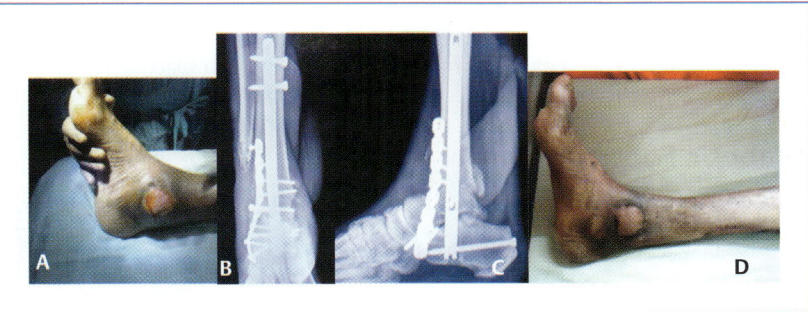

Fig. 12.19 (A-D)   (A) Diabetic Charcot ankle with nonhealing ulcer on the medial side **(B)** and **(C)** AP and lateral radiographs showing postoperative healing following tibiotaloc- alcaneal fusion with the use of tibiotalocalcaneal nail, and **(D)** final clinical picture.

Diabetic Amputations

Tips and Tricks

For diabetic amputations, the following points need to be considered:

◆ Preserve proximal phalanx of great toe to preserve flexor hallucis longus (FHL)
◆ Level of amputation should be distal to flexor hallucis brevis (FHB) insertion
◆ Plantar fascia and intrinsic muscles of metatarsal heads must be sutured to bony ends at toe disarticulation
◆ Try to preserve first ray
◆ For nonviable second toe, a ray amputation is preferred
◆ In fifth toe amputation, trim the lateral condyle of metatarsal to prevent secondary ulcer formation
◆ While performing amputation, shave the head of metatarsal from dorsal distal to proximal plantar direction
◆ In cases with more than one lesser toe involvement, amputation of all rays is advisable
◆ For fifth ray amputation, preservation of base is aimed at to protect insertion of peroneus brevis
◆ Whenever first ray is not salvageable, transmetatarsal amputation should be done
◆ Percutaneous tenotomy of tendo-Achilles is done in all forefoot- and midfoot-level amputations
   Prevention is better than cure!

Ten Commandments of Diabetic Foot Care

◆ Do not walk barefoot
◆ Inspect foot daily
◆ Do not apply hot or cold fomentations or strong ointments
◆ Use correct footwear
◆ Do not walk bearing weight on affected foot
◆ Do not sit cross legged for long time
◆ Do not remove footwear for long time during travel
◆ Cut the nails regularly and trim the square
◆ Do not cut corns or calluses with blades or knives
◆ Clean the feet twice a day with soap and water. Wipe web spaces and apply softening agent

Diabetic Footwear

In diabetics, footwear should do what foot cannot do!

Characters of good diabetic footwear are as follows:

◆ Wide toe box
◆ Extra depth
◆ Appropriate insole
◆ Heel counter

♦ Rigid outsole
♦ Rocker adjustment

Foot deformity has a direct relation with the level of activity. More strenuous activity has more severe deformity (**Fig. 12.20**).

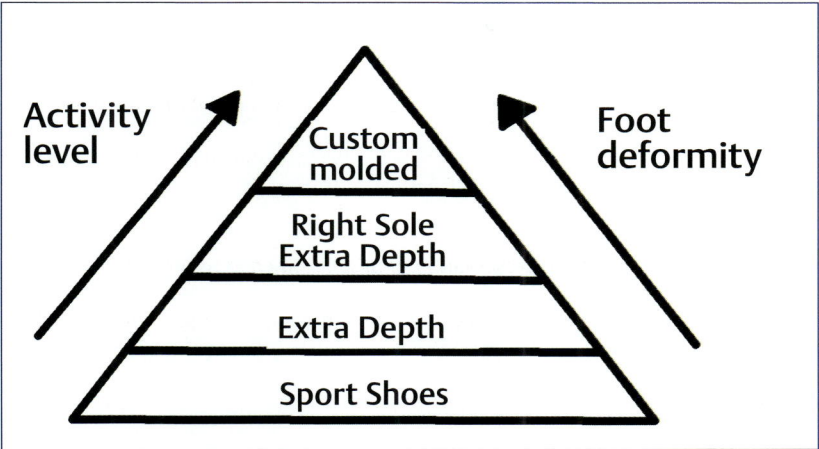

Fig. 12.20   Pyramid of relation between activity level and foot deformity in diabetic foot versus type of footwear.

Chapter 13

Common Foot and Ankle Infections: Diagnosis and Management

Modern-day infections are different with respect to type of organisms, resistance pattern, pattern of presentations, and unique state of immune compromised cases!

Introduction

Fig. 13.1 shows armamentarium of clinicians to battle with modern-day infections.

How Foot and Ankle Infections Are Different?

Foot infections are different from infections elsewhere in the body owing to the specific anatomic and physiologic features of the foot. These features cause easy spread of infection which is explained in **Fig. 13.2**.

Pathogenesis of Foot and Ankle Infections

Pathogenesis of infections of foot and ankle is illustrated in **Flowchart 13.1**.
   Flowchart 13.2 displays causes and conditions that predisposes host to infection.

Spectrum of Infections

♦ The foot can be affected by a wide range of conditions ranging from a relatively mild foreign body granuloma to a limb- or life-threatening gangrene.
♦ Etiologies: Traumatic or nontraumatic.

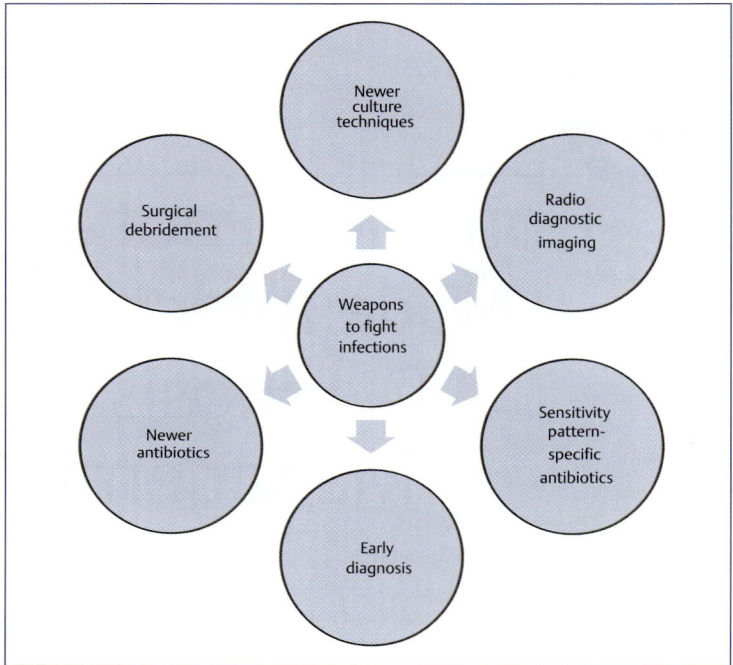

Fig. 13.1 Techniques of dealing with modern-day infections.

♦ Either of the etiologies can result in the following:
  • Cellulitis
  • Fasciitis
  • Osteomyelitis
  • Infective arthritis
♦ Soft-tissue infections can be following:
  • Ingrowing toe nail
  • Paronychia
  • Erythrasma
  • Foreign body impaction
  • Puncture wounds
  • Cellulitis
  • Peripheral vascular disease (PVD)
♦ Bone infection (osteomyelitis): Acute, chronic, or posttraumatic. Osteomyelitis may be pyogenic or tubercular in nature.
♦ Diabetic foot: A variety in itself.
♦ Usual bacteria that cause infection in the foot include:
  • *Staphylococcus aureus*
  • Group A *Streptococci*
  • *Pseudomonas aeruginosa*

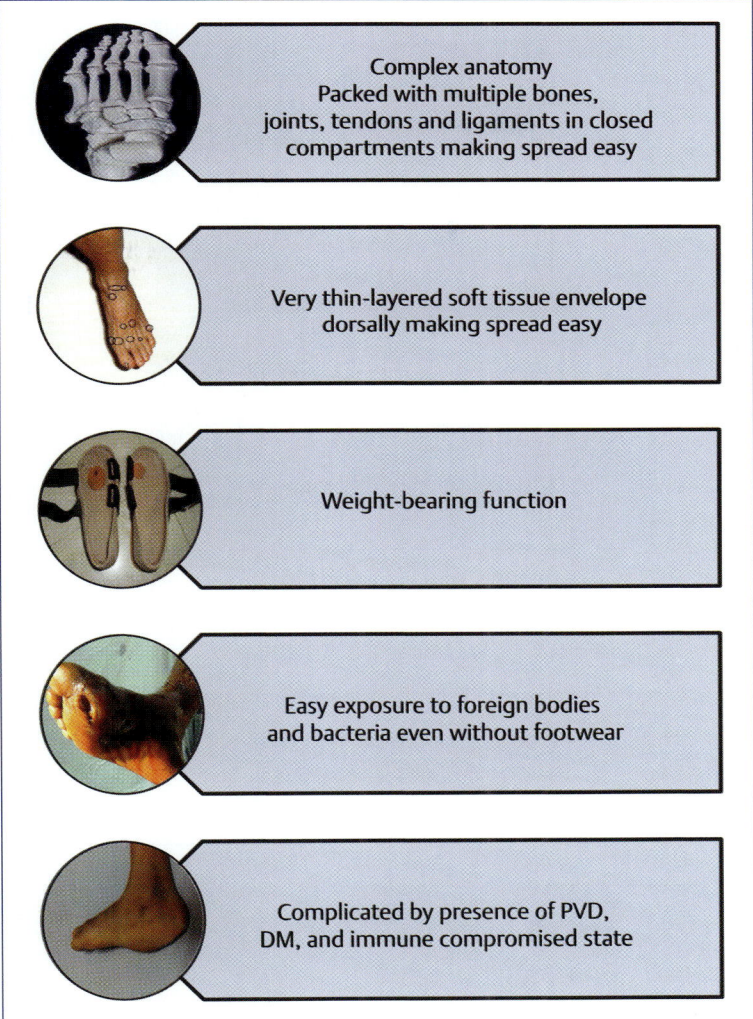

Fig. 13.2   Factors that lead to the spread of foot infections.

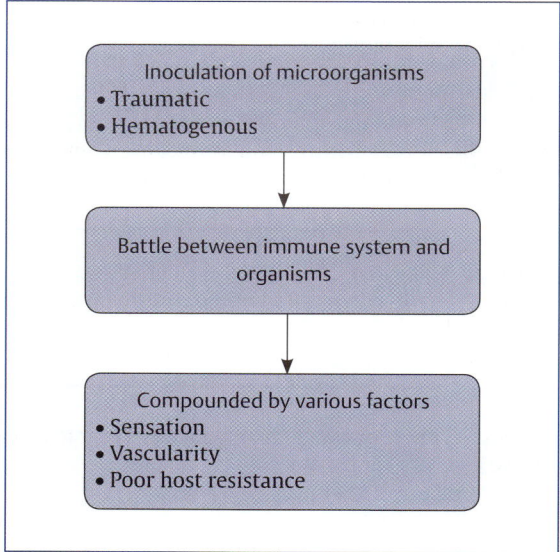

Flowchart 13.1 Pathogenesis of foot and ankle infections.

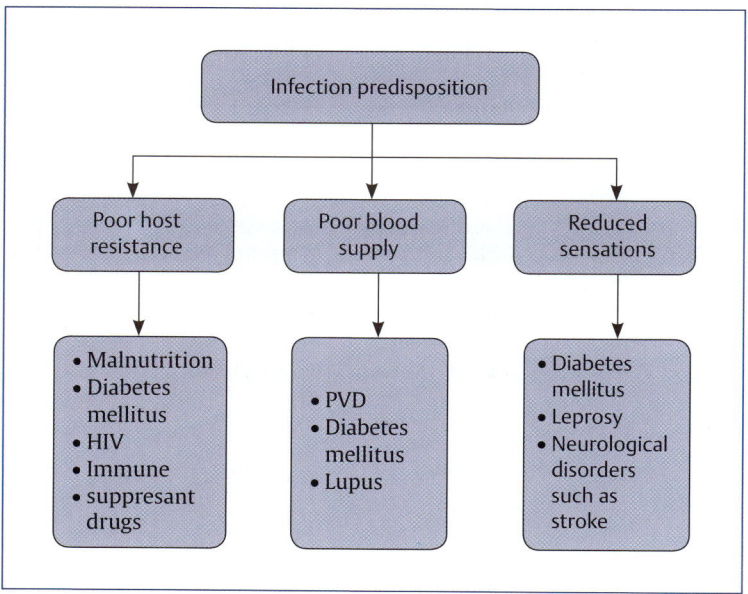

Flowchart 13.2 Reasons for predisposition to infections.

♦ Uncommon pathogens or conditions such as actinomycosis, nocardiosis, and fungi need to be kept in mind.

Diagnosis

To reach at correct diagnosis, proper history of the patient along with evaluation of the signs and symptoms should be carried out.

History

♦ A detailed history is essential, more so in foot infections. A trivial trauma thought to be insignificant by the patient could be significant in the context of the clinical scenario.
♦ Details of the type of trauma (low or high energy) and the environment in which it occurred (e.g., farm yard) could give a clue regarding the organism that one is dealing with.
♦ Medical history to rule out compounding factors such as diabetes, peripheral vascular disease, and smoking.

Symptoms

♦ Pain: For example, throbbing pain suggests case of pyogenic infection or inflammation
♦ Swelling
♦ Constitutional symptoms such as fever, nausea, or vomiting are indicative of septicemia or bacteremia
♦ Discharge: Look for color and presence of bone pieces

Signs

♦ Redness
♦ Edema: Leads to loss of skin wrinkles
♦ Sinus: Probe the sinus to feel the base and confirm whether it is bony or soft tissue. Palpating bone when probing the lesion is highly specific and has a high positive predictive value for diagnosis of osteomyelitis.
♦ Discharge: Smell and color of discharge can give an indication of the organisms involved (**Fig. 13.3**).
♦ Neurovascular examination is necessary to diagnose associated neuropathy and vascular disease.

Pain in the presence of neuropathy is indicative of underlying infection.

Investigations

The following investigations are to be carried out prior to starting the treatment.

Hematology

♦ CBC may not be raised in severe infection or diabetes
♦ ESR and CRP are indicators of infection and are also used to assess improvement after antibiotics and/or debridement

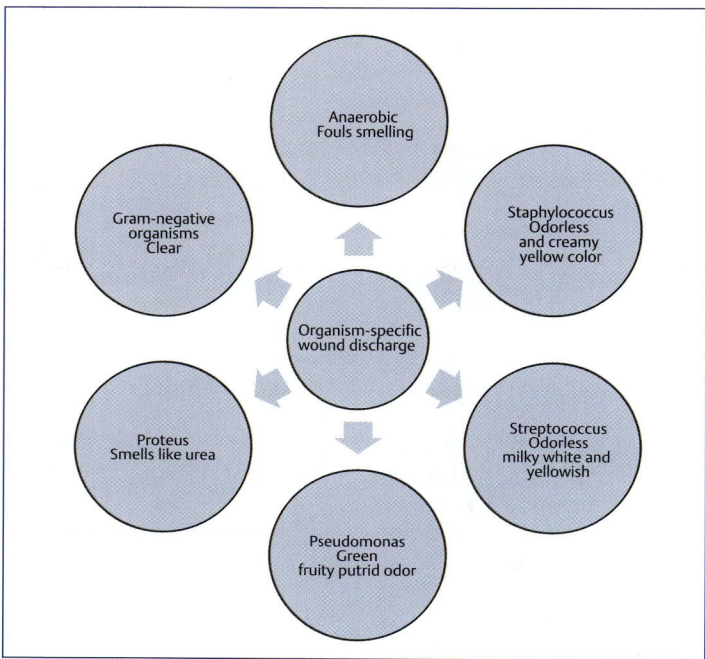

Fig. 13.3 Organism-specific wound discharge.

♦ Liver and renal functions must be assessed prior to starting antibiotics.
♦ Serum albumin levels are necessary to correct malnutrition.

Plain Radiograph

♦ Might show increased soft tissue shadow
♦ Gas could be due to gas gangrene
♦ Foreign body could be seen. For example, radiopaque objects such as metal, gravel, and glass can be identified easily with plain films
♦ Osteolytic lesions in bone, periosteal reaction, sequestrum, involucrum, etc., indicate osteomyelitis. Changes are seen after 2 weeks of infection

Ultrasonography

♦ Radiolucent objects such as glass, rubber, and wood could be seen easily
♦ It helps to define the extent of abscess

MRI

♦ It is the most sensitive investigation. One study demonstrated MRI to be significantly more sensitive and accurate, with equal specificity in comparison to plain radiographs, technetium-99m MDP, and gallium-67 scans in osteomyelitis. With bone infection, marrow is replaced by fluid and inflammatory cells, which are displayed as regions of reduced signal intensity on T1-weighted images and as increased signal intensity on T2-weighted images and short tau inversion recovery (STIR) sequences

♦ It best detects changes in soft tissues
♦ Extent of involvement of muscles, ligaments, joints, and fascial planes could also be assessed
♦ It differentiates viable tissue from necrotic tissue
♦ General consensus exists that MRI is a superior study to CT scan when assessing for nonviable tissue or drainable fluid collections

CT scan

♦ It is ideal for detecting bony changes
♦ It also detects cortical breaks and osteolytic lesions
♦ It is useful in involucrum and sequestrum
♦ It can detect pus pocket within the medullary canal
♦ It delineates abscess cavity
♦ It detects gas in deep tissues in cases of gas gangrene or necrotizing fasciitis

Scintigraphy

♦ Scintigraphic studies can be useful in the diagnosis of bone infections in the foot, bone infection versus soft tissue infection, and bone infection versus Charcot osteoarthropathy
♦ The three common nuclear medicine studies in this group include the radioactive forms of technetium, gallium, and indium
♦ Technetium-99m methylene diphosphonate (MDP)
  • MDP detects infection 24 to 48 hours after its onset
  • It is a three-phase test
  • Uptake in all three phases indicates osteomyelitis
  • No or minimum uptake in last phase suggests soft tissue infection
  • This is not very specific as high uptake is seen following surgery, following trauma, bone tumors, and Charcot's osteoarthropathy
♦ Gallium-67
  • Gallium accumulates in bone
  • It is false negative in case of antibiotics administration
  • It is false positive in case of soft tissue infection, hematoma, fracture, surgery, and tumor
♦ Leukocyte-labeled indium-111
  • This is more sensitive and specific
  • It cannot detect chronic osteomyelitis
  • It is time consuming (3 days)
♦ Leukocyte-labeled technetium-99m hexamethyl propylamine oxime (HMPAO)
  • HMPAO is completed in 3 to 4 hours
  • It is useful in differentiating osteomyelitis from postfracture or postsurgical state
  • It is useful in differentiating osteomyelitis from Charcot's osteoarthropathy

Wound Culture

♦ Deep tissue sample is ideal for culture
♦ Superficial swab is contaminated with normal flora and hence should be avoided.
♦ Biopsy is also very useful for diagnosing bone infections. Bone biopsy remains the standard criterion in the diagnosis of osteomyelitis
♦ Gram and Zeil–Neihlson staining can help in starting empirical antibiotics
♦ Various culture media are used to identify the organism

Management of Infections

Flowchart 13.3 gives a brief overview of the surgical management of infections of foot and ankle.

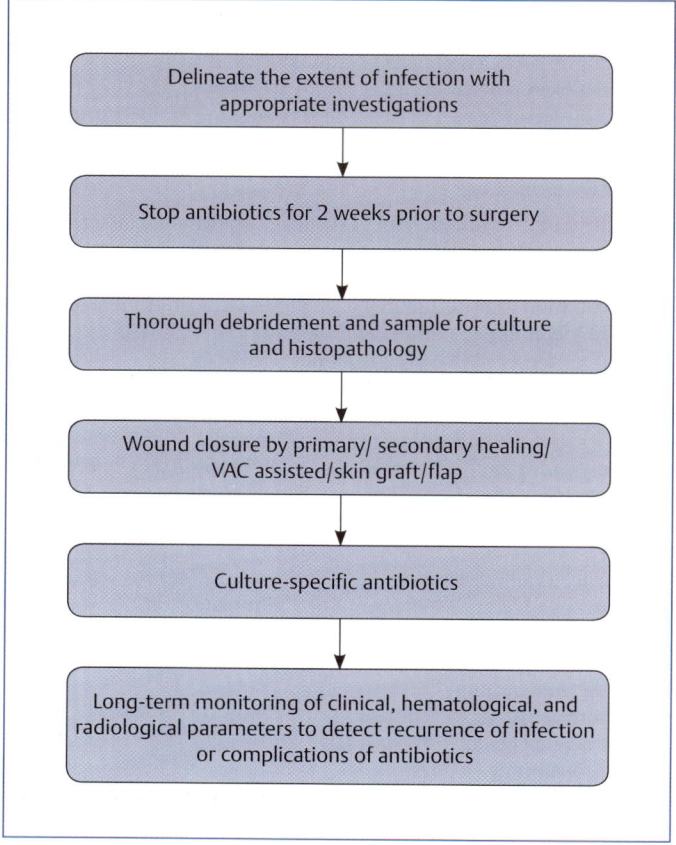

Flowchart 13.3 Overview of the surgical management of infections.

Nonsurgical Management

♦ Done for superficial infection and cellulitis. Generally, this is caused by *Staphylococcus aureus, Staphylococcus epidermidis,* or *Streptococci*
♦ It includes rest and elevation
♦ It also includes oral antibiotics (amoxicillin and clavulanate, first-generation cephalosporins, levofloxacin, or clindamycin)
♦ If the condition becomes significantly worse, intravenous therapy should be considered
♦ Small wound dressings need following important considerations:
  • Saline dressing moists environment, debrides necrotic tissue, helps drainage, inhibits bacterial growth, and stimulates granulation tissue formation
  • Avoid topical povidone iodine, hydrogen peroxide, EUSOL, cetrimide as these are harmful for normal granulation tissue
  • They should be used only when there is a lot of necrotic tissue
♦ Hygroscopic dressings should be used when there is extensive discharge from the wound
♦ Negative pressure wound therapy is a relatively newer modality of occlusive dressing, which has showed encouraging results. It has the following advantages:
  • Stabilization of the wound environment
  • Removal of extracellular fluid
  • Speeds wound healing
  • Increases in blood flow around wounds
  • Reduces bacterial burden
  • Changes in wound biochemistry and systemic response
  • Improves wound bed preparation
  • Helps avoid surgical intervention or reduces the extent of surgery required for wound coverage
  • Should be preceded by extensive debridement

Principles of Debridement

♦ Necrotic and devitalized tissues should be excised until only normal tissue remains because they provide a favorable environment for bacterial growth
♦ Moderate-to-severe infections should be aggressively debrided with excision of all nonviable skin, soft tissue, and bone
♦ Soft tissue and bony debridement should extend till we achieve a fresh bleeding margin, which ensures removal of all the nonviable tissue
♦ Sufficient representative deep tissue samples must be sent for culture and histopathological examination
♦ Avoid primary closure as a new margin of demarcation between viable and nonviable tissue may appear in 2 to 3 days, which would require serial debridement
♦ Sinus tract must be excised as a whole and sent for histopathology to rule out carcinoma

Table 13.1 demonstrates the difference between viable and nonviable components such as fat, tendon, muscle, and bones.

Table 13.1 demonstrates the difference between viable and nonviable components such as fat, tendon, muscle, and bones.

	Viable	Nonviable
Fat	Soft, resilient, shiny yellow	Nonpliable, hard, gray- white
Tendon	White and shiny	Dull, soft, stringy
Muscle	Beefy red and bleeds when cut, contracts when stimulated	Dull, dark, falls apart easily when handled, does not contract when stimulated
Bone	Firm, bleeds when cut	White, soft, does not bleed when cut

Diagnosis-specific Treatment Protocol

Specific treatment is required for some specific diseased conditions. Their characteristic etiology and clinical features, and specific treatment options are listed in **Table 13.2.** These conditions are mentioned as follows:

1. Cellulitis
2. Paronychia
3. Abscess
4. Puncture wounds
5. Acute, chronic, and posttraumatic osteomyelitis
6. Necrotizing fasciitis
7. Tuberculosis
8. Fungal infections
9. Diabetic foot

Infections in Special Situations

Infection in immunocompromised individuals like those who are suffering from HIV, systemic lupus erythematosus (SLE), rheumatoid arthritis (RA), high-dose corticosteroid use, diabetes, and asplenia is described.

HIV

♦ Patients with HIV are more susceptible to fungal and viral pedal infections.
♦ Tinea pedis and onychomycosis are often observed in this population.
♦ Human papilloma virus, manifesting itself as verruca plantaris, occurs at a higher rate than in the non-HIV population.

Systemic Lupus Erythematosus

♦ Skin and soft tissue infections in SLE most commonly are caused by *S. aureus*.
♦ These are caused less commonly by *Group A Streptococci*.

Table 13.1   Diagnosis-specific treatment protocol for various conditions

Disease condition	Etiology	Important/clinical features	Treatment
Cellulitis	• Group A *Streptococci* • *Staphylococcus aureus*	• Blanching erythema • Bright red skin • Increased temperature • Can lead to deep infection, gout, PVD	Responds to antibiotics, rest, and elevation
Paronychia	• Periungal infection • Ingrowing toe nail is the most common cause		• Antibiotics • Partial or total matrixectomy • Scalpel matrixectomy • Chemical matrixectomy
Abscess			• Drainage • Antibiotics
Puncture wounds	• *Staphylococcus aureus* • Beta hemolytic *Streptococci* • Anaerobic organisms	• Barefoot walking • Plantar aspect • Missed often • Can develop late • Mimicks Kochs	• Removal of contamination and foreign bodies • *In toto* excision of foreign body granuloma • Antibiotics
Acute, chronic, and posttraumatic osteomyelitis		• Acute, chronic, posttraumatic • Thin soft tissue layer involved • Direct extension	• Antibiotics • Surgical debridement
Necrotizing fasciitis	• Many bacteria involved (polymicrobial)	• Surgical emergency • Limb and life threatening • Spreads in fascia and deeper structures • Skin involved late • Cutaneous gangrene	• Repetitive aggressive debridements • Reconstruction
Tuberculosis	Common suspicion	• Diagnosis by clinical and radiological signs, biopsy, and TB culture	• Anti-TB drugs • Surgery for sinuses, cavities, sequestrum
Fungal infections	• Exogenous traumatic inoculation or colonization of altered skin • Systemic spread with secondary cutaneous involvement	• Missed diagnosis • Penetrating wound • Colorful discharge • Poor response to antibiotics or anti-TB treatment • Fungal culture	• Excision • Anti-fungal treatment for 6 months
Diabetic foot	Refer to chapter on Diabetic foot		

Rheumatoid Arthritis

♦ Patients with systemic arthropathies such as RA are often on long-term corticosteroid therapy that suppresses cell-mediated immunity and puts them at higher risks for infection.
♦ Rheumatoid nodules frequently occur over pressure areas in the foot, which can rupture, causing skin breakdown, erythema, and infection.

Asplenia

♦ People with asplenia are at particular high risk of infection with encapsulated bacterial organisms.
♦ Antibiotic coverage should be directed toward the encapsulated pathogens and consist of third- or fourth-generation cephalosporins.
♦ If hardware is present and has become colonized, it should be removed for complete resolution of the infection because of the organisms' affinity for seeding these areas.

Peripheral Vascular Disease

♦ Ischemic foot in PVD is prone to more frequent and severe infections due to low oxygen tension.

Case Discussion

Case I

A 43-year-old man presented with discharging sinus over dorsum of foot from past five months. Following were his clinical and radiological pictures (**Fig. 13.4**).

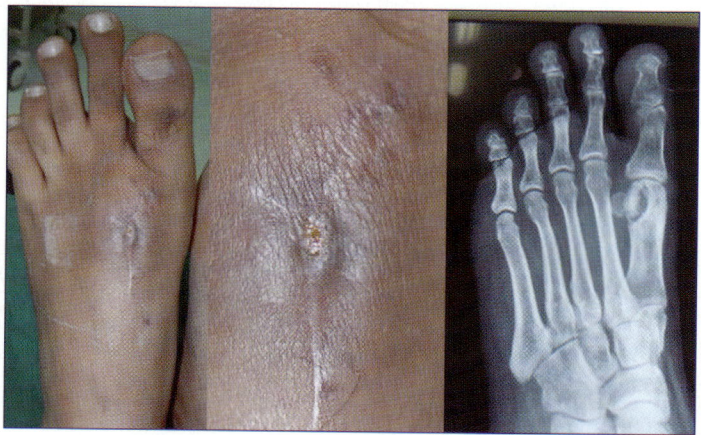

Fig. 13.4   Clinical and X-ray picture of case I.

He was operated for exploration for tuberculosis of the first metatarsal. Culture was positive and susceptible first-line antituberculous medications were started. Even after 3 months of this treatment, there was no healing. X-ray shows that sequestrum was not removed.

MRI showed signal intensity at the distal end of the first metatarsal (**Fig. 13.5**).

Decision to reexplore was taken and sequestrum was removed at surgery (**Fig. 13.6**).

Culture at reexploration was negative. Primary lines of antituberculous drugs were continued. Sinus healed in 3 weeks. Total healing occurred and is depicted in **Fig. 13.7**.

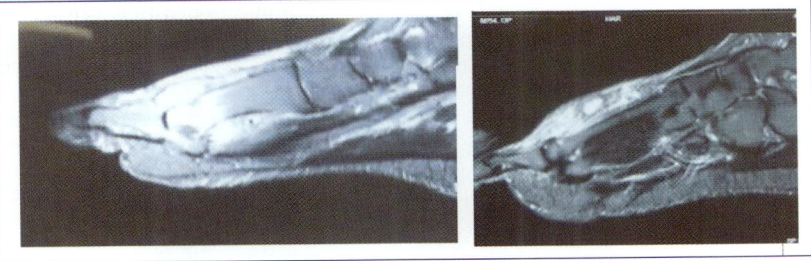

Fig. 13.5   MRI showing signal intensity in the first metatarsal.

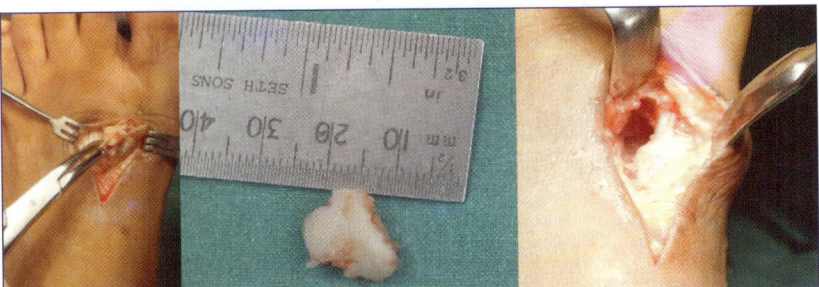

Fig. 13.6   Surgical exploration pictures.

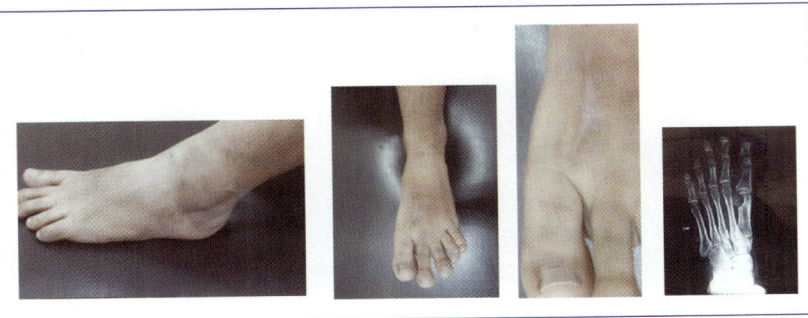

Fig. 13.7   Final pictures after discontinuation of drugs after 10 months.

Case II

A 35-year-old man presented with discharging sinus for many years despite anti-tuberculous drugs taken twice. On detailed history taking, there was a history of penetrating injury. Clinically, the condition is shown in **Fig. 13.8**.

CT scan and MRI demonstrated a bony cavity (**Figs. 13.9** and **13. 10**).

Patient was taken for surgical exploration and sinus excision. On exploration, wooden bone pieces were found from cavity (**Fig. 13.11**).

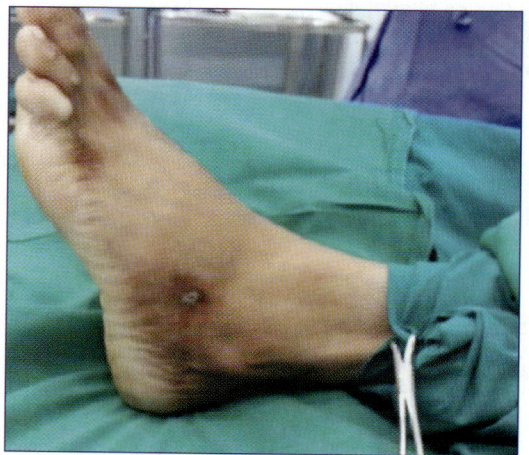

Fig. 13.8 Clinical picture of case II.

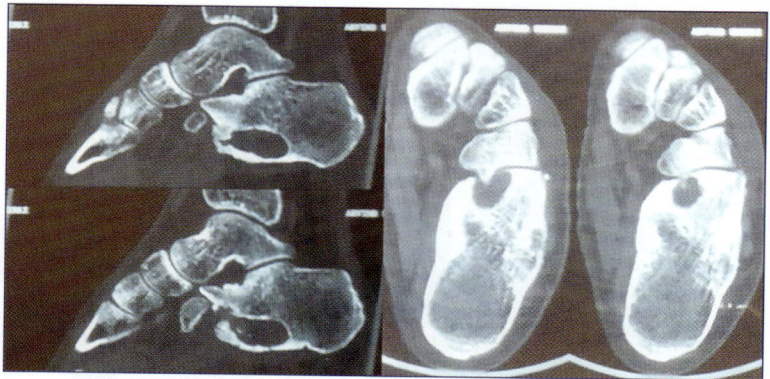

Fig. 13.9 CT pictures of this patient showing a bony cavity.

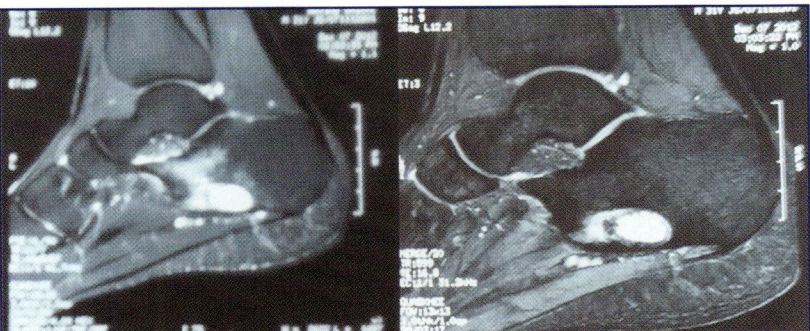

Fig. 13.10   MRI of the same patient.

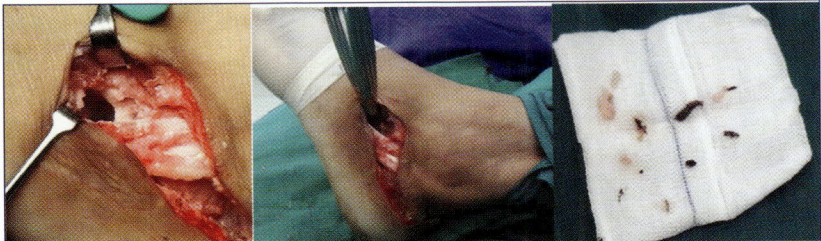

Fig. 13.11   Final operative pictures of the same patient showing wooden bone pieces.

Case III

An adult female patient came with constitutional symptoms with dirty infected raw area at the base of foot (**Fig. 13.12**).

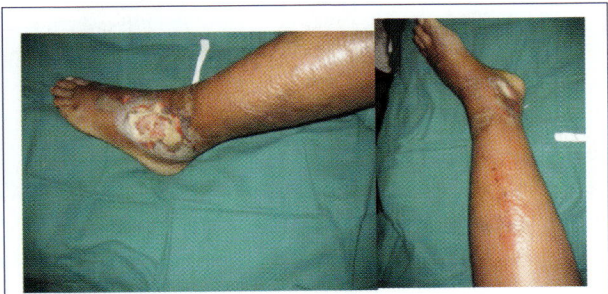

Fig. 13.12   Clinical pictures of infected raw area with cellulitis.

Patient was taken for emergency surgery as a case of necrotizing fasciitis (**Fig. 13.13**).

Serial dressings were done and susceptible antibiotics were given. Wound became healthy and was later on skin grafted (**Figs. 13.14** and **13.15**).

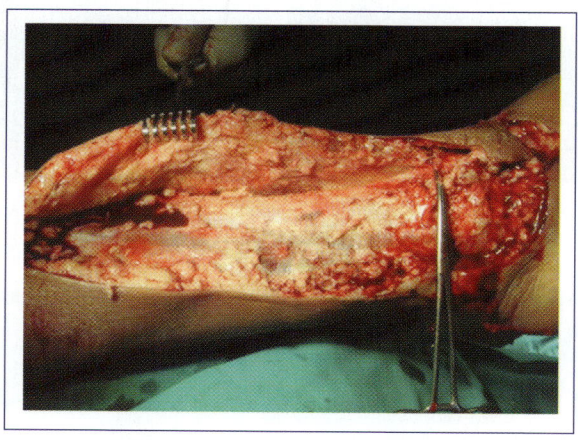

Fig. 13.13 Surgical picture showing spread of infection in deeper planes.

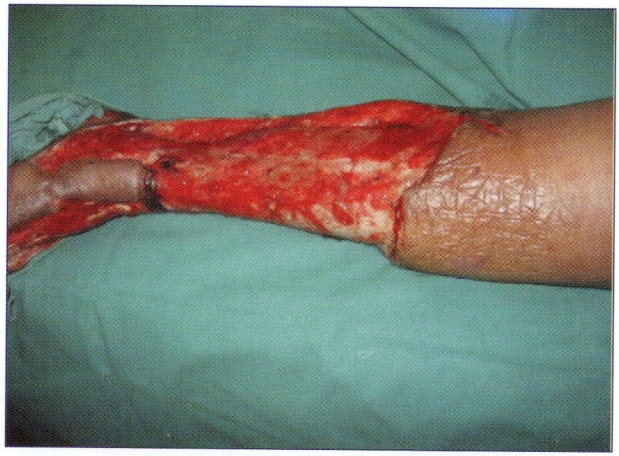

Fig. 13.14 Clinical picture before skin grafting.

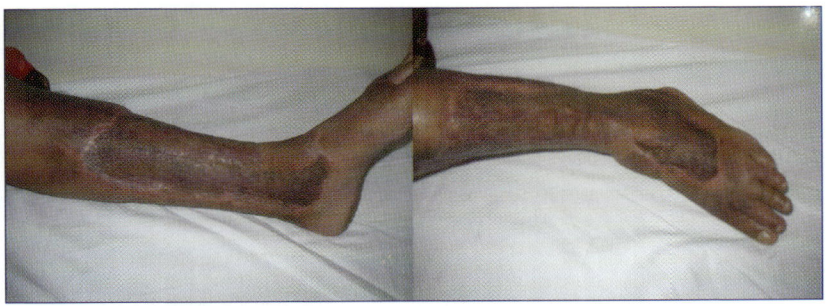

Fig. 13.15 Clinical pictures of final healing.

Art of Arthrodesis in Foot and Ankle

Arthrodesis is an art, let us live it!

Principles of Arthrodesis

The aims of arthrodesis are as follows:

♦ Creation of broad, cancellous, bleeding surfaces
♦ To restore a plantigrade foot
♦ Rigid fixation and compression across the arthrodesis site
♦ Filling of defects with bone grafts or bone substitutes
♦ Augmentation of healing if needed using orthobiologics

Tips and Tricks

♦ Generous release of soft tissues and soft tissue balancing
♦ Correction proceeds from proximal to distal
♦ Arthrodesis is always done in a corrected position
♦ Removal of bone to correct deformity must precede removal of articular cartilage
♦ Release of tendo Achilles or contracted muscles must accompany arthrodesis, if needed
♦ Tissue force balancing by suitable tendon transfer may be required as an adjunct procedure
♦ Spare as many joints as you can
♦ Drilling of articular surface is done to increase vascularity
♦ Feathering of arthrodesis surfaces is done to increase the vascularity
♦ Arthrodesis in grossly infected cases shall follow generous debridement
♦ Arthrodesis in low-grade infection cases can be done as a single-stage procedure where debridement precedes arthrodesis

◆ Use of plate and screws is justified in cases with good bone stock and good soft tissue envelope
◆ Use of external or ring fixator is justified in cases with poor bone stock, poor soft tissue envelope, and comorbid conditions
◆ For a case with nonunion, fusion mass must extend to stabilize nonunion site
◆ Proximal or distal corrective osteotomy will be needed as an adjunct procedure in cases with severe deformity
◆ In neuropathic fusions, longer and stronger combination fixations are used. These fixations must cross multiple joints to augment stability
◆ Neuropathic arthrodesis needs extended period of immobilization and no weight bearing. Postunion protection with brace is done for a long duration
◆ Use of lamina spreaders of various sizes and Hintermann retractor of various sizes is a must for midfoot and forefoot arthrodesis

Ankle Arthrodesis

Position: Position of fusion is neutral dorsi/plantar flexion, 5° to 10° of external rotation of foot with hindfoot in neutral; 5° of valgus with talus slightly posterior. The specific indications for arthroscopic ankle arthrodesis and open-ankle arthrodesis are mentioned in **Flowchart 14.1**.

Ankle for arthrodesis could be approached anteriorly, posteriorly, or laterally (**Flowchart 14.2**).

Depending on the severity of the deformity, arthrodesis procedure changes with the addition of other adjuvant procedures (**Flowchart 14.3**).

In case of associated infection, treatment of infection is done prior to arthrodesis (**Flowchart 14.4**).

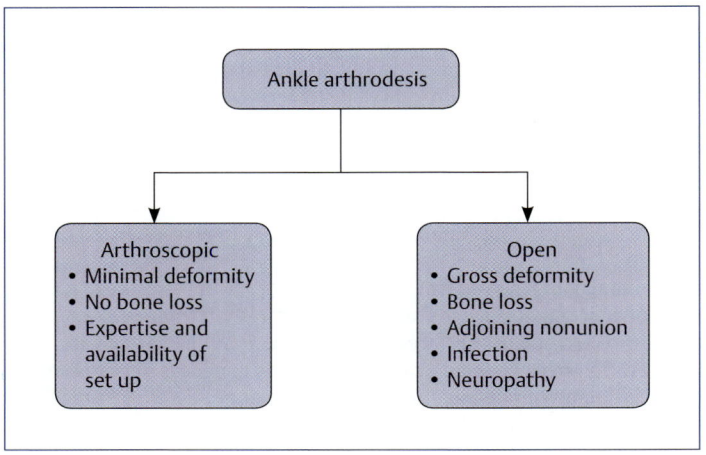

Flowchart 14.1   Indications for arthroscopic and open ankle arthrodesis.

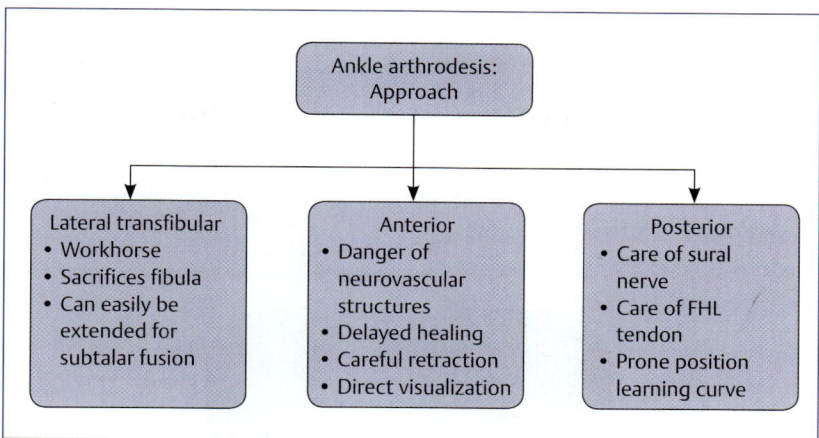

Flowchart 14.2   Comparisons of indications of various approaches.

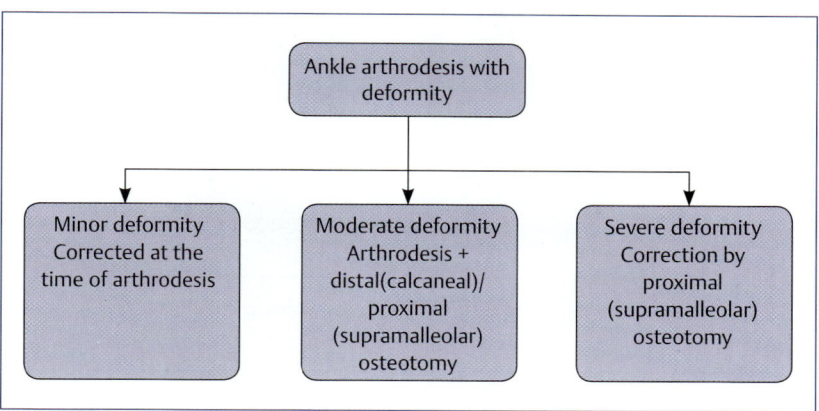

Flowchart 14.3   Ankle arthrodesis with deformity.

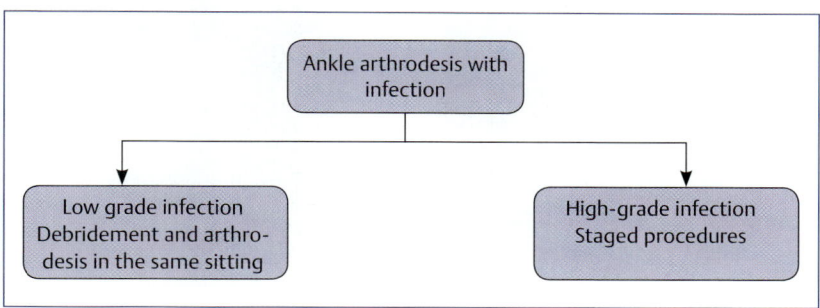

Flowchart 14.4   Ankle arthrodesis with infection.

Tips and Tricks

♦ Always assess preoperative movements of transverse tarsal and subtalar joint
♦ Assess vascular status of the limb
♦ Assess the neurological status of the limb
♦ Vascularity of the talus must be confirmed preoperatively for successful fusion (**Fig. 14.1**)
♦ Presence of deformity must be noted and corrected during ankle fusion (**Fig. 14.2**)

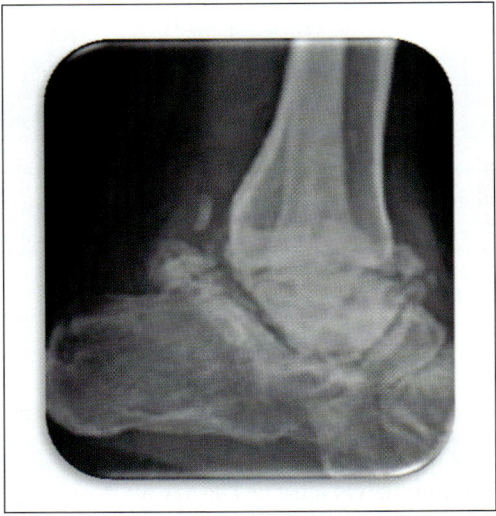

Fig. 14.1   X-ray showing ankle arthritis with avascular talus.

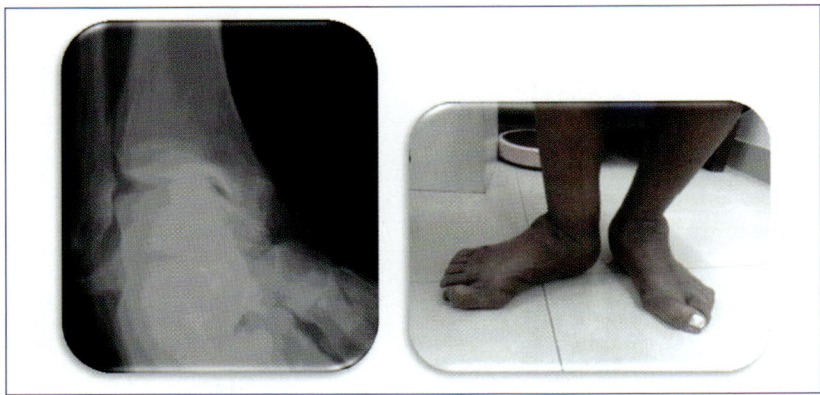

Fig. 14.2   X-ray and clinical picture of a case showing gross varus deformity with ankle arthritis.

♦ Tendo Achilles tightness must be assessed and, if needed, release of tendo Achilles should be done
♦ Previous scars and badly healed incisions would mandate change of approach (**Fig. 14.3**)

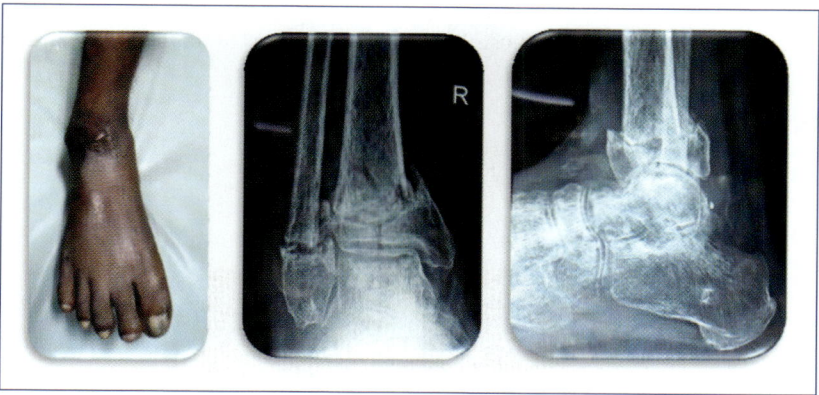

Fig. 14.3 Clinical and radiological pictures of a case with poor skin condition on the lateral aspect of ankle mandating anterior approach for fusion.

♦ Poor host conditions such as diabetes, medical comorbidities, and osteoporosis shall be dealt with augmentation, additional fixations, external fixation, prolonged protection over and above medical management (**Fig. 14.4**)
♦ Care of subcutaneous nerves must be taken while doing surgery to prevent future neurological complications
♦ Take full-thickness flaps and avoid vigorous retraction of soft tissues

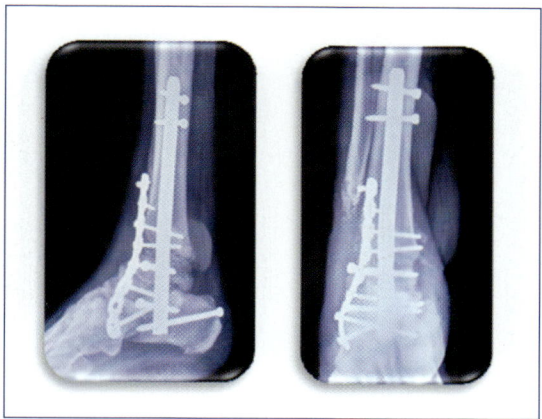

Fig. 14.4 Diabetic ankle fusion done with hindfoot nail with addition of plate.

♦ Excision of anterior osteophytes of tibia is a must (**Fig. 14.5**)
♦ Transfibular approach is preferred as far as possible
♦ Fibular osteotomy is done 2.5 cm above lateral malleolus and fibula is cut in a proximal lateral to distal medial direction

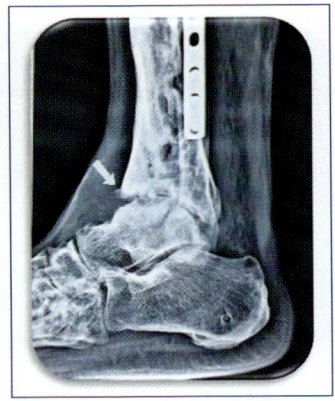

Fig. 14.5   X-ray showing ankle arthritis with anterior osteophyte.

♦ Fibula should be used as a biological plate and is fixed with two 4 mm screws, one in tibia and the other in talus (**Fig. 14.6**)
♦ Compression at arthrodesis site must be generated before placement of plate
♦ All screw threads should cross the arthrodesis site
♦ Crossing of compression screws should not be at the level of arthrodesis site
♦ For cases with minimal deformity and no bone loss, arthroscopic ankle fusion is the best alternative

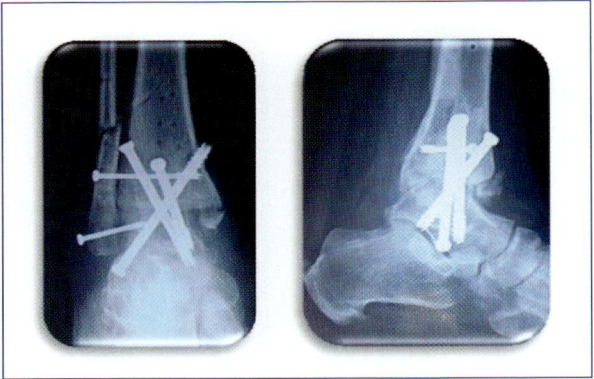

Fig. 14.6   AP and lateral projections of a case operated by transfibular ankle fusion in a case of infected ankle arthritis. Fibula is used in this case as a biological plate.

♦ Try to save the fibula in younger patients for feasibility of future total ankle replacement (**Fig. 14.7**)
♦ For an ununited pilon fracture with ankle arthritis, fusion mass must extend upward to cover fracture problem (**Fig. 14.8**)

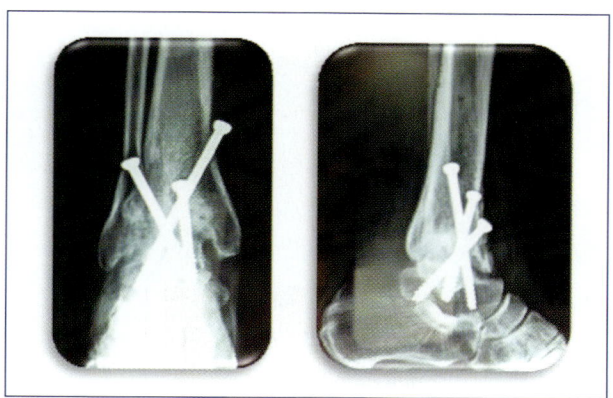

Fig. 14.7 Case where fibula was preserved for possibility of future ankle replacement.

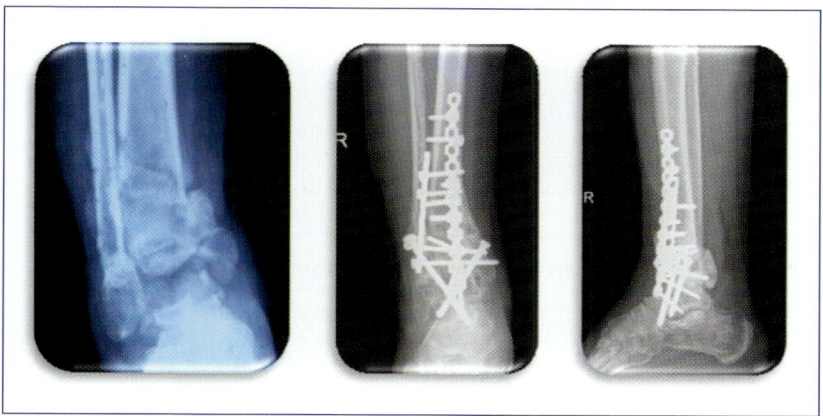

Fig. 14.8 Series of X-ray images of a patient with ununited pilon fracture with infective ankle arthritis treated with extension of fusion above to cover up ununited pilon fracture.

Subtalar Arthrodesis

Position is 5 to 10 degrees of valgus with transverse tarsal joints in 0 degree of abduction or adduction.

Indications for subtalar arthrodesis are post calcaneal malunion and other causes. Their respective treatment modalities are mentioned in **Flowchart 14.5**.

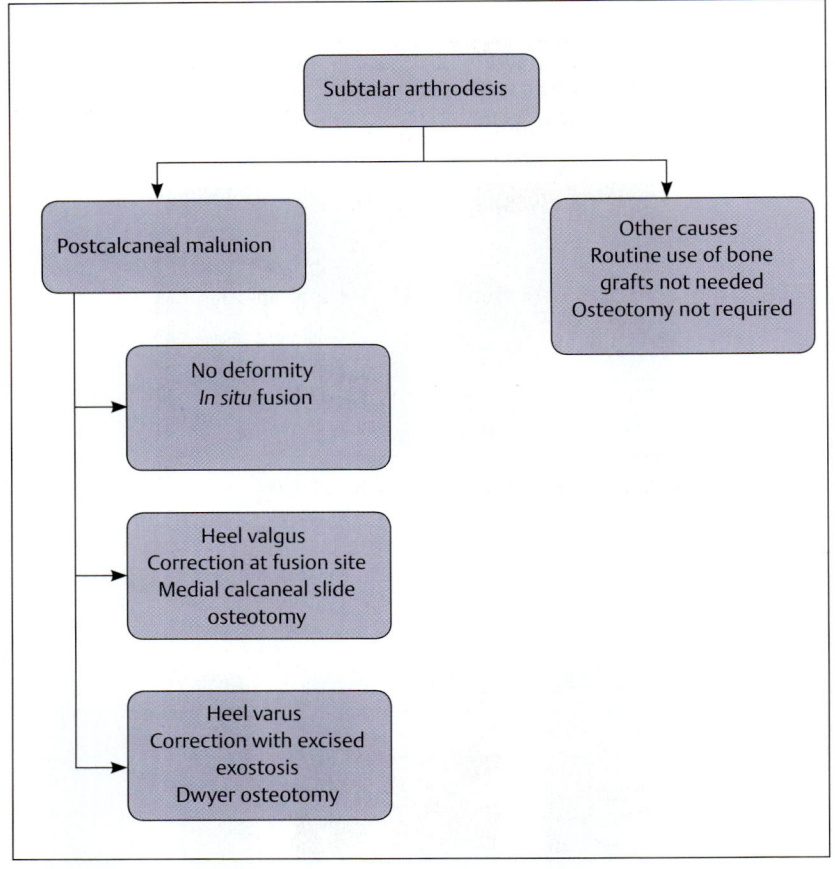

Flowchart 14.5 Indications for subtalar arthrodesis and their respective treatment modalities.

Tips and Tricks

◆ Motion of joints proximal and distal must be assessed
◆ Use four bent K-wires as retractors for sural nerve dorsally and peroneal tendons plantarward (**Fig. 14.9**)
◆ Often, osteophytes obscure visualization of the joint and need to be excised to reach the joint
◆ Lamina spreader is positioned in the sinus tarsi for mobilization of joints (**Fig. 14.10**)
◆ Flexor hallucis longus (FHL) marks the medial limit of joint preparation

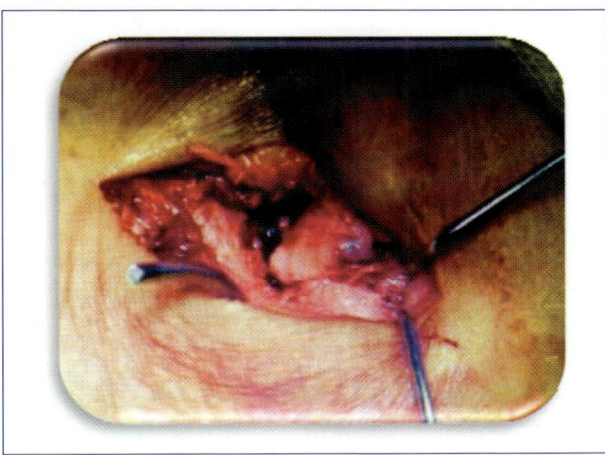

Fig. 14.9 Intraoperative picture showing bent K-wires acting as retractors.

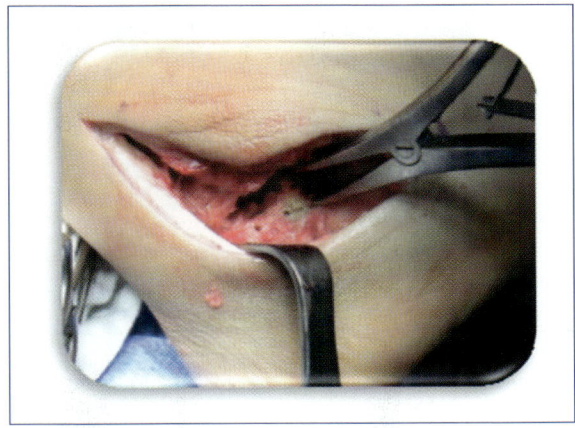

Fig. 14.10 Lamina spreader positioned in sinus tarsi for visualization of joint as well as opening of the joint.

♦ Screws are passed from non-weight-bearing area of heel. These screw heads should be countersunk to avoid implant impingement issues (**Fig. 14.11**)
♦ Use short-threaded screws for threads not crossing the arthrodesis site
♦ Anterior screw from anterior process of calcaneus to talar neck can increase stability in osteoporotic situations (**Fig. 14.12**)

Radiographs for distraction and postcalcaneal fixation subtalar arthrodesis are shown in **Figs. 14.13** and **14.14**.

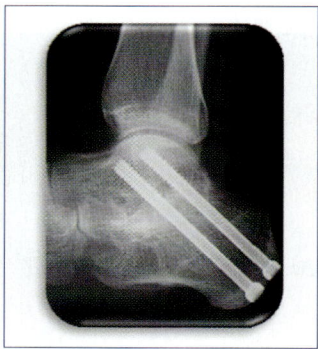

Fig. 14.11 Postoperative image of subtalar fusion showing passage of screws from non-weight-bearing area of heel.

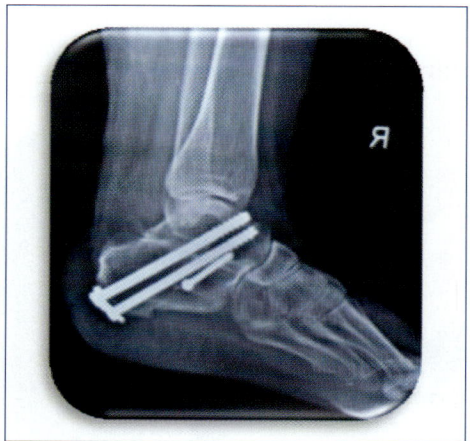

Fig. 14.12 Use of anterior screw for enhancing fusion.

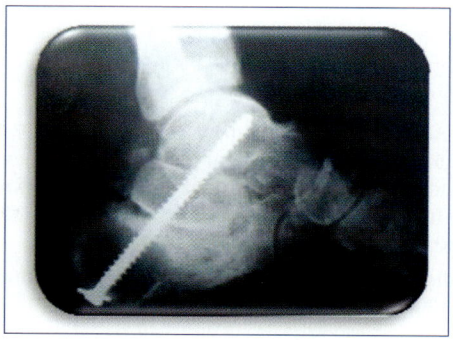

Fig. 14.13 Distraction subtalar arthrodesis following calcaneal malunion.

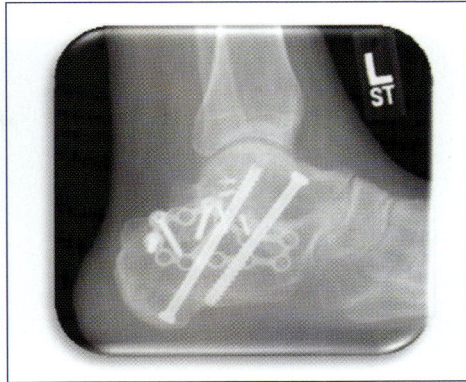

Fig. 14.14   X-ray picture of postcalcaneal fixation subtalar arthrodesis.

Tibiotalocalcaneal Arthrodesis

Position: Subtalar joint in 5 to 10 degrees of valgus and ankle in 0 to 5 degrees of dorsiflexion, neutral rotation with talus pushed backward.

Box 14.1 shows specific indications of tibiotalocalcaneal arthrodesis.

Box 14.1 Specific indications of tibiotalocalcaneal arthrodesis.
◆ Arthritis of ankle and subtalar joint ◆ Revision cases ◆ Neuropathy ◆ Big varus/valgus deformities ◆ AVN talus ◆ Bone loss ◆ Failed total ankle replacement

Tips and Tricks

◆ Incision needs to be extended up to the base of the fourth metatarsal for reaching out to subtalar joint
◆ Preparation of subtalar joint is equally important as that of ankle joint
◆ Pattern of hindfoot deformity (varus or valgus) would necessitate change in the way intramedullary nailing is performed. For valgus deformity, medialization of hindfoot should be done to hit the canal in center
◆ A well-fitting nail is a must for better stability; hence, use a largest-diameter nail
◆ Hybrid technique in the form of combination of IM nail and low-profile locking compression plate (LCP) may be better for Charcot (**Fig. 14.15**)

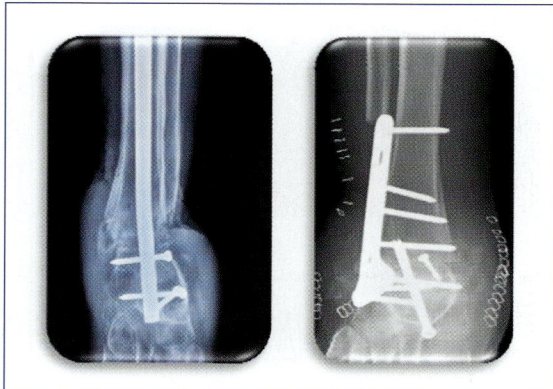

Fig. 14.15 Radiological image of a case treated by tibiotalar arthrodesis by nail and by plate, respectively.

♦ Compression at both the joint site with specially devised compression facility in the nail is a must

Triple Arthrodesis

Position: Subtalar joint in 5 to 10 degrees of valgus, talonavicular and calcaneocuboid joints in neutral abduction and adduction.

Tips and Tricks

♦ Correction of equinus contracture must precede surgery to get anatomical reduction
♦ Analysis and correction of coexisting ankle deformity is a must for successful end result
♦ Most important part of surgery is centering of calcaneus under the talus, and it should be done first followed by talonavicular fixation
♦ Use of lamina spreader in sinus tarsi would help in correction of deformities
♦ Long incisions and generous soft tissue releases would help in correcting the deformity
♦ For a single medial approach for triple arthrodesis, a separate lateral approach for reaching lateral side of talonavicular joint is needed
♦ For subtalar joint, fusion of posterior, middle, and anterior facet is done
♦ Most meticulous preparation is needed for fusion of talonavicular joint, which is one of the most difficult joint of body to fuse
♦ While reducing talonavicular joint, put fingers, one medially and other laterally fingers on either side of the navicular through both the approaches to make sure about reduction (**Fig. 14.16**)
♦ While correcting planovalgus deformity err on the side of navicular over correction over talar head
♦ Ream medial most overhanging portion of medial cuneiform for having entry for medial talonavicular screw fixation

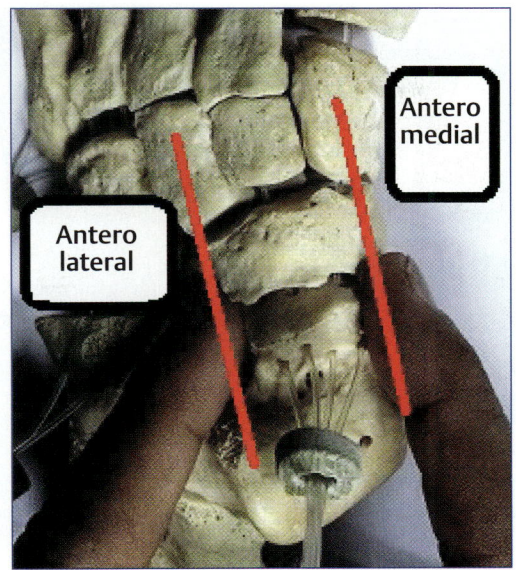

Fig. 14.16 Method of assessing reduction of talonavicular joint during triple fusion.

♦ Removal of small bone from anterior process of calcaneus gives a resting area for compression screw for calcaneocuboid arthrodesis (**Fig. 14.17**)
♦ For having a proper trajectory for screw fixation in the calcaneocuboid joint, proximal entry is made through the soft tissues behind the peroneal tendons (**Fig. 14.18**)

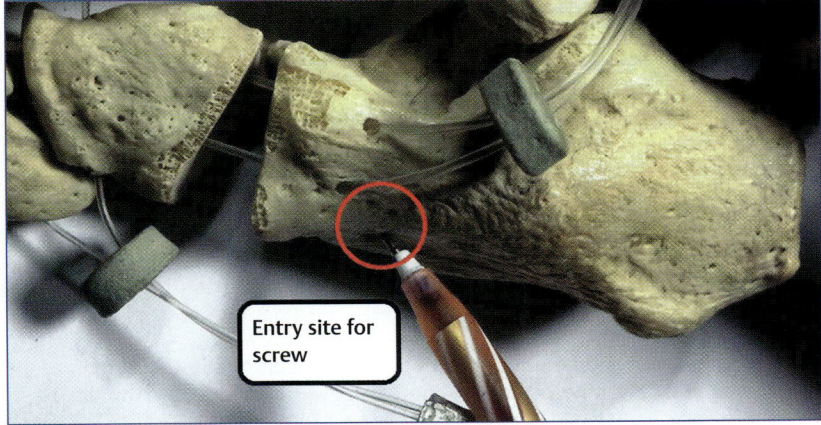

Fig. 14.17 Removal of bone from anterior process of calcaneus for facilitation of screw passage.

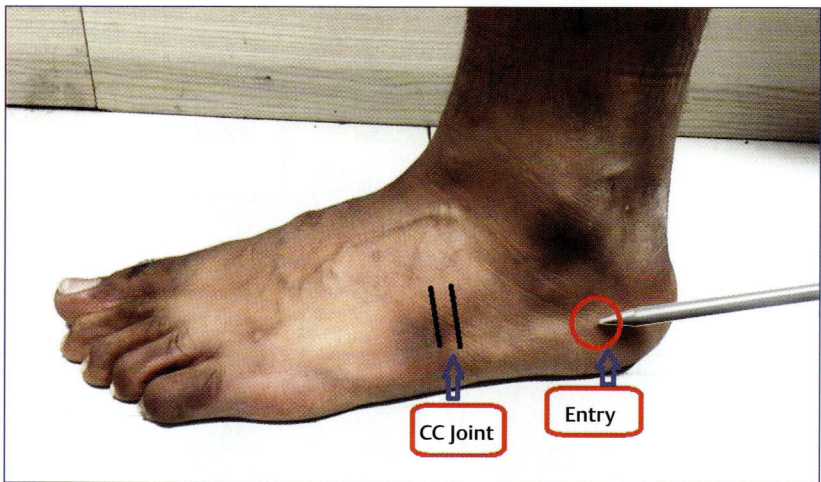

Fig. 14.18 Proximal subcutaneous entry for better trajectory for calcaneocuboid joint arthrodesis.

♦ Do not drill screws for full length for best purchase
♦ Screw placement chronology is subtalar screws followed by talonavicular screws followed by calcaneocuboid screws
♦ For greater stability, a third talonavicular screw may be pushed from lateral navicular to talus to calcaneus
♦ Full-thickness skin flaps, avoiding vigorous retraction and spacing between incisions would prevent skin problems
♦ Care of nerves is of paramount significance while doing triple fusion
♦ Do not give saline wash after drilling of articular cartilage as this contains osteogenic material
♦ Put bone grafts at the junction of talus, calcaneus, navicular, and cuboid —"quadruple arthrodesis site" for successful end result (**Figs. 14.19** and **14.20**)
♦ Screws should be placed through the stab incisions
♦ Tourniquet must be released before skin closure

Midfoot and Lisfranc Arthrodesis

Position: Neutral abduction or adduction and neutral dorsiflexion or plantar flexion.

Tips and Tricks

♦ Preoperative use of differential injectioning helps identify the affected joints
♦ In cases with deformity, osteotomy should also be planned with arthrodesis
♦ Achilles lengthening and plantar fascia release may also be needed
♦ Transverse approach is not universally accepted and can damage superficial nerves and tendons

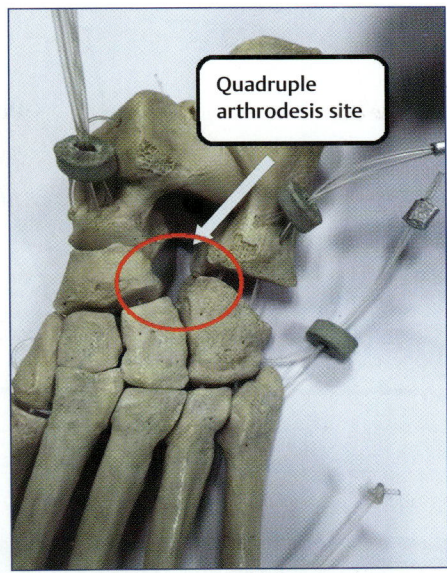

Fig. 14.19 Figure shows quadruple arthrodesis site.

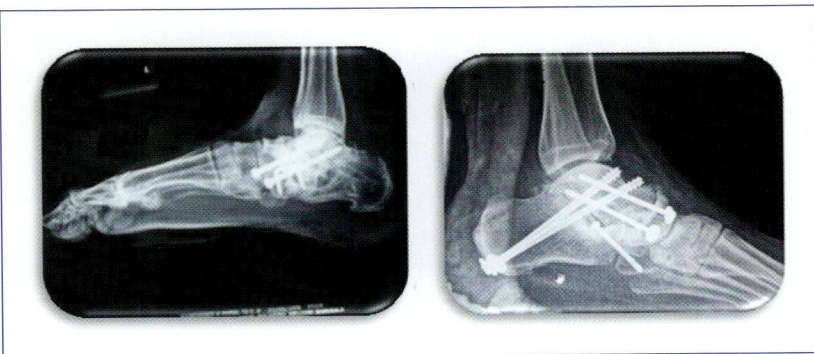

Fig. 14.20 X-ray pictures after triple fusion.

♦ Great care is needed to protect damage to nerves, tendons, and vessels
♦ Joints are obscured by the presence of osteophytes and they need to be excised
♦ Intraoperative use of C-arm is a must to delineate joint surfaces
♦ Toes are dorsiflexed fully while tightening the screws (**Fig. 14.21**)
♦ Compression screws are followed by plate fixation
♦ All screws must be pushed after forming a pocket hole (**Fig. 14.22**)

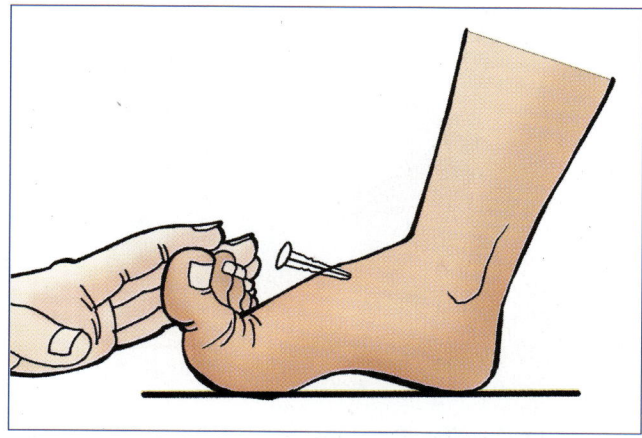

Fig. 14.21   Dorsiflexion of toes while tightening screws used for Lisfranc joint arthrodesis.

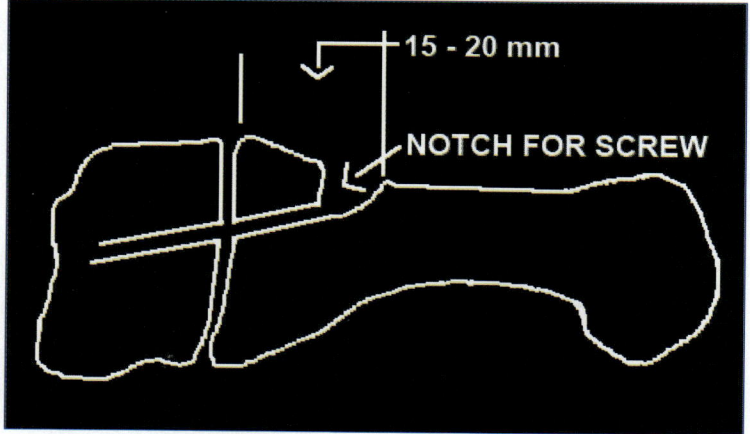

Fig. 14.22   Pocket hole for passage of screws.

♦ Plate needs to be precontoured
♦ Fusion of lateral rays is avoided
♦ Longitudinal arch must be maintained by realigning talo first metatarsal axis in both AP and lateral planes
♦ Tarsometatarsal (TMT) joints must be prepared till its bases to avoid dorsiflexion malunion
♦ Relative positioning of metatarsal heads must be checked with flat plate put on the plantar aspect of foot after temporary fixation. Head of first metatarsal must be plantar to the heads of other metatarsals (**Fig. 14.23**)

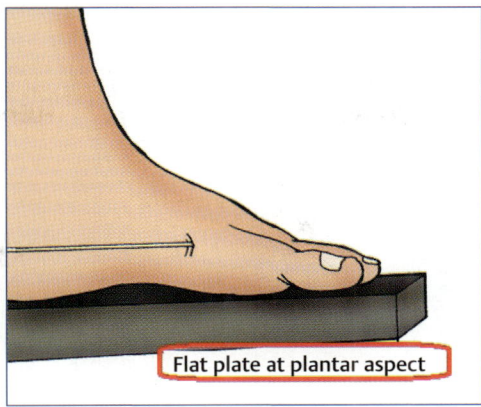

Fig. 14.23 Plate at the plantar aspect helps for assessing the position of metatarsal heads after arthrodesis.

♦ For correcting forefoot abduction, a plate should initially be fixed on medial cuneiform and then first metatarsal base should be reduced to plate
♦ Stability can be augmented by spanning plate or by crossing screws where the latter gives stability at the cost of articular damage (**Fig. 14.24**)

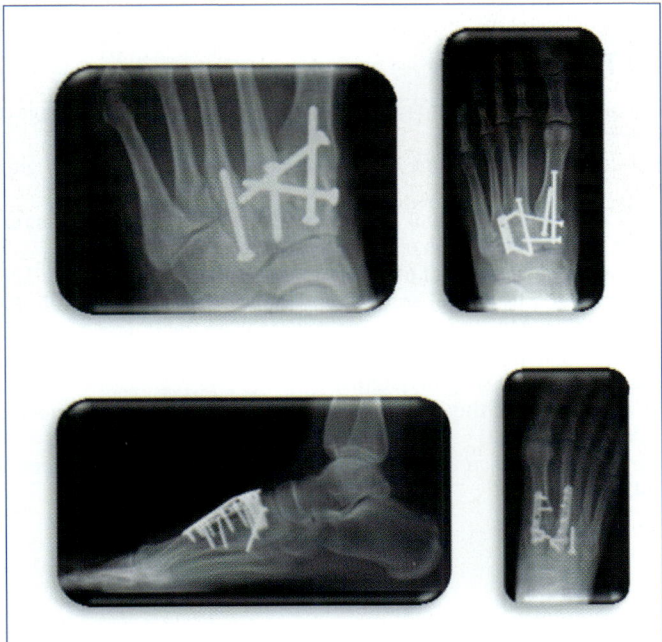

Fig. 14.24   X-ray images of midfoot and Lisfranc arthrodesis.

First MTP Arthrodesis

Position: Ideal position for non–high-heel-wearing population is 10 to 15 degrees of dorsiflexion and 10 to 15 degrees of valgus with neutral rotation of hallux (**Fig. 14.25**).

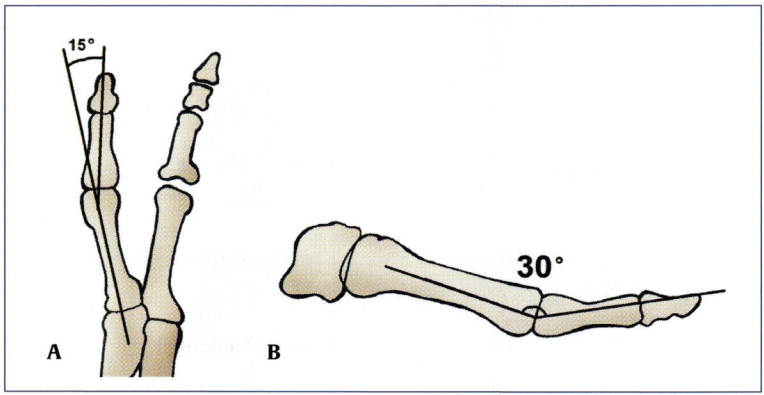

Fig. 14.25   Diagrammatic representation of positioning of hallux at arthrodesis.

Tips and Tricks

♦ Look for arthritis of TMT joint preoperatively as this would be a relative contraindication to procedure
♦ Preoperative assessment of neurological status and tendo Achilles tightness is a must
♦ Endpoint of release of medial and lateral capsuloligamentous structures is on achieving full plantar flexion of phalanx over metatarsal head
♦ Care of superficial nerve is of utmost importance
♦ In case of nonavailability of concave and convex reamers, removal of articular cartilage must be done in such a manner that the original shape of both articulating surfaces is maintained and minimal bone is removed
♦ Allowable shortening is up to 6 mm
♦ Use of a flat plate at the bottom of the foot guides for proper positioning of arthrodesis (**Fig. 14.23**)
♦ Use of a compression screw and low-profile dorsal plate gives maximum stability (**Fig. 14.26**)

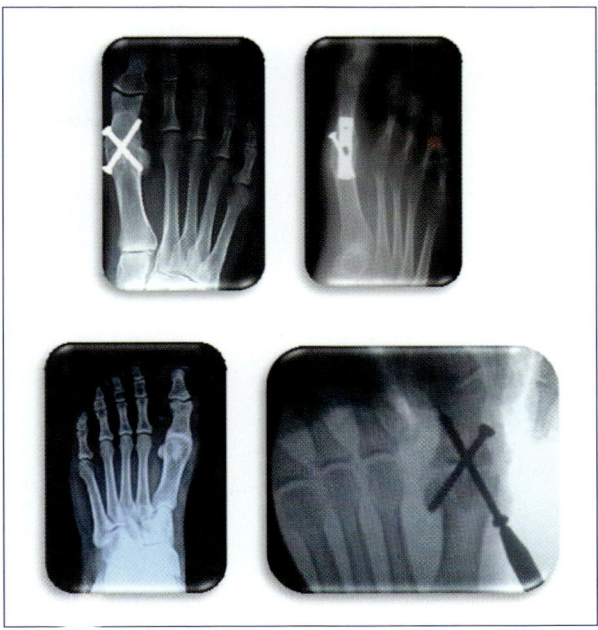

Fig. 14.26   X-ray images of first MTP joint arthrodesis.

Dealing with Tendo Achilles Problems!

Tendo Achilles is the strongest tendon of body contributing significantly in gait cycle!

Disorders of Tendo Achilles

The following are the common disorders of tendo Achilles tendon:

♦ Acute rupture
♦ Chronic (neglected) rupture
♦ Noninsertional tendo Achilles tendinopathy
♦ Insertional tendo Achilles tendinopathy: Tendon problems, bursal problems, bony spurs, and ruptures

Basic Science

Typical anatomical considerations for disorders of tendo Achilles tendon include the following:

♦ Tendon twists 90 degrees onto itself at insertion so gastrocnemius inserts posterolaterally and soleus inserts posteromedially (**Fig. 15.1**).
♦ Tensioning in twisted fibers causes "wringing effect," compromising blood flow, promoting ischemic degeneration.
♦ Tendon has a very thin paratenon (**Fig. 15.2**).
♦ Tendon inserts slightly medially on heel inverting it on its action.
♦ Insertion of Achilles: Half way between the dorsal and plantar aspects of the posterior tuberosity.
♦ Tendon has two bursas at insertion: Retrocalcaneal bursa in front and Achilles tendon bursa behind (**Fig. 15.3**).
♦ There is a hypovascular zone 2 to 6 cm proximal to its insertion surrounded by thin paratenon, making it vulnerable to injuries and degeneration (**Fig. 15.4**).
♦ Talocalcaneal joint movements and hyperpronation increase this wringing effect.

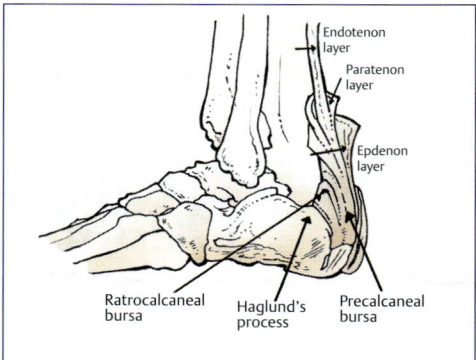

Fig. 15.1 Picture showing anatomy of tendo Achilles with typical rotation of tendo Achilles tendon during its course.

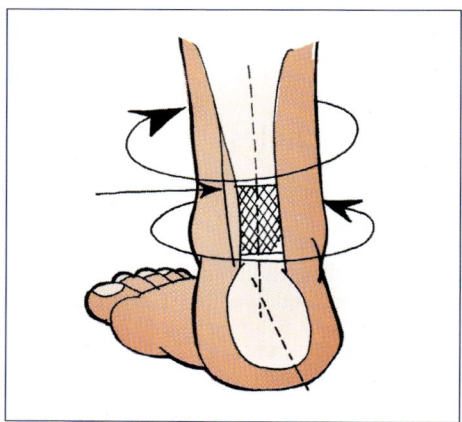

Fig. 15.2 Tendon has a thin paratenon with wringing effect.

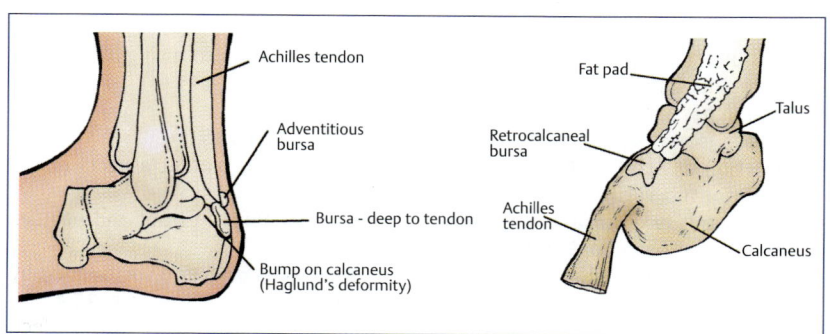

Fig. 15.3 Pictures showing the location of both the bursa with tendo Achilles tendon.

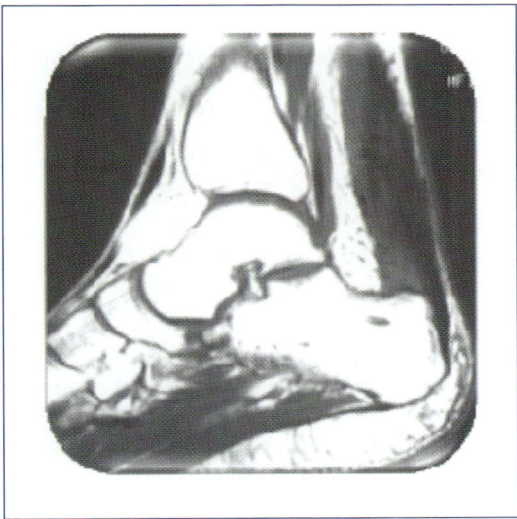

Fig. 15.4   MRI showing hypovascular zone of tendon.

Biomechanics

There are high stresses at the insertion.

♦ While running, the tendo Achilles tendon bears five to seven times of body weight
♦ Subtalar motion will produce rotational forces
♦ Malalignments of the foot and ankle will eccentrically load the tendon
♦ When the knee is straight and the ankle is dorsiflexed, there are high stresses at insertion
♦ Repetitive loads will lead to early tendon degeneration

Acute and Chronic Tendo Achilles Rupture

Diagnosis of rupture can be missed because of action of other active ankle flexors!

♦ Rupture can be at various sites, which are as follows:
  • High (musculotendinous junction)—9%
  • Midportion—72%
  • Calcaneal insertion—19%
♦ Predisposing factors leading to ruptures are as follows:
  • Preexisting tendinosis
  • Trauma
  • Leg muscle imbalance
  • Training errors
  • Pronation of foot
  • Use of steroids
  • Use of fluoroquinolones

Diagnosis

Diagnosis could be made easily if the answers to the following points are positive.

♦ History of "pop" or "snap" in the area
♦ Inability to bear weight ±.
♦ Palpable gap
♦ Positive Thompson's test
♦ Repetitive tip toe raise may not be possible
♦ USG
♦ MRI

Management

Management of acute Achilles rupture is full of controversies!

   Box 15.1 lists the criteria for the selection of conservative and operative treatment.

Box 15.1   Criteria for the selection of conservative and operative treatment.

♦ Conservative treatment: It is selected as per the following criteria:
  • Elderly patients
  • Sedentary patients
  • Diabetics
  • Smokers
  • Patients on steroids
♦ Operative treatment: It is selected as per the following criteria:
  • Young patients
  • Active patients
  • Sports population

Tips and Tricks for Management of Tendo Achilles Ruptures

♦ Nonoperative care should be started as early as possible, within 48 hours of injury
♦ While doing nonoperative management, it is imperative to check preoperatively by USG that both the ruptured tendon ends meet with each other
♦ At conservative treatment, gradual reduction of plantarflexed position of ankle must be followed
♦ A midline incision may give a painful scar, while a lateral incision may damage the sural nerve; hence, a medial incision should be preferred
♦ At open repair, it is imperative not to create a plane between skin and tendon sheath
♦ Care of sural nerve is of utmost significance
♦ Continuous pull over tendon for 5 minutes will release the slackness and result in length gain up to 2 cm (**Fig. 15.5**)
♦ Put a pillow under the dorsum of foot while repairing the tendon to maintain the required plantarflexion

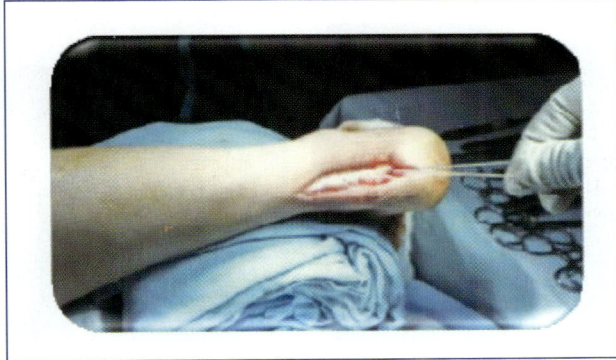

Fig. 15.5 Pull-over tendon at heel end gains length.

♦ Always drape both the legs at surgery for intraoperative comparison and accurate length restoration (**Fig. 15.6**)
♦ Avoid strangulating locking sutures as these may compromise tendon healing and may increase scarring
♦ Like repairs of flexor tendon in hand, reinforce repair with direct additional sutures
♦ Paratenon must be meticulously repaired for better healing process (**Fig. 15.7**)
♦ Postoperative cast is given in gravity-assisted dorsiflexion (**Fig. 15.8**)
♦ Early mobilization gives better functional outcome after surgery
♦ Primary repair may need augmentation where excision of a grossly degenerated tendon creates gap

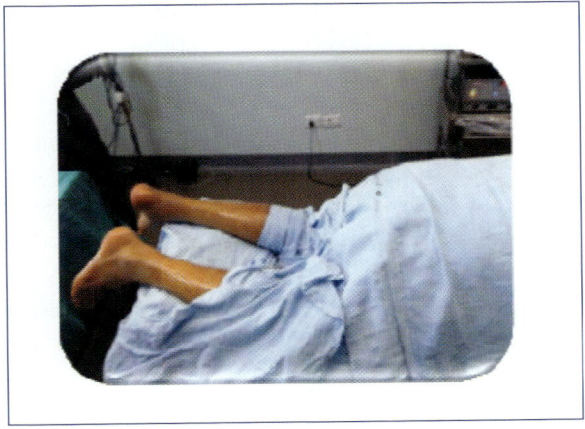

Fig. 15.6 Positioning at surgery showing a pillow under foot and draping of both the limbs.

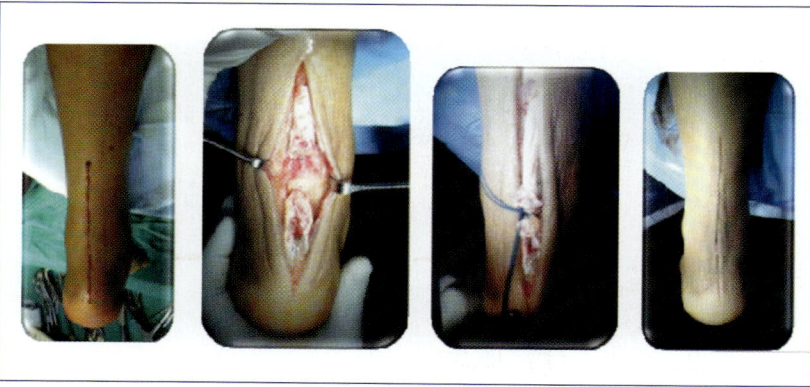

Fig. 15.7   Sequential intraoperative pictures of acute Achilles rupture repair.

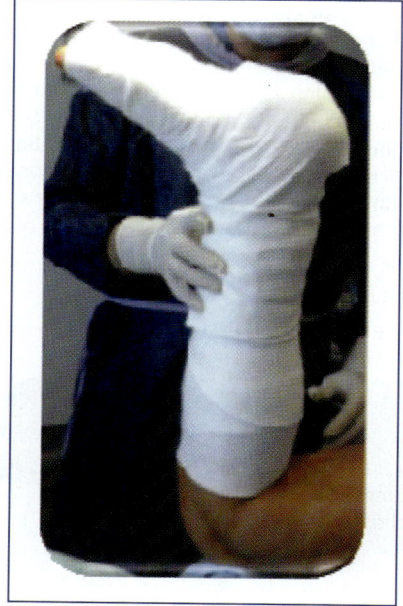

Fig. 15.8   Position of ankle and foot while tying plaster.

Chronic or Neglected Rupture

About 20% to 25% of acute ruptures are missed by clinicians initially!

♦ It is defined as 4 to 6 weeks posttrauma rupture and consists of all neglected cases, late presentations, and delayed repairs.

◆ Diagnosis is by history, palpable gap, poor strength of plantar flexion, and by using USG and MRI (**Fig. 15.9**).

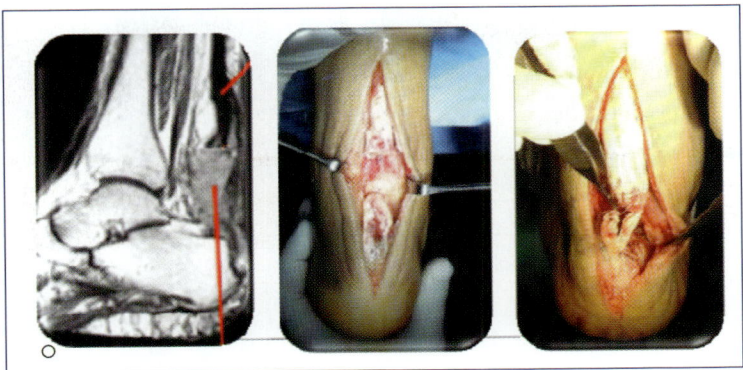

Fig. 15.9   MRI and intraoperative pictures of chronic Achilles rupture.

Management

◆ Conservative care should be selected in patients with high medical risk factors, poor distal circulation, and impaired wound-healing potential due to conditions such as smoking, diabetes, peripheral vascular disease (PVD), immune compromise, and patients on steroids.
◆ Conservative care is in the form of physiotherapy and orthotics.

An aggressive calf-strengthening exercise program can enable a patient to function adequately with impaired Achilles function!!

◆ The following are the surgical options:
   • Primary repair—This is controversial!
   • Augmentation—By fascia lata, gracilis, semitendinosus, patellar tendon, and peronei.
   • Fascial advancements—V–Y plasty and central turn down.
   • Local tendon transfers—Flexor hallucis longus (FHL), flexor digitorum longus (FDL), plantar longus (PL), plantar brevis (PB), and plantaris.
   • Synthetic or allograft—Polyglycol threads, Marlex mesh, Dacron vascular graft, carbon fiber, and allograft substitution.

FHL transfer has advantages such as being in phase transfer; it has 30% of Achilles strength. Moreover, it is close to tendo Achilles and increases blood supply.

FHL can be harvested by single/double/triple incisions (**Figs. 15.10–15.12**).

Flowchart 15.1 shows the operative management of chronic Achilles ruptures.

Tips and Tricks for Management of Chronic Ruptures

◆ Generous excision of fibrosis and dead tendon is a must (**Fig. 15.13**)! Mobilization of tendon proximally is a must to gain length
◆ Drape and prepare both the lower extremities and put a pillow under the dorsum of foot

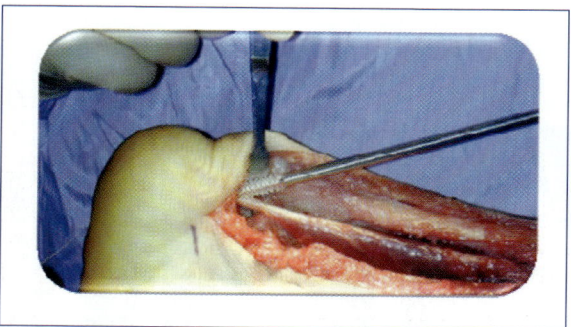

Fig. 15.10 Single-incision FHL transfer.

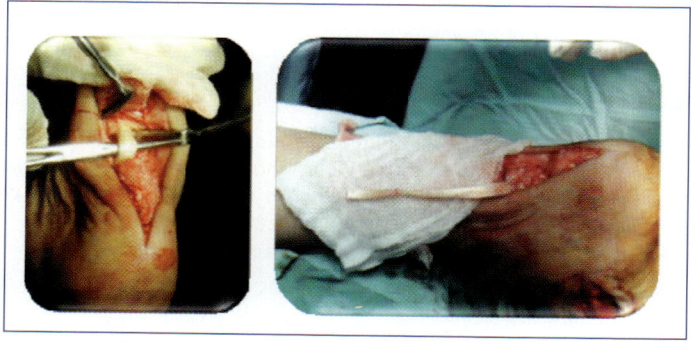

Fig. 15.11 Double-incision FHL transfer.

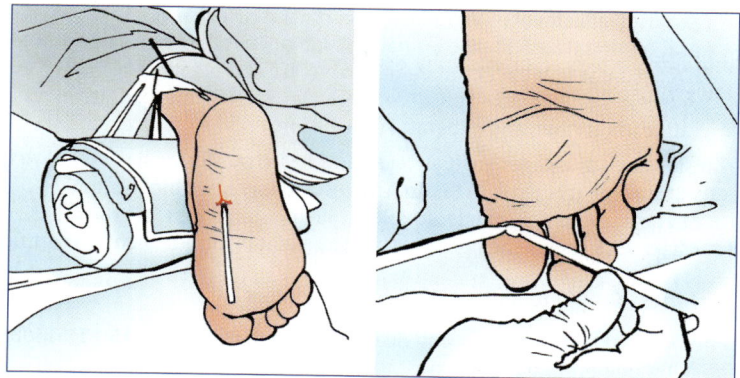

Fig. 15.12 Triple-incision FHL transfer.

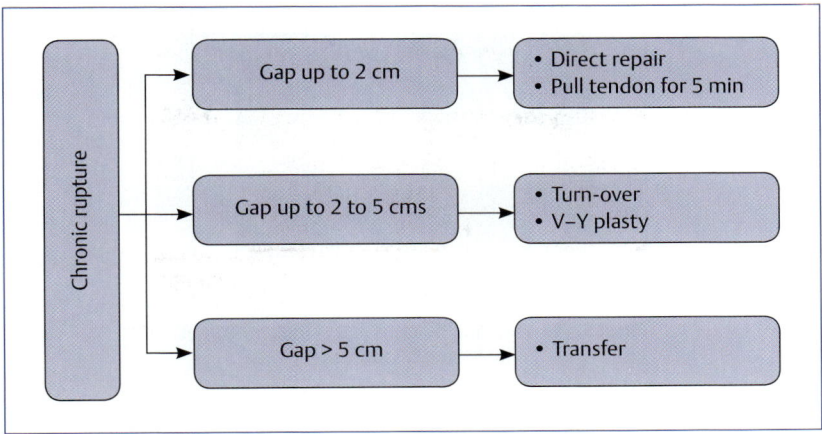

Flowchart 15.1   Operative management of chronic Achilles ruptures.

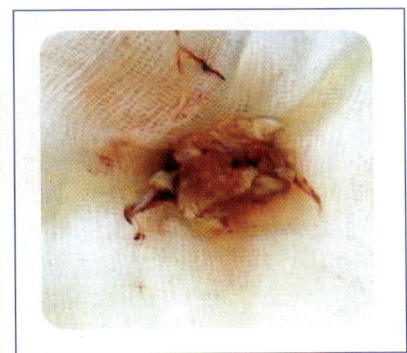

Fig. 15.13   Amount of excised degenerated tendon.

- Sural nerve needs to be carefully dissected and separated as it may be caught between fibrosis
- At V–Y advancement, make limbs twice as long as gap is to be filled (**Fig. 15.14**)
- While planning a central turn down, calculation of length lost due to turn down is a must (**Fig. 15.15**)
- For identification of FHL, simultaneous check by flexion of great toe is a must to avoid inadvertent excision of the posterior tibial nerve
- FHL is buried dorsal to insertion of the tendo Achilles
- While drilling the tunnel, the ankle is dorsiflexed to make the tunnel nearer to the insertion of Achilles tendon
- Suturing of FHL muscle belly with tendo Achilles should be done as it forms an additional source of vascularity
- Anterior dissection of the tendo Achilles from sheath should be avoided to prevent damage to the vascular supply of the tendo Achilles

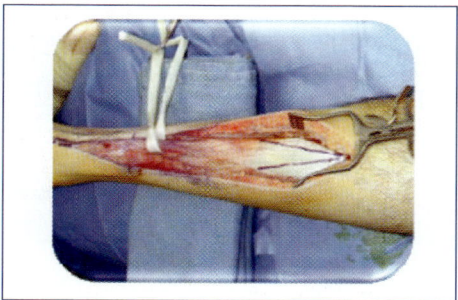

Fig. 15.14   Planning of limbs at V–Y advancement.

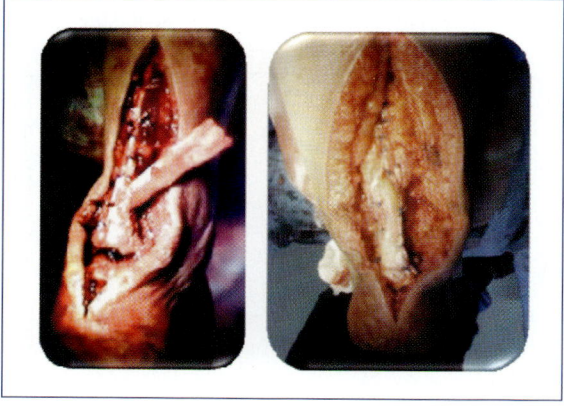

Fig. 15.15   Operative pictures of central turn down.

Achilles Tendinopathy

♦ Problems/pathologies could be any of the following (**Fig. 15.16**):
  • Non-Achilles tendinopathy
  • Insertional Achilles tendinopathy
  • Retrocalcaneal bursitis and Haglund's deformity
  • Insertional Achilles tendinopathy with insertional spur
  • Retrocalcaneal bursitis, Haglund's deformity, insertional spur, insertional tendinopathy
  • All above + rupture

It is most imperative for the clinician to precisely diagnose the condition he/she is dealing with!

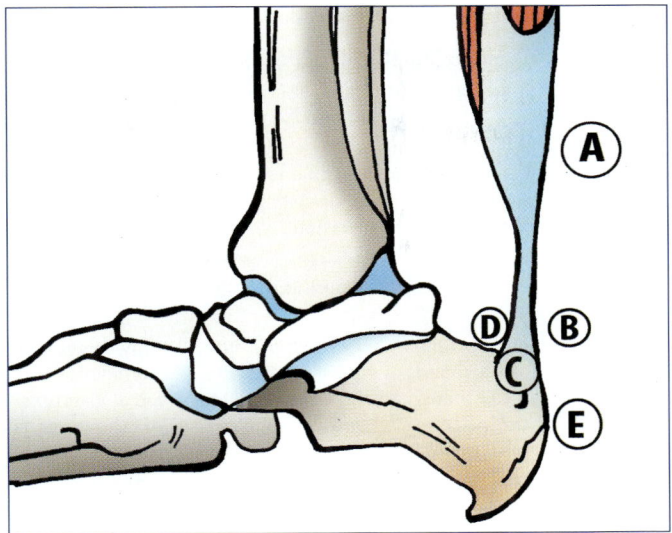

Fig. 15.16 Location of various tendo Achilles pathologies. A, Non-insertional achilles tendinopathy; B, Insertional achilees tendinopathy; C, Haglund's deformity; D, Retrocalcaneal bursitis; E, Insertional spur.

Differential Diagnosis

Since pathologies are numerous, it becomes imperative for the clinician to be able to rule out the wrong ones and come to a correct diagnosis. Various Achilles tendinopathies are briefly described and compared in **Tables 15.1** and **15.2**.

Differentiating features of various elements of noninsertional tendinopathy is shown in **Flowchart 15.2**.

Table 15.1	Comparative clinical and radiological differentiation between insertional and noninsertional tendinopathy	
Criteria	**Noninsertional tendinopathy**	**Insertional tendinopathy**
Location	2 to 6 cm above the insertion	At insertion
Age group affected	Most common in sports population	Middle-aged population
Diagnosed by	• X-ray shows calcification in the course of tendon. • USG and MRI will show features of tendon degeneration.	• X-ray shows calcification at the insertion of tendon. • USG and MRI will show features of tendon degeneration at other places.

Table 15.2   Comparative analysis of various tendo Achilles pathologies

Criteria	Retrocalcaneal bursitis and Haglund's deformity	Insertional spur and insertional tendinitis	Retrocalcaneal bursitis, Haglund's deformity, insertional spur, and insertional tendinitis
Clinical features	Fullness and tenderness anterior to tendon and at/or above bone	Tenderness at insertion	• Generalized, tenderness anterior and posterior to tendon and at insertion. • Gap, if ruptured
Investigative findings	• X-ray shows prominent posterosuperior angle of calcaneus. • MRI shows no tendon involvement	• X-ray shows bony spur at insertion. • MRI shows tendinosis	X-ray shows bony prominence anterior and at insertion. MRI shows tendinosis
Treatment	• Open/MIS • Paratenon or posterior approach • No tendon procedures	• Open • Transtendon posterior approach • Tendon anchorage procedures	• Open • Posterior approach • ± Augmentation procedures

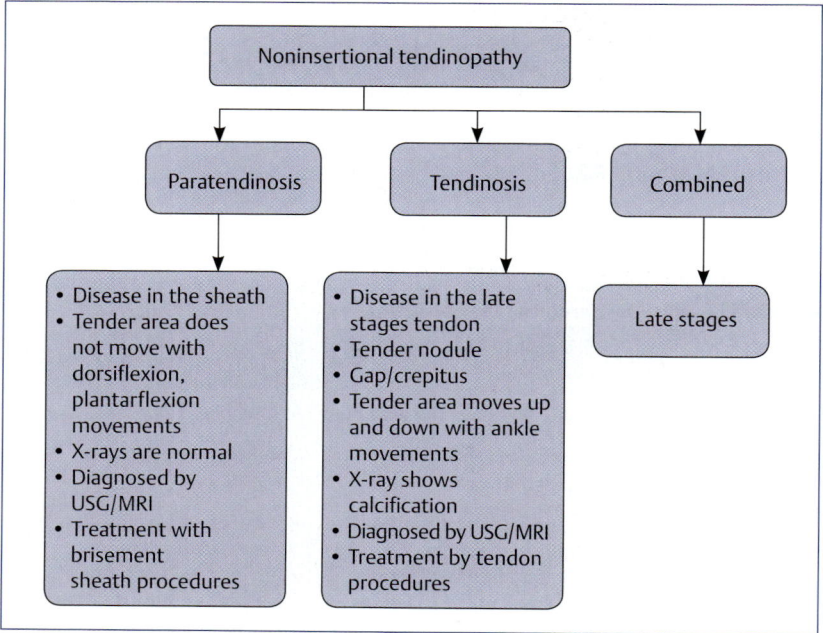

Flowchart 15.2   Differentiating features of various elements of noninsertional tendinopathy.

Management of Noninsertional Achilles Tendinopathy

Conservative Management

♦ Rest to tendon by activity restriction and modifications
  • Role of NSAIDS is questionable
  • Eccentric strengthening exercises
  • Modalities like ultrasound, laser and iontophoresis.
  • Orthotics with heel lift
  • Brisement—injecting 5 to 10 ml of saline in paratenon
  • Radiofrequency coblation (open or closed) (**Figs. 15.17** and **15.18**)
  • Extracorporeal shock wave therapy (**Fig. 15.19**)

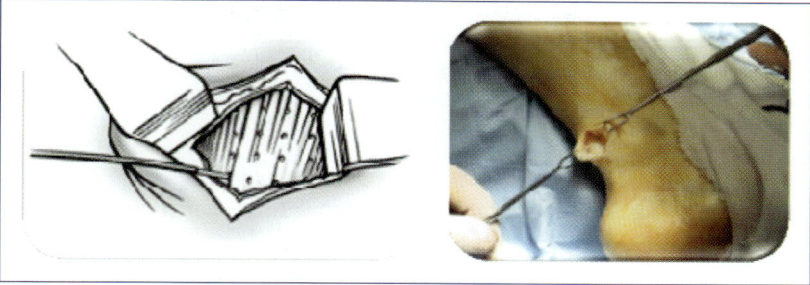

Fig. 15.17   Open radiofrequency coblation procedure.

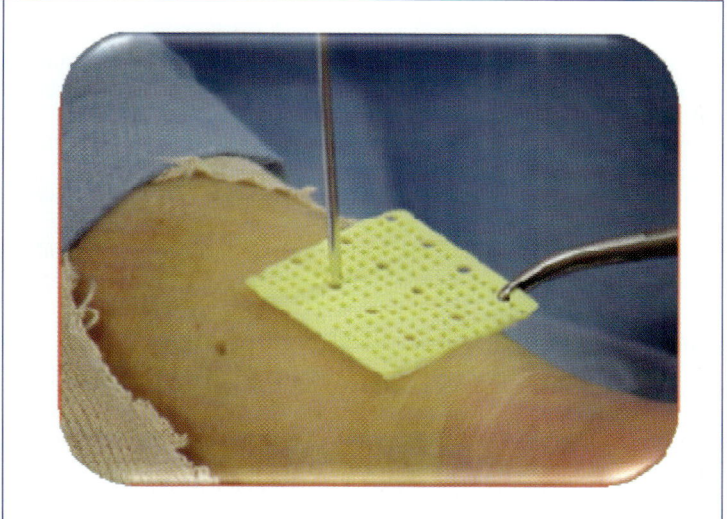

Fig. 15.18   Closed/percutaneous radiofrequency coblation.

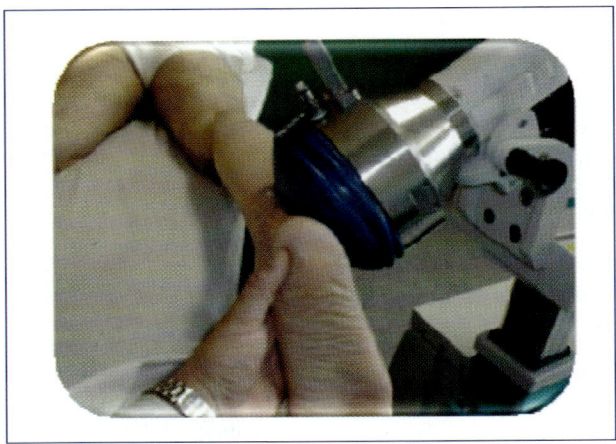

Fig. 15.19 Extracorporeal shockwave therapy being applied to a patient with noninsertionaltendinopathy.

Tips and Tricks for Surgery of Noninsertional Achilles Tendinopathy

◆ Surgical treatment is advised after 3 to 6 months of failure of conservative treatment
◆ Removal of degenerated tendon is the surgical aim
◆ For cases with restriction of disease in paratenon, only excision of paratenon and lysis of adhesions is done
◆ Care must be taken not to debride the anterior paratenon as it the source of blood supply to the tendon
◆ Clinician should be prepared to change the procedure, if, on exploration, disease is also found in tendon in the form of tendinosis, degenerated tendon is also excised
◆ Excise all degenerated tendon fearlessly as failure of surgery is due to inadequate excision of degenerated tendon
◆ If more than 50% of tendon is excised, then augmentation procedure like tendon transfer is needed
◆ Early postoperative range-of-motion exercises are a must to get good clinical function

Management of Insertional Achilles Tendinopathy

◆ Initial management is conservative management, which is the same as with noninsertional tendinopathy.
◆ Failure of such measures for more than 3 to 6 months is an indication for surgery.

Tips and Tricks of Surgical Management of Insertional Achilles Tendinopathy

It is most imperative to diagnose before surgery that what elements are there in a given case!

- Care of sural nerve is of paramount significance while taking the lateral approach
- Inadequate excision of the offending bone is a reason for failure
- Generous excision of degenerated tendon is a must
- Excision of calcification is equally important at surgery
- Do not separate tendon sheath from the skin to prevent wound complications
- Periodic release of self-holding retractors at surgery is must to prevent tendon ischemia
- Take incision as down as possible for proper surgical exposure
- A midline incision has a better blood supply than medial or lateral incision and hence it is the most preferred incision
- The same principles of defect management apply as those for chronic tendon rupture
- Leaving behind a few medial and lateral tendon fibers at insertion will help in guiding surgeon about the resting tendon tension
- Be generous in bone, tendon, and bursa excision
- Intraoperative C-arm imaging helps to guide about adequacy of bone excision.
- Closure of paratenon is a must
- Adequate tension in the reattached tendon is a must
- At surgery, be prepared to change the procedure as per the demand of the case.
- Full-thickness flap and gentle retraction would prevent skin problems
- In cases with only Haglund's deformity and retrocalcaneal bursitis, paratendon approach should be taken from the most tender and most prominent side (**Figs. 15.20–15.25**)
- Prepare both the limbs for comparative evaluation of tendon tension
- Addition of gastrocnemius release is done if preoperative gastrocnemius tightness is observed
- Closed method or minimally invasive surgery (MIS) are applicable to cases where clinician is sure that the disease is not in the tendon and it is in bursa with the prominence of bone
- Immobilization is done with adequate tension in the tendon, and gravity-assisted dorsiflexion
- Wound can break open as late as 4 weeks and hence it should be closely observed

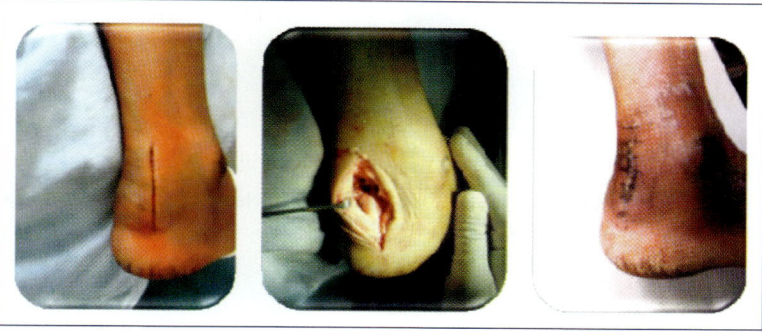

Fig. 15.20 Case showing retrocalcaneal bursitis with Haglund's deformity treated with nontendon procedures with lateral incision.

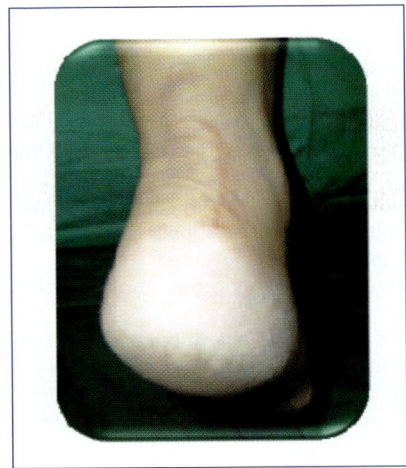

Fig. 15.21 Case showing retrocalcaneal bursitis with Haglund's deformity operated through the medial incision.

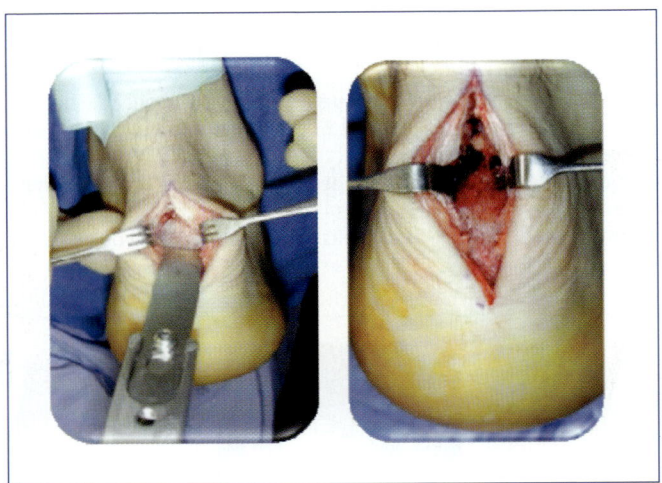

Fig. 15.22 Case showing retrocalcaneal bursitis with Haglund's deformity operated through the posterior incision.

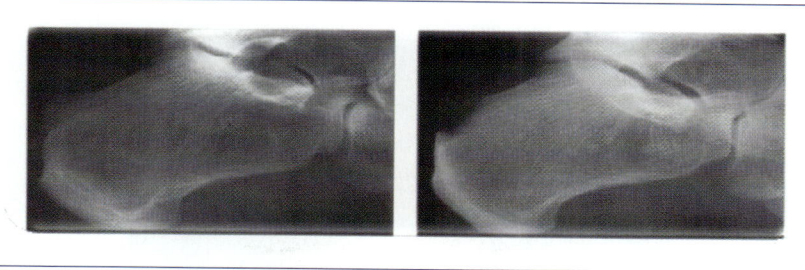

Fig. 15.23 Pre- and postoperative X-rays of a case of Haglund's deformity treated with minimally invasive method.

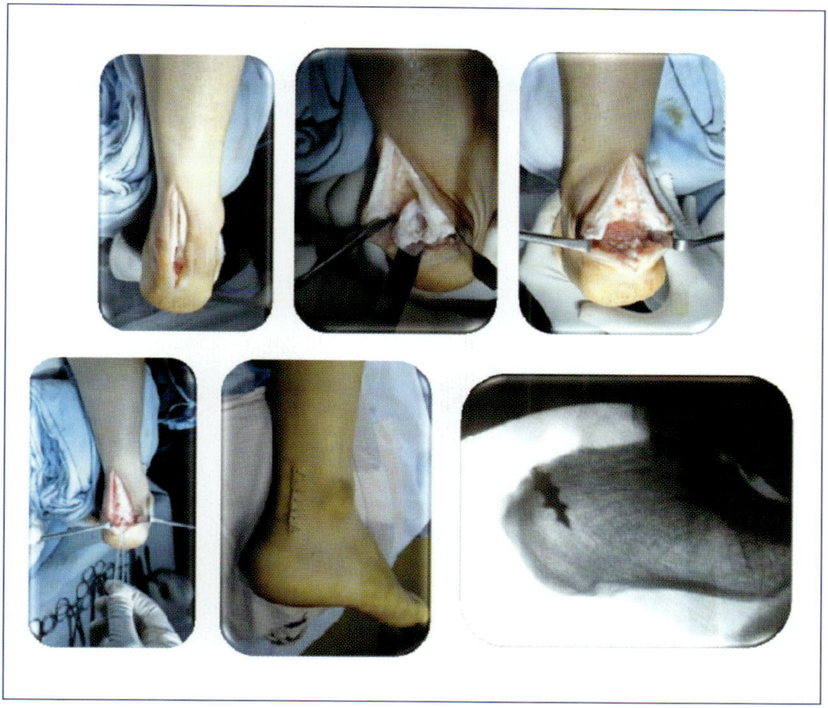

Fig. 15.24 Intraoperative pictures and postoperative X-ray of a patient operated for excision of insertional spur, tendinosis, Haglund's deformity, and retrocalcaneal bursa. Note that reattachment of tendon is done with suture anchor.

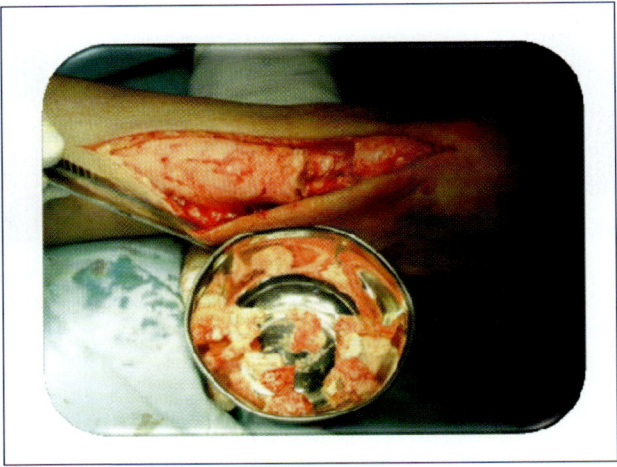

Fig. 15.25 Intraoperative picture after excision of degenerated tendo Achilles showing amount of gap in the tendon as well as amount of excised tendon.

Setting Up of Foot and Ankle Practice

Tomorrow belongs to foot and ankle orthopedics!

Why Choose Foot and Ankle?

♦ It is the specialty where every orthopedic subspecialty comes into action. The spectrum of foot and ankle consists of traumatic conditions, cold orthopedics, pediatric orthopedics, sports orthopedics, arthroscopy and endoscopy, arthroplasty, and deformity corrections.
♦ With increase in lifestyle diseases in addition to increased longevity, well-being of foot and ankle has become mandatory.
♦ Even in developing countries, people have started using footwear obliging orthopedic surgeons to solve issues related to same.
♦ Aggressive sports population competing globally demand great need for care of foot and ankle.
♦ Ratio of specialized foot and ankle surgeons versus total number of orthopedic specialists is too small.

Making of a Foot and Ankle Surgeon

♦ After qualifying as an orthopedic surgeon, further exposure in foot and ankle surgery is a must.
♦ Looking at the scarce opportunities in the developing countries, advanced training in the Western as well as Eastern world is a must.
♦ Specialized training must focus on orthotics, footwear, and physiotherapy as conservative care has a great role play in foot and ankle.
♦ Hands-on training in a cadaver laboratory is a must and so is hands-on exposure of an oculomotor laboratory for performing arthroscopy, endoscopy, and tendoscopy.
♦ There is a great scope for foot and ankle practice in the developing countries because of a huge number of suffering cases.

◆ However, foot and ankle surgeons of developing countries comes across many challenges such as ignorance; delayed presentations; poorly managed cases; limited resources; and nonavailability of proper instruments, equipment, and implants.

◆ There always is a great platform for practicing indigenous techniques and developing newer innovations!

Setting Up of Foot and Ankle Practice

A dedicated foot and ankle center is the need of the day to comprehensively treat foot and ankle disorders under one roof.

Six Milestones of Foot and Ankle Practice

The six milestones of foot and ankle practice are depicted in **Fig. 16.1**.
Milestone 1: Setting up of a foot and ankle center.
Milestone 2: Patient and surgeon education.
Milestone 3: Branding, image building, and marketing of the center.
Milestone 4: Activities of social obligations.
Milestone 5: Research, publications, and training.
Milestone 6: Expansion of centers.

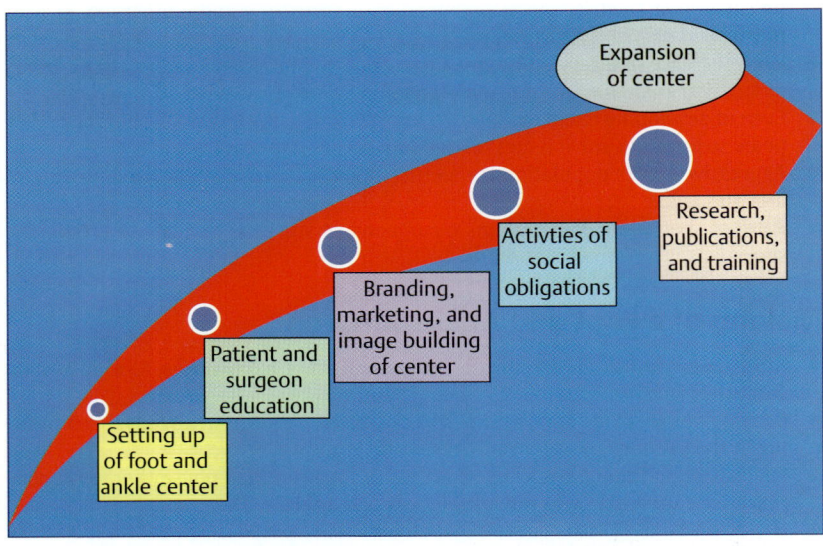

Fig. 16.1   Six milestones of foot and ankle practice.

Milestone 1: Setting Up of Foot and Ankle Center

Building and Floor Planning

- Center can be on any floor with facility of elevators.
- Total floor space needed is 750 to 900 square feet.
- Space for consulting room should be 15×15 feet with walking space and low-height examination couch.
- Space for waiting room should be 10×10 feet with charts and visual display facility, and audio visual display facility.
- Space for dressing cum procedure room should be 12×12 feet with low-height dressing table, digital radiology, pedicure area, and X-ray viewing box.
- Space for the foot laboratory should be 12×12 feet with foot laboratory equipment, foot scan, and low-height tables.

Infrastructure, Equipment, and Instruments

- Digital radiography machine and cassettes
- Stands for getting standing foot and ankle radiographs
- Dressing trolley
- Plaster instruments
- Orthotic devices
- Physiotherapy equipment
- Computers
- Monofilament, hammer, and tuning fork
- Harris met
- Biothesiometer
- Vascular Doppler
- Foot scan (optional)
- Mini saw and bur device
- General orthopedic surgical instruments
- Special foot and ankle instrument set consisting of lamina spreaders, Hintermann retractors, mini-osteotome, gauge, and chisel set and special distractors
- A 2.7-mm and a 1.9-mm 30-degree scopes for arthroscopy, endoscopy, and tendoscopy (1.9 mm)
- Extracorporeal shockwave device (optional)
- Radiofrequency coblation unit (optional)

Manpower and Medical Team

- Receptionist
- Technician trained for dressing, radiology, and foot laboratory
- Part-time medical social worker cum counsellor
- Medical team consisting of general physician, dialectologist/endocrinologist, plastic surgeon, vascular surgeon, and general surgeon
- Paramedical team consisting of physiotherapist and orthotist

Services

♦ Adult foot and ankle clinic
♦ Senior citizen's foot and ankle clinic
♦ Pediatric foot and ankle clinic
♦ Sports foot and ankle clinic
♦ Diabetic foot and ankle clinic
♦ Foot and ankle physiotherapy clinic
♦ Foot and ankle orthotic clinic

How Much Would It Cost?

♦ Erection cost of INR 5,00,000
♦ Infrastructure cost (minimum) of INR 5,00,000
♦ Rent up to INR 30,000 per month
♦ Running cost of INR 80,000 per month
♦ Business development cost of INR 30,000 per month

Milestone 2: Patient and Surgeon Education

♦ Educating patients as well as doctors for foot and ankle ailments and availability of advanced treatment for the same is the need of the day.
♦ In developing countries, several myths prevail regarding foot and ankle disorders, which need to be addressed by the center.
♦ Education can be imparted with literatures, print and electronic media communications, awareness talks, exhibitions, etc.
♦ At our center, we have devised a novel media titled "Foot School," which is an interactive educational symposium of 90 minutes where, through the audio visual medium and demonstrations, knowledge of foot and ankle with its disorders is imparted. This is followed by an open house discussion.

Milestone 3: Branding, Image Building, and Marketing of the Center

♦ Branding and image building of a center shall be done through print, electronic, and social media. Every effort of visibility of the center is practiced.
♦ An educative and interactive website of the center is a portal of branding. Success stories must be shared through these tools.

Milestone 4: Activities of Social Obligations

♦ There are numerous cases suffering from foot and ankle problems. With very few foot and ankle surgeons in India, the society requires continuous help from an expert to prevent these ailments. Diabetics, sports, leprosy, and school population are in need of such a help.
♦ The author at his center run two such programs of social obligations, "Save the foot" for diabetics and "We walk" for leprosy patients.
♦ Diagnostic camps could also be one such activity of social obligation.

Milestone 5: Research, Publication, and Training

♦ *Foot and ankle problems in developing countries need tailor-made solutions obtained on the strong platform of innovations. There is tremendous scope for research and publications by the center.*

♦ Looking at the demand and supply gap in developing countries, more and more foot and ankle surgeons need to be trained by such "Regional centers of excellence" in foot and ankle orthopedics.

♦ Short-term and long-term fellowships by such a center must be structured in such a manner that it gets local accreditation as well.

♦ *Future of foot and ankle orthopedics in developing countries must be crafted by its own breed of foot and ankle surgeons and not by the counterparts from developed countries!*

Milestone 6: Expansion of Center

♦ Foot and ankle center of excellence must expand, leading to the formation of chain of such centers to actually bridge the gap.

♦ Stimulation of private equity and venturing of capital funds to enter in such an investment portal should be the goal.

Appendix

14 Step Calcaneal Fracture Fixation Surgery

Prerequisites:

♦ Lateral position Radiolucent table Tourniquet C-arm in proper position
♦ Incision: Vertical limb is taken more posterior with gentle apical curve
♦ Flap lifting: Calcaneofibular ligament (CFL), sural nerve, and peronei goes inside the flap
♦ Flap retraction: Three or more bent K-wires in talus, fibula, and cuboid

Step 1: Lateral wall dissection and hinging it down.

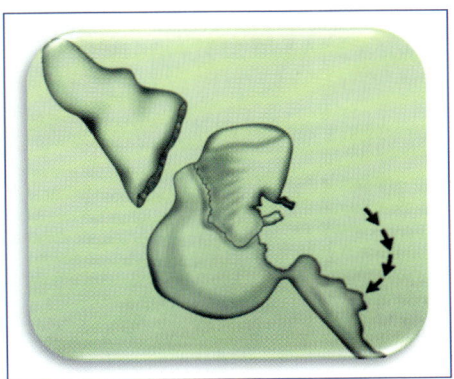

Step 2: ST pin passage.

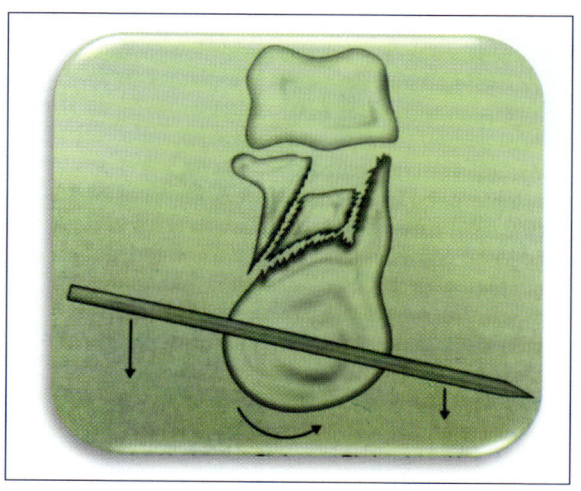

Step 3: Removal of articular fragment.

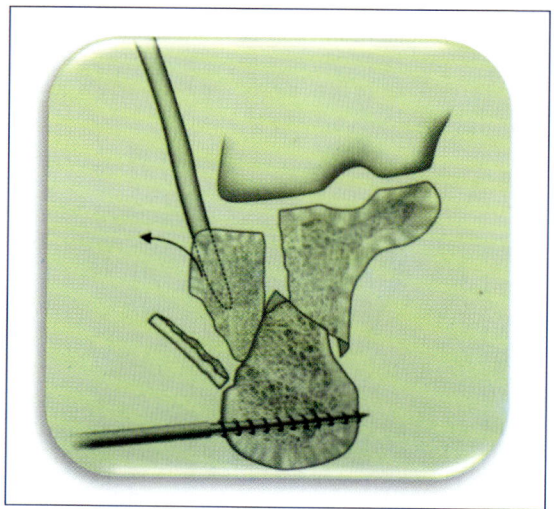

Step 4: Medial wall/sustentacular reduction.

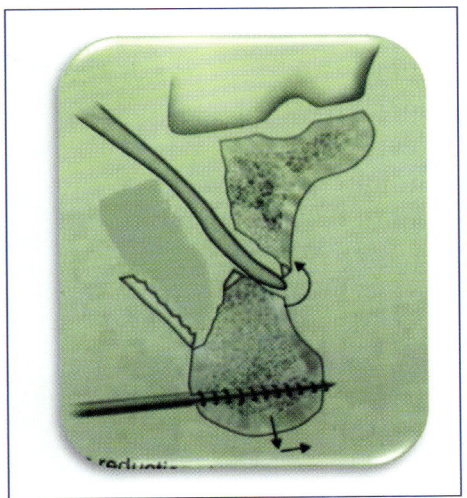

Step 5: Heel height and heel axis restoration.

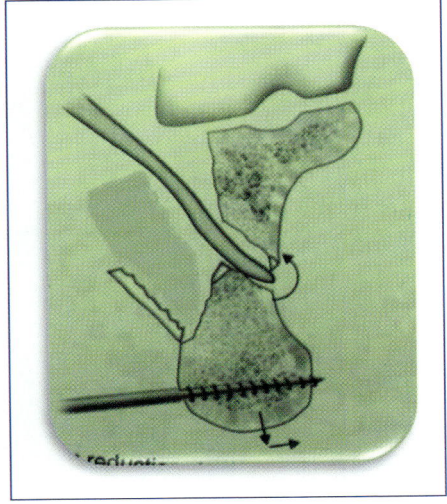

Step 6: Articular fragment back in reduced position.

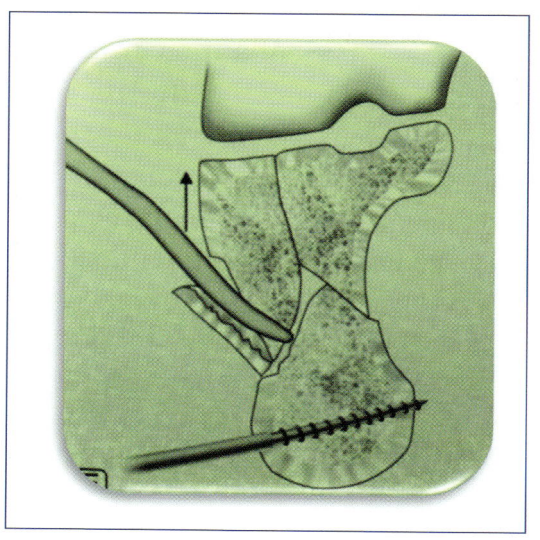

Step 7: Articular fragment fixation with 1/2 temporary K-wires.

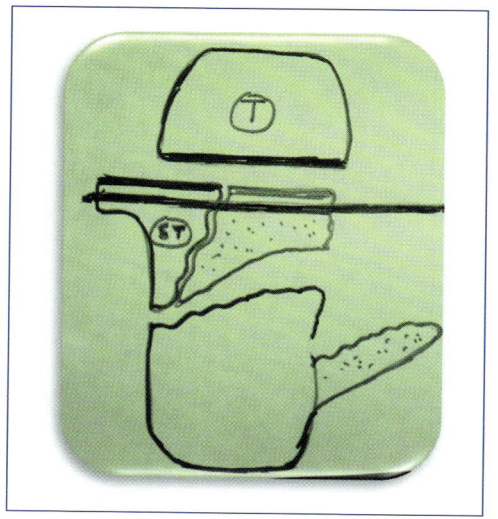

Step 8: Fixation of heel tuberosity with proximal fragment with two temporary K-wires.

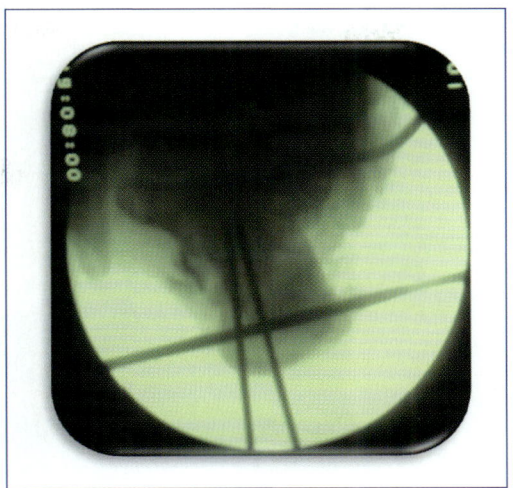

Step 9: Restoration of Gissane angle.

Step 10: Heel length restoration and temporary K-wire fixation from heel tuberosity to anterior fragment.

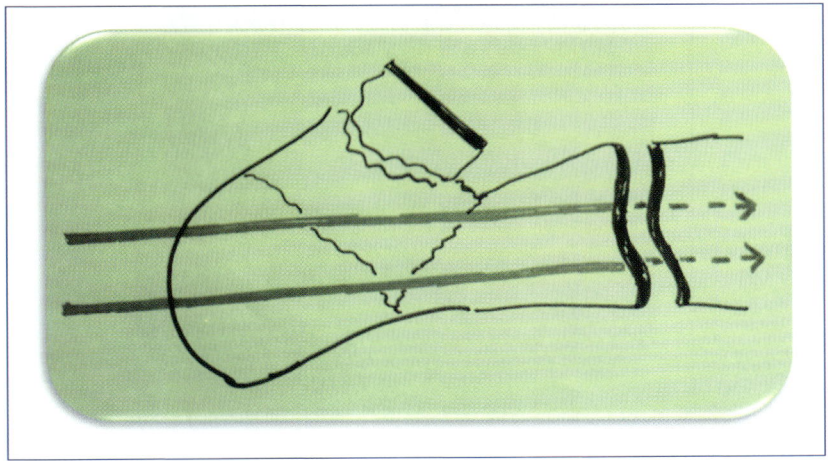

Step 11: Final anteroposterior, axial, and Broden fluro check.

Step 12: Articular fragment fixation: outside the plate or through the plate one or two 5-mm cannulated cancellous (CC) screws.

Step 13: Repositioning of lateral wall.

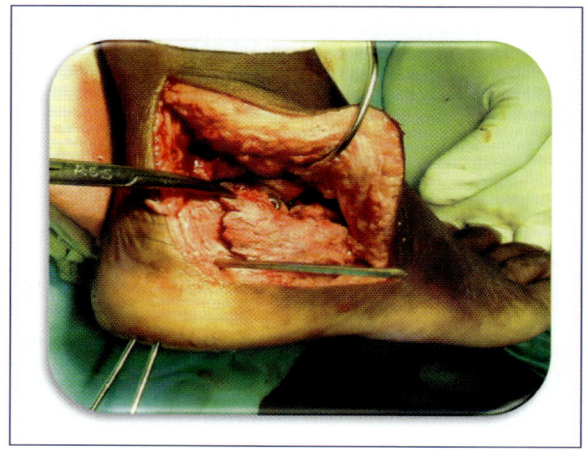

Step 14: Neutralization with plate.

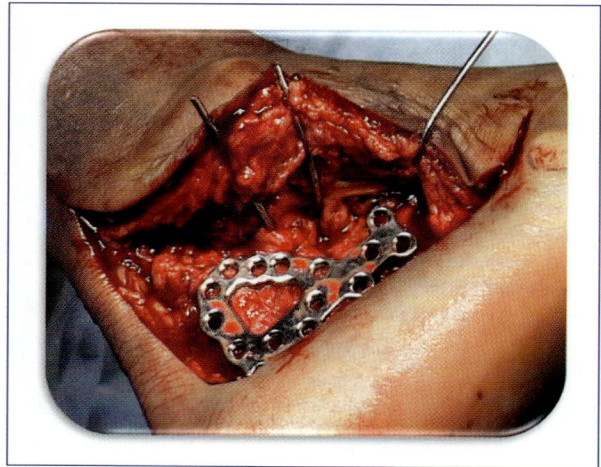

Optional steps

♦ Use of dry subtalar arthroscopy for articular reduction check.
♦ Filling up of void with bone grafts or bone graft substitutes.
♦ Closure in two layers and it starts from the end and goes towards the apex.

Index